THE LEARNING HEALTH SYSTEM SERIES

W9-BGK-205

EFFECTIVE CARE
FOR HIGH-NEED PATIENTS

OPPORTUNITIES FOR IMPROVING OUTCOMES, VALUE, AND HEALTH

Peter Long, Melinda Abrams, Arnold Milstein, Gerard
Anderson, Katherine Lewis Apton, Maria Lund
Dahlberg, and Danielle Whicher, *Editors*

 NATIONAL ACADEMY OF MEDICINE

WASHINGTON, DC
NAM.EDU

NATIONAL ACADEMY OF MEDICINE • 500 FIFTH STREET, NW • WASHINGTON, DC 20001

NOTICE: This publication has undergone peer review according to procedures established by the National Academy of Medicine (NAM). Publication by the NAM signifies that it is the product of a carefully considered process and is a useful contribution worthy of public attention, but does not represent formal endorsement of conclusions and recommendations by the NAM. The views presented in this publication are those of individual authors and do not represent formal consensus positions of the authors' organizations; the NAM; or the National Academies of Sciences, Engineering, and Medicine.

Support for this activity was provided by the Peterson Center on Healthcare, which is dedicated to identifying proven solutions that improve care quality, lower costs, and accelerate the adoption of these solutions on a national level.

Library of Congress Cataloging-in-Publication Data

Names: Long, Peter (Peter V.), editor. | National Academy of Medicine (U.S.), publisher. | Leadership Consortium for a Value & Science-Driven Health System, issuing body. | Models of Care for High-Need Patients (Workshop) (2015-2016 : Washington, D.C.)
Title: Effective care for high-need patients : opportunities for improving outcomes, value, and health / Peter Long, Melinda Abrams, Arnold Milstein, Gerard Anderson, Katherine Lewis Apton, Maria Lund Dahlberg, and Danielle Whicher, editors ; Leadership Consortium for a Value & Science-Driven Health System.
Description: Washington, DC : National Academy Of Medicine, [2017] | Report on issues discussed over the course of 3 public workshops held between July 2015 and October 2016 at the National Academy of Medicine, Washington, DC. | Includes bibliographical references.
Identifiers: LCCN 2017041343 (print) | LCCN 2017042253 (ebook) | ISBN 9781947103078 (Ebook) | ISBN 9781947103061 (pbk.)
Subjects: | MESH: Health Services Needs and Demand | Health Services--utilization | Delivery of Health Care--utilization | Delivery of Health Care--economics | Patient Care Management--economics | United States | Congresses
Classification: LCC RA425 (ebook) | LCC RA425 (print) | NLM W 84 AA1 | DDC 362.1--dc23
LC record available at https://lccn.loc.gov/2017041343

Suggested citation: Long, P., M. Abrams, A. Milstein, G. Anderson, K. Lewis Apton, M. Lund Dahlberg, and D. Whicher, Editors. 2017. *Effective Care for High-Need Patients: Opportunities for Improving Outcomes, Value, and Health*. Washington, DC: National Academy of Medicine.

"Knowing is not enough; we must apply.
Willing is not enough; we must do."

—GOETHE

LEADERSHIP
INNOVATION
IMPACT

for a healthier future

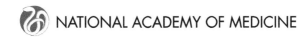
NATIONAL ACADEMY OF MEDICINE

ABOUT THE NATIONAL ACADEMY OF MEDICINE

The **National Academy of Medicine** is one of three academies constituting the National Academies of Sciences, Engineering, and Medicine (the National Academies). The National Academies provide independent, objective analysis and advice to the nation and conduct other activities to solve complex problems and inform public policy decisions. The National Academies also encourage education and research, recognize outstanding contributions to knowledge, and increase public understanding in matters of science, engineering, and medicine.

The **National Academy of Sciences** was established in 1863 by an Act of Congress, signed by President Lincoln, as a private, nongovernmental institution to advise the nation on issues related to science and technology. Members are elected by their peers for outstanding contributions to research. Dr. Marcia McNutt is president.

The **National Academy of Engineering** was established in 1964 under the charter of the National Academy of Sciences to bring the practices of engineering to advising the nation. Members are elected by their peers for extraordinary contributions to engineering. Dr. C. D. Mote, Jr., is president.

The **National Academy of Medicine** (formerly the Institute of Medicine) was established in 1970 under the charter of the National Academy of Sciences to advise the nation on issues of health, medical care, and biomedical science and technology. Members are elected by their peers for distinguished contributions to medicine and health. Dr. Victor J. Dzau is president.

Learn more about the National Academy of Medicine at NAM.edu.

PLANNING COMMITTEE FOR THE WORKSHOP SERIES ON MODELS OF CARE FOR HIGH-NEED PATIENTS

PETER V. LONG (*Chair*), President and Chief Executive Officer, Blue Shield of California Foundation

MELINDA K. ABRAMS, Vice President, Delivery System Reform, The Commonwealth Fund

GERARD F. ANDERSON, Director, Center for Hospital Finance and Management, Johns Hopkins Bloomberg School of Public Health

TIM ENGELHARDT, Director, Federal Coordinated Health Care Office, Centers for Medicare & Medicaid Services

JOSE FIGUEROA, Instructor of Medicine, Harvard Medical School; Associate Physician, Brigham and Women's Hospital

KATHERINE HAYES, Director, Health Policy, Bipartisan Policy Center

FREDERICK ISASI, Executive Director, Families USA; former Health Division Director, National Governors Association

ASHISH K. JHA, K. T. Li Professor of International Health & Health Policy, Director, Harvard Global Health Institute, Harvard T.H. Chan School of Public Health

DAVID MEYERS, Chief Medical Officer, Agency for Healthcare Research and Quality

ARNOLD S. MILSTEIN, Professor of Medicine, Director, Clinical Excellence Research Center, Center for Advanced Study in the Behavioral Sciences; Stanford University

DIANE STEWART, Senior Director, Pacific Business Group on Health

SANDRA WILKNISS, Program Director, Health Division, National Governors Association

NAM Staff

Development of this publication was facilitated by contributions of the following NAM staff, under the guidance of Michael McGinnis, NAM Leonard D. Schaeffer Executive Officer and Executive Director of the Leadership Consortium for a Value & Science-Driven Health System:

KATHERINE LEWIS APTON, Program Officer, National Academy of Medicine (*until January 2017*)

MARIA LUND DAHLBERG, Associate Program Officer, National Academies of Sciences, Engineering, and Medicine (*until April 2017*)

ELIZABETH MALPHRUS, Associate Program Officer, National Academy of Medicine (*until June 2015*)

DANIELLE WHICHER, Senior Program Officer, National Academy of Medicine

MINA BAKHTIAR, Senior Program Assistant, National Academy of Medicine (*until May 2016*)

GWEN HUGHES, Research Coordinator, National Academy of Medicine

CARRIE WOLF, Senior Program Assistant, National Academy of Medicine (*until March 2016*)

BROOKE KEANE, Intern, National Academy of Medicine (*until August 2017*)

DANIEL BEARSS, Senior Librarian, National Academies of Sciences, Engineering, and Medicine

LAURA DESTEFANO, Director of Communications, National Academy of Medicine

KYRA E. CAPPELUCCI, Communications Specialist, National Academy of Medicine

MOLLY DOYLE, Communications Specialist, National Academy of Medicine

Consultant

JOE ALPER, Science Writer and Rapporteur

TAXONOMY WORKGROUP

MELINDA K. ABRAMS, Vice President, Delivery System Reform, The Commonwealth Fund

GERARD F. ANDERSON, Director, Center for Hospital Finance and Management, Johns Hopkins Bloomberg School of Public Health

MELINDA J. BEEUWKES BUNTIN, Chair, Department of Health Policy, Vanderbilt University School of Medicine

DAVE A. CHOKSHI, Assistant Vice President, New York City Health and Hospitals Corporation

HENRY CLAYPOOL, Policy Director, Community Living Policy Center, University of California San Francisco

DAVID A. DORR, Professor & Vice Chair, Medical Informatics, Department of Medical Informatics & Clinical Epidemiology, Oregon Health & Science University

JOSE FIGUEROA, Instructor of Medicine, Harvard Medical School; Associate Physician, Brigham and Women's Hospital

ASHISH K. JHA, K.T. Li Professor of International Health and Health Policy, Director, Harvard Global Health Institute, Harvard T.H. Chan School of Public Health

DAVID LABBY, Founding Chief Medical Officer & Health Strategy Adviser, Health Share of Oregon

PRABHJOT SINGH, Director, Arnhold Institute for Global Health, Mount Sinai Health System

POLICY WORKGROUP

GERARD F. ANDERSON, Director, Center for Hospital Finance and Management, Johns Hopkins Bloomberg School of Public Health

TIM ENGELHARDT, Director, Federal Coordinated Health Care Office, Centers for Medicare & Medicaid Services

KATHERINE HAYES, Director, Health Policy, Bipartisan Policy Center

SANDRA WILKNISS, Program Director, Health Division, National Governors Association

REVIEWERS

This special publication has been reviewed in draft form by individuals chosen for their diverse perspectives and technical expertise, in accordance with review procedures established by the NAM. We wish to thank the following individuals for their review of this publication:

BRUCE CHERNOF, The SCAN Foundation
BRUCE HANSON, First Lutheran Church
JULIAN HARRIS, Cigna
GAIL WILENSKY, Project HOPE

Although the reviewers listed above have provided many constructive comments and suggestions, they were not asked to endorse the content of this publication, nor did they see the final draft before it was published. Review of this publication was overseen by **Danielle Whicher,** senior program officer, NAM; **Gwen Hughes,** senior program assistant, NAM; and **Michael McGinnis,** Leonard D. Schaeffer Executive Officer, NAM. Responsibility for the final content of this publication rests entirely with the authors and the NAM.

FOREWORD

Health care expenditures are rising, yielding far too little value for the health of Americans, and are placing serious economic strains on individuals, families, states—and the nation. In the context of these urgent circumstances, the National Academy of Medicine (NAM) and the Peterson Center on Healthcare have partnered to present, in this NAM special publication, approaches and priorities for improving care for the 5 percent of patients who account for 50 percent of health care spending. *Effective Care for High-Need Patients: Opportunities for Improving Outcomes, Value, and Health* is the product of a series of stakeholder meetings—clinicians, patients, economists, researchers, and policy leaders—led by the NAM Leadership Consortium for a Value & Science-Driven Health System, conducted in collaboration and coordination with policy assessment activities of the Bipartisan Policy Center and research activities at Harvard University, and planned by a committee of national experts.

The publication offers several new contributions that can be applied to provide more effective and efficient care to those who need it most:

- Understanding the key characteristics of high-need patients;
- Using a patient taxonomy as a tool to inform and target care;
- Identifying promising care models and attributes to better serve this patient population, linking clinical and community engagement; and
- Promising areas of policy-level actions to support the spread and scale of evidence-based programs.

We are hopeful that this publication will help sharpen the national discussion to improve health and health care for patients with the greatest need and improve treatment at the point of care/service. With the stakes as high as they are, both for the individuals who require tailored, high-intensity services, and for a nation that urgently seeks more efficient care models, the NAM and the Peterson Center are already engaging in follow-up activities to engage the health care community, including webinars and podcasts showcasing successful implementation; patient and caregiver testimonials to illustrate the impact of successful care models; and stakeholder briefs that identify actions specific groups can take to improve care for high-need patients.

In releasing *Effective Care for High-Need Patients*, we would like to underscore our gratitude to the members of the project steering group, chaired by Peter Long, President of the Blue Shield of California Foundation, as well as members of a five-foundation coalition—The Commonwealth Fund, John A. Hartford Foundation, Robert Wood Johnson Foundation, Peterson Center on Healthcare, and SCAN Foundation—committed to improving care and outcomes for patients with high needs. The health and economic well-being of the nation depends on their success.

Michael McGinnis, MD, MPP
Executive Officer
National Academy of Medicine

Jay Want, MD
Executive Director
Peterson Center on Healthcare

PREFACE

The National Academy of Medicine's Leadership Consortium for a Value & Science-Driven Health System provides a trusted venue for national leaders in health and health care to work cooperatively toward effective, innovative care that consistently adds value to patients and society. Consortium members are leaders from stakeholder communities brought together by their common commitment to steward advances in science, value, and culture necessary for a health system that continuously learns and improves in fostering healthier people.

It has been known for some time that a small percentage of patients with complex health and social needs use a disproportionate share of medical care at significant cost to them, the healthcare system, and broader society. There is also substantial evidence that the standard of care provided to these individuals, while costly, often does not meet their expectations. That said, there exists a number of successful programs and models in health systems and communities across the country that are providing excellent care and producing positive results. To date, they have remained positive exceptions to the norm rather than become the standard of care. Beyond the inherent challenges of scaling and spreading promising care models, there is a growing recognition that some federal and state health policies and payment models inhibit rather than facilitate the delivery of more effective and lower cost care and services for high-need patients.

The National Academy of Medicine (NAM) hosted three public workshops exploring high-need patients in more depth to inform future policy and practice. Through our inquiry, we found that bold policy action and care delivery reform is needed to improve care for high-need patients and reduce costs. The high-need patient population is diverse, complex, expensive, and dynamic. Addressing their needs will require the appropriate balance between standardized and customized approaches to care. Segmenting high-need patients into smaller homogeneous subgroups using a "taxonomy" represents one promising tool to inform and target care and should be rapidly tested in real-world settings in conjunction with care models that have been shown to work. It is clear that effective tools, care models, and policies must extend beyond strictly medical approaches to address social and behavioral factors. In order to be actionable, policy solutions must account for existing system constraints and complexities such as the integration of medical and social approaches and the financing of care models.

I want to recognize the Peterson Center on Healthcare, who funded these activities at the NAM in order to advance our knowledge and actions around this critical issue. The Center also supported associated research projects at the Harvard T. H. Chan School of Public Health and the Bipartisan Policy Center to provide quantitative and policy analysis used to inform these workshops. Those teams provided invaluable input and shared important perspectives throughout the process, as did Melinda Abrams from The Commonwealth Fund.

Thanks also to the hundreds of individuals who participated in the three public workshops. In particular, I want to recognize the patients and caregivers who shared their personal stories at the beginning of each workshop. Their stories provided a powerful reminder why this effort is so important and focused our attention on improving outcomes from their perspectives.

Thank you to the planning group, who remained committed, curious, and engaged throughout the process. The process produced a publication that is both comprehensive in its scope and focused on practical policy solutions. Beyond planning the three workshops, two subgroups addressed specific issues that were raised as gaps in our knowledge. The taxonomy and policy workgroups greatly enhanced the utility of this publication.

Finally, I would like to acknowledge the leadership demonstrated by the dedicated staff at the NAM (Elizabeth, Katie, Maria, Danielle, Gwen, Emma, Michelle, Marianne, Michael, Daniel Bearss of the National Academies of Science, Engineering, and Medicine Research Center, and Joe Alper) who shepherded this project from its inception through the release of this publication. They organized the three public workshops, supported the working groups, and assisted in the drafting of this publication.

As our nation once again debates health care financing approaches that could fundamentally alter people's access to health insurance coverage and medical care, it is critical to focus attention on those individuals who are the heaviest users of health care and commit to improving their outcomes while reducing spending. There are currently major policy barriers to broad implementation of what we already know does work. Future policies and funding proposals that either ignore what we know works or inhibit us from implementing effective care models will be detrimental to the health of these vulnerable populations. If our goal is to improve the health of our most vulnerable neighbors, we must take effective actions now.

—Peter V. Long, PhD
Chair, Planning Committee

CONTENTS

BOXES, FIGURES, AND TABLES

Tables

ACRONYMS AND ABBREVIATIONS

ACE	Adverse Childhood Experiences
ACO	accountable care organization
AHRQ	Agency for Healthcare Research and Quality
BPC	Bipartisan Policy Center
CMMI	Center for Medicare & Medicaid Innovation
CMS	Centers for Medicare & Medicaid Services
CRG	clinical risk group
D-SNP	Dual Eligible Special Needs Plan
DME	Durable Medical Equipment
EHR	electronic health record
EMDR	eye-movement desensitization and reprocessing
FPL	federal poverty line
FQHC	federally qualified health center
HCH	Health Care Home program (Minnesota)
HIPAA	Health Insurance Portability and Accountability Act of 1996
HRP	Health Resilience Program
HSPH	Harvard T.H. Chan School of Public Health
IMPACT	Improving Mood: Promoting Access to Collaborative Treatment
IOCP	Intensive Outpatient Care Program
LTC	Long-Term Care
LTSS	long-term services and supports

MEPS   Medical Expenditure Panel Survey
MIND   Maximizing Independence at Home
at Home

NAM   National Academy of Medicine

OECD   Organisation for Economic Co-operation and Development

PAC   Post-Acute Care
PACE   Program of All-Inclusive Care for the Elderly
PBGH   Pacific Business Group on Health
PMPM   per-member per-month
PRAPARE   Protocol for Responding to and Assessing Patients' Assets,
              Risks, and Experiences
PRISM   Predictive Risk Intelligence System
PTSD   Post-Traumatic Stress Disorder

SNP   Special Needs Plan

SUMMARY

Today, 1 percent of patients account for more than 20 percent of health care expenditures, and 5 percent account for nearly half of the nation's spending on health care (Figure S-1) (Mitchell, 2016). Improving care management for this population while balancing quality and associated costs is at the forefront of national health care goals, and reaching this particular goal will require active involvement of a broad range of stakeholders at multiple levels. To advance insights and perspectives on how to better manage the care of this population and to stimulate actions on opportunities for improving outcomes and reducing the costs of health care, the National Academy of Medicine (NAM), through its Leadership Consortium for a Value & Science-Driven Health System (the Leadership Consortium), in partnership with the Harvard T.H. Chan School of Public Health (HSPH), the Bipartisan Policy Center (BPC), The Commonwealth Fund, and the Peterson Center on Healthcare—which funded this initiative—has undertaken a collaborative assessment on strategies for better serving high-need patients.

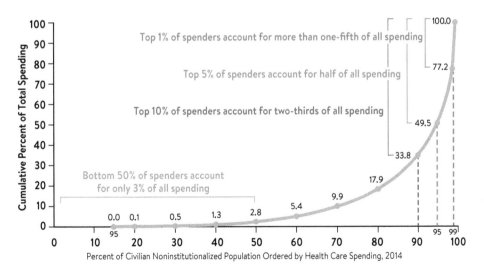

FIGURE S-1 | Distribution of personal health care spending in the US civilian noninstitutionalized population, 2014.
SOURCE: Dzau et al., 2017

1

The NAM was tasked with bringing together experts and stakeholders over the course of three workshops held between July 2015 and October 2016 to consider and reflect upon the key issues for improving care for high-need patients and summarizing the presentations, discussions, and literature for publication. This publication reports and reflects on the following issues: (1) key characteristics of high-need patients; (2) the use of a patient categorization scheme—or a taxonomy—as a tool to inform and target care; (3) promising care models and attributes to better serve this patient population, as well as insights on "matching" these models to specific patient groups; and (4) areas of opportunity for policy-level action to support the spread and scale of evidence-based programs. The publication concludes by exploring common themes and opportunities for action in the field.

KEY CHARACTERISTICS OF HIGH-NEED PATIENTS

To date, little has been written about the characteristics of high-need individuals using empirical data, and, as a result, there is not yet a consistent definition of need. Since understanding the characteristics of high-need patients is the first step in determining how to improve care, chapter 2 explores candidate criteria used to identify high-need patients along with key demographic and experiential characteristics.

While the high-need patient population is diverse, a synthesis of analyses reported in the literature identified three criteria that could form a basis for defining and identifying this population: total accrued health care costs, intensity of care utilized for a given period of time, and functional limitations. Functional limitations include limitations in activities of daily living such as dressing, bathing or showering, ambulating, self-feeding, grooming, and toileting, or limitations in instrumental activities of daily living that support an independent lifestyle such as housework, shopping, managing money, taking medications, using a telephone, or being able to use transportation (Hayes et al., 2016b). In terms of demographics, recent literature demonstrates that high-need individuals are disproportionately older, female, white, and less educated (Cohen et al., 2014; Hayes et al., 2016b; Joynt et al., 2017). They are also more likely to be publicly insured, have fair to poor self-reported health (Hayes et al., 2016c), and be susceptible to lack of coordination within the health care system (Sarnak and Ryan, 2016). Their needs extend beyond care for their physical ailments to social and behavioral services, which are often of central importance to their overall well-being. As a result, addressing clinical needs alone will not improve outcomes or reduce costs for this population. Rather, it will also be necessary to address an individual's functional, social, and behavioral needs, largely through the provision of social and community services that today are not typically the province of health care delivery systems (Blumenthal et al., 2016).

THE PATIENT TAXONOMY AND IMPLICATIONS FOR CARE DELIVERY

Understanding how to effectively care for high-need patients requires knowing which factors drive health care need. Because this patient population is heterogeneous, those factors will differ for different segments of the population. Therefore, a taxonomy that segments individuals in a health system's population based on the care they need as well as how often they might need it can help determine how to serve that population more effectively. Drawing on recent taxonomies developed by two organizations, the Harvard T.H. Chan School of Public Health and The Commonwealth Fund, as well as the workshop series, the assessment of an expert taxonomy working group, and the published literature, chapter 3 provides guidance on the adoption and application of key elements of a patient taxonomy in practice.

Both the taxonomy developed by the Harvard T.H. Chan School of Public Health and the one developed by The Commonwealth Fund segment high-need individuals based on medical characteristics because this is a feasible starting point for most health care systems. Recognizing that a taxonomy focused on medical characteristics may neglect other factors that are key drivers of need, the taxonomy working group built on these efforts to offer a conceptual starter taxonomy that incorporates functional, social, and behavioral factors into a medically oriented taxonomy, not as independent segments but as factors that influence the care model or care team composition most likely to benefit particular patient segments (Figures S-2 and Table S-1). This starter taxonomy can provide guidance for health system leaders and payers on how to embed social risk factors, behavioral health factors, and functional limitations in a taxonomy for high-need patients. Patients would first be assigned to a clinical segment, with follow-on assessment of behavioral health issues and social services needs to determine the specific type of services that are required. Key behavioral health factors most likely to affect care delivery decisions include substance abuse, serious mental illness, cognitive decline, and chronic toxic stress and key social risk factors include low socioeconomic status, social isolation, community deprivation, and house insecurity.

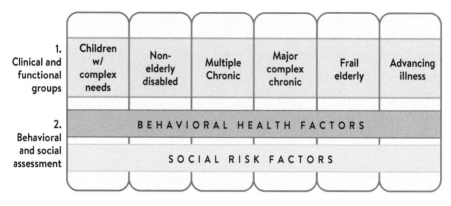

FIGURE S-2 | A conceptual model of a starter taxonomy for high-need patients.

NOTE: For this taxonomy, functional impairments are intrinsically tied to the clinical segments.
SOURCE: Adapted from Abrams presentation, October 21, 2016

TABLE S-1 | Clinical Group Features

CLINICAL GROUP	FEATURES
Children with complex needs	Have sustained severe impairment in at least four categories together with enteral/parenteral feeding or sustained severe impairment in at least two categories and requiring ventilation or continuous positive airway pressure[A]
Non-elderly disabled	Under 65 years and with end-stage renal disease or disability based on receiving Supplemental Security Income
Multiple chronic	Only one complex condition and/or between one and five noncomplex conditions[B,C]
Major complex chronic	Two or more complex conditions or at least six noncomplex conditions[B,C]
Frail elderly	Over 65 years and with two or more frailty indicators[D]
Advancing illness	Other terminal illness, or end of life

a Categories for children with complex needs are: learning and mental functions, communication, motor skills, self-care, hearing, vision

b Complex conditions, as defined in Joynt et al., 2017, are listed in Table 2-1.

c Noncomplex conditions, as defined in Joynt et al., 2017, are listed in Table 2-1.

d Frailty indicators, as defined in Joynt et al., 2017, are gait abnormality, malnutrition, failure to thrive, cachexia, debility, difficulty walking, history of fall, muscle wasting, muscle weakness, decubitus ulcer, senility, or durable medical equipment use.

While this starter taxonomy is useful, additional work is needed to develop an ideal taxonomy that presents holistic guidance on how care and finite resources should be targeted and delivered to improve the health of high-need individuals, and ideally reduce the cost of care. One challenge to achieving this is that most health information technology systems do not support integrated and streamlined data collection of patient's physical and behavioral conditions, their care utilization, and their social challenges. Additionally, multiple payers and varied benefits packages pose administrative and operational hurdles for the implementation of a taxonomy.

CARE MODELS THAT DELIVER

The purpose of taxonomies is to align high-need patients with the care models that target their specific needs. For taxonomies to be actionable, successful care models for different segments of high-need patients must exist. Chapter 4 draws on the workshop series and a review of evidence syntheses and other literature to produce a list of attributes of successful care models and to map successful models to different high-need patient segments.

While the success of even the best care model will depend on the particular needs and goals of the patient group a model intends to serve, which varies for different segments of high-need patients, all successful care models should foster effectiveness across three domains: health and well-being, care utilization, and costs. Care models that have been shown to be successful share a number of common attributes, which can be organized in an analytic framework with the following four dimensions: focus on service setting, care attributes, delivery features, and organizational culture. With respect to service setting, generally, the most successful programs for managing high-need individuals focus on either a targeted age group with broad combinations of diagnoses or individuals classified as high-utilizers. Models tend to fall into several broad, nonmutually exclusive categories related to service settings: enhanced primary care, transitional care, and integrated care (Bleich et al., 2015; Boult et al., 2009). Care and condition attributes and delivery features that are common across many successful care models are described in Boxes S-1 and S-2, respectively. Finally, features of organizational culture identified by various authorities that can contribute to the success of care models include the engagement of leadership across levels, customization of the model to the local context, strong team relationships, including patients and care partners, the implementation of appropriate training, continuous assessment with effective metrics, and the use of multiple sources of data (Hong et al., 2014b).

BOX S–1
Care and Condition Attributes of Successful Care Models

- **Assessment**. Multidimensional (medical, functional, and social) patient assessment
- **Targeting**. Targeting those most likely to benefit
- **Planning**. Evidence-based care planning
- **Alignment**. Care match with patient goals and functional needs
- **Training**. Patient and care partner engagement, education, and coaching
- **Communication**. Coordination and communication among and between patient and care team
- **Monitoring**. Proactive tracking of the health status and adherence to care plans
- **Continuity**. Seamless transitions across time and settings

SOURCES: Anderson et al., 2015; Bodenheimer and Berry-Millett, 2009; Boult and Wieland, 2010; Brown et al., 2012; McCarthy et al., 2015; Nelson, 2012

BOX S–2
Delivery Features of Successful Care Models

- **Teamwork**. Multidisciplinary care teams with a single, trained care coordinator as the communication hub and leader
- **Coordination**. Extensive outreach and interaction among patient, care coordinator, and care team, with an emphasis on face-to-face encounters among all parties and collocation of teams
- **Responsiveness**. Speedy provider responsiveness to patients and 24/7 availability
- **Feedback**. Timely clinician feedback and data for remote patient monitoring
- **Medication management**. Careful medication management and reconciliation, particularly in the home setting
- **Outreach**. The extension of care to the community and home
- **Integration**. Linkage to social services
- **Follow-up**. Prompt outpatient follow-up after hospital stays and the implementation of standard discharge protocols

SOURCES: Anderson et al., 2015; Bodenheimer and Berry-Millett, 2009; Brown et al., 2012; Hasselman, 2013; McCarthy et al., 2015; Nelson, 2012; Rodriguez et al., 2014

Using this analytic framework, the planning committee identified 14 successful care models for high-need patients and cross-referenced those to the segment(s) of the proposed taxonomy that could be served if health systems leaders match the needs of their patients to appropriate models within this "menu" of evidence-based approaches (Figure S–3).

POLICY TO SUPPORT THE SPREAD AND SCALE OF CARE MODELS

A number of barriers currently prevent the spread or sustainability of successful care models including the misalignment between financial incentives and the services that are necessary to care for high-need patients, health system fragmentation, workforce training issues, and disparate data systems that cannot easily share data. Chapter 5 explores areas in which policy initiatives could accelerate the spread and scale of care models for high-need patients—particularly the programmatic integration of social supports and medical care—through expanding and realigning payment policies, improving the organization of care, developing a workforce to deliver comprehensive health care, and improving the data infrastructure.

PROGRAM \ SEGMENT	Children w/ complex needs	Non-elderly disabled	Multiple chronic	Major complex chronic	Frail elderly	Advancing illness
Care Management Plus				*		*
Commonwealth Care Alliance		*				
Complex Care Program at Children's National Health System	■					
GRACE				*		
Guided Care				■		
Health Quality Partners			■	■		
Health Services for Children with Special Needs	*					
Hospital at Home						■
H-PACT		*				
IMPACT			*		*	
Partners HealthCare Integrated Care Management Program	■			■		
MIND at home					*	
Naylor Transitional Care Model (Penn)					■	
PACE					*	

FIGURE S–3 | A sample of 14 care models which have evidence of success, matched to the six population segments identified in the taxonomy showing that each segment has been matched to at least one program. A subset of these care models also targets social and/or behavioral risk factors faced by high-need patients and is marked with an (*).

NOTE: Many of these programs could be matched and/or adapted to other patient segments.

SOURCE: Models of Care for High-Need Patients Planning Committee, National Academy of Medicine

Perhaps the most prominent barrier to the adoption of successful care models is payment policies that misalign financial incentives—particularly those that reimburse providers on a fee-for-service basis for discrete medical interventions at the expense of a broader assessment and engagement of medical and social needs. While many insurers, including states and the federal government, are starting to embrace value-based purchasing that includes paying for care delivered outside of the traditional medical silo (Bachrach et al., 2014), further progress could be made by combining Medicare and Medicaid funding streams for dual-eligible patients[1] into an integrated benefit and care delivery structure that allows flexibility in benefit design to address the full range of patient needs (Hayes et al., 2016a). Virtually all high-need patients have challenging social support needs that determine the success of their care management. To be effective, value-based payment models for high-need patients require supporting and rewarding the seamless integration of medical, behavioral, and social services including, where appropriate, support for the delivery of these services in home and community settings (Barnett et al., 2015). This is the aim of shared savings approaches structured to ensure that any savings from the implementation of successful care models accrue to both payers and providers (Hong et al., 2014a).

To improve the organization of care, federal and state governments, working with their local partners, will need to engage in a strategy coordinated to incentivize the provision of evidence-based social support services in conjunction with the delivery of medical services. State efforts may be informed by a policy framework developed by McGinnis and colleagues at The Commonwealth Fund to help states establish the infrastructure necessary to support ongoing integration of health and social services, particularly for Medicaid beneficiaries (McGinnis et al., 2014). It is also necessary to prepare the workforce to deliver team-based, comprehensive health care. To accomplish this, academic health centers and professional societies should collaborate on developing new training and certification opportunities that focus on the treatment and social support needs of high-need patients, including training on team-based care and care coordination across health and social sectors (Thomas-Henkel et al., 2015). In addition, credentialing programs, particularly for nontraditional health workers such as community health workers and peer support providers, could be developed.

Finally, reliable monitoring and continuous improvement of effective models of care for high-need patients depend on high-quality data and analytics that

---

1 Dual eligible patients are low-income Medicare beneficiaries who are eligible for Medicare and Medicaid.

can be used to match high-need individuals with specific interventions (Bates et al., 2014; Bradley et al., 2016; Dale et al., 2016; Rajkumar et al., 2015). High-quality data are also required for quality measurement to determine the impact that care models are having on care coordination, utilization, and cost. Currently, there are many disparate systems that cannot easily share information, making it difficult to assess the requirements of high-need individuals and whether they are getting appropriate care. Coordinated federal, state, and local government initiatives must identify barriers that currently inhibit data flow among the clinicians and organizations treating high-need populations and work to minimize those barriers while respecting patient privacy and data security.

COMMON THEMES AND OPPORTUNITIES FOR ACTION

Common to the presentations and discussions among workshop participants was the notion that improving the care management of high-need patients will require bold policy action and system and payment reform efforts by a broad range of stakeholders at multiple levels. Chapter 6 describes important lessons from this initiative and opportunities for action for each relevant stakeholder group: health systems, payers, providers, patients and family or unpaid caregivers, and the research community.

Three key care requirements stem from the fact that the population of high-need patients is diverse: segmenting patients based on factors that drive health care need is essential for targeting care; effective care models must address the social and behavioral factors in play for a given patient; and finally, policy action should focus on addressing the existing constraints and complexities preventing the integration of medical, behavioral, and social services and with the way the United States finances care models.

Based on these lessons, overarching opportunities for action include:

- Refining the starter taxonomy based on real-world use and experience to facilitate the matching of individual need and functional capacity to specific care programs;
- Integrating and coordinating the delivery of medical, social, and behavioral services in a way that reduces the burdens on patients and caregivers;
- Developing approaches for spreading and scaling successful programs and for training the workforce capable of making these models successful;
- Promoting payment reform efforts that further incentivize the adoption of successful care models and the integration of medical and social services;

- Establishing a small set of proven quality measures appropriate for assessing outcomes, including return on investment, and continuously improving programs for high-need individuals; and
- Creating road maps and tools to help organizations adopt models of care suitable for their particular patient populations.

While each stakeholder sector individually may impact a patient's life, a community, or even a regional health delivery system, one of the most expensive and challenging populations for the current health care system will remain underserved until there is a unified effort—rather than small, incremental steps—to improve care for the nation's high-need patients and to reduce the cost of delivering that care.

REFERENCES

Abrams, M. 2016. *Matching patients to tailored care models: a strategy to enhance care, improve outcomes, and curb costs.* Presentation at the October 21st NAM Models of Care for High-Need Patients meeting, Washington, DC.

Anderson, G. F., J. Ballreich, S. Bleich, C. Boyd, E. DuGoff, B. Leff, C. Salzburg, and J. Wolff. 2015. Attributes common to programs that successfully treat high-need, high-cost individuals. *American Journal of Managed Care* 21(11):e597-600.

Bachrach, D., S. Anthony, and A. Detty. 2014. *State strategies for integrating physical and behavioral health services in a changing medicaid environment.* New York, NY: The Commonwealth Fund.

Barnett, M. L., J. Hsu, and J. M. McWilliams. 2015. Patient characteristics and differences in hospital readmission rates. *JAMA Intern Med* 175(11):1803–1812.

Bates, D. W., S. Saria, L. Ohno-Machado, A. Shah, and G. Escobar. 2014. Big data in health care: Using analytics to identify and manage high-risk and high-cost patients. *Health Affairs* 33(7):1123–1131.

Bleich, S. N., C. Sherrod, A. Chiang, C. Boyd, J. Wolff, E. Chang, C. Salzberg, K. Anderson, B. Leff, and G. Anderson. 2015. Systematic review of programs treating high-need and high-cost people with multiple chronic diseases or disabilities in the United States, 2008–2014. Preventing Chronic Disease 12:e197.

Blumenthal, D., G. Anderson, S. Burke, T. Fulmer, A. K. Jha, and P. Long. 2016. *Tailoring complex-care management, coordination, and integration for high-need, high-cost patients.* Vital Directions for Health and Health Care Series. Discussion Paper, National Academy of Medicine, Washington, DC.

Bodenheimer, T., and R. Berry-Millett. 2009. Follow the money—controlling expenditures by improving care for patients needing costly services. *New England Journal of Medicine* 361(16):1521–1523.

Boult, C., A. F. Green, L. Boult, J. T. Pacala, C. Snyder, and B. Leff. 2009. Successful models of comprehensive care for older adults with chronic conditions: Evidence for the institute of medicine's "retooling for an aging america" report. *Journal of the American Geriatrics Society* 57(12):2328–2337.

Boult, C., and G. D. Wieland. 2010. Comprehensive primary care for older patients with multiple chronic conditions: "Nobody rushes you through". *JAMA* 304(17):1936–1943.

Bradley, E. H., M. Canavan, E. Rogan, K. Talbert-Slagle, C. Ndumele, L. Taylor, and L. A. Curry. 2016. Variation in health outcomes: The role of spending on social services, public health, and health care, 2000–09. *Health Affairs* 35(5):760–768.

Brown, R. S., D. Peikes, G. Peterson, J. Schore, and C. M. Razafindrakoto. 2012. Six features of medicare coordinated care demonstration programs that cut hospital admissions of high-risk patients. *Health Affairs* 31(6):1156–1166.

Cohen, S. B. 2014. *The concentration and persistence in the level of health expenditures over time: Estimates for the US Population, 2011–2012.* Statistical Brief 449 Agency for Healthcare Research and Quality. http://meps.ahrq.gov/mepsweb/data_files/publications/st449/stat449.pdf

Dale, S. B., A. Ghosh, D. N. Peikes, T. J. Day, F. B. Yoon, E. F. Taylor, K. Swankoski, A. S. O'Malley, P. H. Conway, R. Rajkumar, M. J. Press, L. Sessums, and R. Brown. 2016. Two-year costs and quality in the comprehensive primary care initiative. *New England Journal of Medicine* 374(24):2345–2356.

Dzau, V. J., M. B. McClellan, J. McGinnis, and et al. 2017. Vital directions for health and health care: Priorities from a national academy of medicine initiative. *JAMA* 317(14):1461–1470.

Hasselman, D. 2013. *Super-Utilizer Summit: Common Themes from Innovative Complex Care Management Programs.* Center for Health Care Strategies, Inc.

Hayes, K., G. W. Hoadland, N. Lopez, M. Workman, P. Fise, K. Taylor, R. Meltzer, and S. Seong. 2016a. *Delivery system reform: Improving care for individuals dually eligible for medicare and medicaid.* Washington, DC: Bipartisan Policy Center.

Hayes, S. L., C. A. Salzburg, D. McCarthy, D. C. Radley, M. K. Abrams, T. Shah, and G. F. Anderson. 2016b. *High-need, high-cost patients: Who are they and how do they use health care?* New York: The Commonwealth Fund.

Hong, C. S., M. K. Abrams, and T. G. Ferris. 2014a. Toward increased adoption of complex care management. *New England Journal of Medicine* 371(6):491–493.

Hong, C. S., A. L. Siegel, and T. G. Ferris. 2014b. *Caring for high-need, high-cost patients: What makes for a successful care management program?* New York, NY: The Commonwealth Fund.

Joynt, K. E., J. F. Figueroa, N. Beaulieu, R. C. Wild, E. J. Orav, and A. K. Jha. 2017. Segmenting high-cost medicare patients into potentially actionable cohorts. *Healthc (Amst)* 5(1-2):62-67.

McCarthy, D., J. Ryan, and S. Klein. 2015. Models of care for high-need, high-cost patients: An evidence synthesis. *Issue Brief (Commonw Fund)* 31:1–19.

McGinnis, T., M. Crawford, S. A. Somers. 2014. *A state policy framework for integrating health and social services.* The Commonwealth Fund.

Mitchell, E. M. 2016. *Statistical Brief #497: Concentration of Health Expenditures in the US Civilian Noninstitutionalized Population, 2014.* Agency for Healthcare Research and Quality.

Nelson, L. 2012. *Lessons from medicare's demonstration projects on disease management, care coordination, and value-based payment.* Congressional Budget Office

Rajkumar, R., M. J. Press, and P. H. Conway. 2015. The cms innovation center—a five-year self-assessment. *New England Journal of Medicine* 372(21):1981–1983.

Rodriguez, S., D. Munevar, C. Delaney, L. Yang, and A. Tumlinson. 2014. *Effective Management of High-Risk Medicare Populations.* Avalere Health.

Sarnak, D. O., and J. Ryan. 2016. How high-need patients experience the health care system in nine countries. Issue Brief (The Commonwealth Fund) 1:1–14.

Thomas-Henkel, C., A. Hamblin, and T. Hendricks. 2015. *Opportunities to improve models of care for people with complex needs.* Princeton, NJ: Robert Wood Johnson Foundation & Center for Health Care Strategies.

1

INTRODUCTION AND OVERVIEW

The exceptionally high expenditures associated with providing care for a relatively small but growing number of individuals with significant medical needs disproportionately drive the escalating cost of medical care in the United States. This population of high-need individuals includes an increasingly heterogeneous group of people with multiple chronic diseases, members of an aging population, and patients with varying levels of medical, functional, social, and behavioral complexity. Today, 1 percent of patients account for more than 20 percent of health care expenditures, and 5 percent account for nearly half of the nation's spending on health care (Mitchell, 2016). Improving care management for this population while balancing quality and associated costs is at the forefront of national health care goals, and reaching this particular goal will require the active involvement of a broad range of stakeholders at multiple levels. Health care systems have implemented several successful strategies with the hope of improving health outcomes, improving the patient experience, and lowering costs, but a "best practice" for high-need patient management has proven elusive; the majority of care remains fragmented, uncoordinated, reactive, and often poorly matched to individuals' circumstances. The nation needs a better understanding of how to best utilize its resources to care for this growing population.

To advance insights and perspectives on how to better manage the care of high-need patients and to stimulate actions on opportunities for improving outcomes and reducing the costs of health care for these vulnerable populations, the National Academy of Medicine (NAM), through its Leadership Consortium for a Value & Science-Driven Health System (the Leadership Consortium), in partnership with the Harvard T.H. Chan School of Public Health (HSPH), the Bipartisan Policy Center (BPC), The Commonwealth Fund, and the Peterson Center on Healthcare—which funded this initiative—has undertaken a collaborative assessment on strategies for better serving high-need patients. The project activities were overseen by an independent planning committee and included (1) planning three workshops to explore the state of knowledge and action;

(2) conducting a literature review of the key studies on the care of high-need patients; and (3) synthesizing the work and proceedings that reflected critical needs and common themes on effective approaches, care models, and possible policy actions to address those needs. This publication synthesizes information and insights gleaned from the workshop presentations and discussions, as well as concurrent and supplemental work led by the partnering organizations, the workshop planning committee, and other external experts and stakeholders, to move the field forward.

PARTNER ORGANIZATIONS

The five-way partnership involving the Leadership Consortium, the HSPH, the BPC, the Peterson Center on Healthcare, and The Commonwealth Fund has driven this project, with each partner taking on a specific role. The Peterson Center on Healthcare is dedicated to identifying proven solutions that improve care quality, lower costs, and accelerate the adoption of these solutions on a national level. With the aim of identifying programs that successfully serve the growing number of high-need individuals and potential policy solutions to bring these models to scale, the Peterson Center initiated and provided support for the contributions of the NAM, the BPC, and the HSPH.

The BPC examined different policy approaches that might address barriers and accelerate the adoption of proven models for improving care and reducing costs for high-need patients. Its work culminated in a report that was presented at the final workshop and contained draft policy recommendations and areas of opportunity to improve care and outcomes for high-need patients (Hayes et al., 2016a). These recommendations aimed to better align financial incentives, specifically those targeting care for dual-eligible[2] high-need patients.

HSPH's role in this project has been to provide an analysis of data to define both clinically and socially meaningful segments of this heterogeneous group of people as a means of identifying subgroups that might benefit from specific types of programs (Joynt et al., 2017). This analysis addressed three key questions relevant to controllable costs:

• What are the specific characteristics associated with high-need, high-cost patients within these segments?

---

2 Dual-eligible patients are low-income Medicare beneficiaries who are eligible for Medicare and Medicaid.

- How do utilization patterns differ between these segments and within the segments?
- What proportion of the spending and utilization might be reduced for each segment?

HSPH's project team has attempted to identify characteristics of providers and health systems that are more effective at caring for high-need, high-cost patients and reducing the costs associated with preventable health care issues. The project team, with the help of The Commonwealth Fund, examined data from the Medicare population and a set of commercial patients. The team has also worked with colleagues at the Peterson Center on Healthcare to examine data on the dual-eligible population.

The Commonwealth Fund has placed a primary emphasis on these issues and has served as a strategic adviser and contributor throughout the initiative, leveraging its extensive portfolio of work focused on improving care for high-need, high-cost patients. A research and funding institution that aims to promote a high-performing health care system, particularly for the most vulnerable, The Commonwealth Fund is also part of a consortium of five national foundations along with the John A. Hartford Foundation, the Robert Wood Johnson Foundation, the Peterson Center on Healthcare, and The SCAN Foundation—all focused on furthering efforts to improve care for high-need patients. The collaboration works to develop resources to understand the diverse high-need population, to identify evidence-based programs that offer high-quality integrated care at a lower cost, and to accelerate the adoption of these programs nationally.[3]

THE NATIONAL ACADEMY OF MEDICINE

As the convening body for this initiative, the National Academy of Medicine— through its Leadership Consortium for a Value & Science-Driven Health System—brought together experts and stakeholders to reflect upon the key issues for improving care for high-need patients, synthesize the information and insights gathered, and summarize the presentations, discussions, and literature for publication.

Broadly, the Leadership Consortium convenes national experts and executive-level leaders from key stakeholder sectors for collaborative activities to

---

3   For more information on this consortium, see www.commonwealthfund.org/publications/ newsletters/the-commonwealth-fund-connection/2016/aug/aug-2-2016/whats-new/five-health-care-foundations (accessed December 21, 2016). For an example of resources pulled together, see "the Playbook," at http://www.bettercareplaybook.org (accessed December 21, 2016).

foster progress toward a continuously learning health system in which science, informatics, incentives, and culture are aligned for enduring improvement and innovation; best practices are seamlessly embedded in the care process; patients and families are active participants in all elements; and new knowledge is captured as an integral by-product of the care experience. Priorities in this respect include advancing the development of a fully interoperable digital infrastructure, the application of new clinical research approaches, and a culture of transparency on outcomes and cost.

Participants in the Leadership Consortium have set a goal that, by 2020, 90 percent of clinical decisions will be supported by accurate, timely, and up-to-date clinical information and reflect the best available evidence. The Leadership Consortium's approach to meeting this goal is to serve as a forum to facilitate the collaborative assessment and action around issues central to achieving its vision and goal. To address the challenges of improving both evidence development and evidence application, as well as improving the capacity to advance progress on each of those dimensions, Leadership Consortium members (all leaders in their fields) work with their colleagues to identify the issues not being adequately addressed, the nature of the barriers and possible solutions, and the priorities for action. They then work to marshal the resources of the sectors represented on the Leadership Consortium to work for sustained public-private cooperation for change.

A common commitment to certain principles and priorities guides the activities of the Leadership Consortium and its members. These include the commitment to the right health care for each person; putting the best evidence into practice; establishing the effectiveness, efficiency, and safety of medical care delivered; building assessment and accountability into care; advancing clinical data as a public resource for health improvement; shared responsibility distributed equitably across stakeholders, both public and private; collaborative stakeholder involvement in priority setting; transparency in executing activities and reporting results; and individual stakeholder perspectives subjugated to the common good.

SCOPE AND ACTIVITIES

The independent planning committee organized the three workshops (see Appendix B for the agendas) in accordance with the procedures of the National Academies of Sciences, Engineering, and Medicine. The planning committee's members were Peter V. Long, Chair (Blue Shield of California Foundation), Melinda K. Abrams (The Commonwealth Fund), Gerard F. Anderson (Johns

Hopkins Bloomberg School of Public Health), Tim Engelhardt (Centers for Medicare & Medicaid Services), Jose Figueroa (Harvard Medical School), Katherine Hayes (Bipartisan Policy Center), Frederick Isasi (National Governors Association), Ashish K. Jha (Harvard T.H. Chan School of Public Health), David Meyers (Agency for Healthcare Research and Quality), Arnold S. Milstein (Stanford University), Diane Stewart (Pacific Business Group on Health), and Sandra Wilkniss (National Governors Association).

The workshops brought together national experts and stakeholders to explore commonalities and differences among the subpopulations of high-need patients, to consider the lessons learned from targeted intervention activities, to discuss and inform the approach of the ongoing study by the HSPH on the high-cost Medicare population, and to review policy issues and options, including those suggested by the BPC.

The first workshop, held in July 2015, laid the groundwork for this project and the subsequent workshops. The presentations and discussions identified the key characteristics of high-need patient populations and subgroups of these heterogeneous populations that offer the greatest opportunity for impact. This workshop also examined the factors that are most important in determining which care models are most effective for particular subgroups of high-need patients; the types of active care coordination and providers of social and behavioral health services and supports in different circumstances; and the lessons from past experiences with high-need patients that can inform efforts to spread and scale successful care models.

The second workshop, convened in January 2016, built on the insights from the first workshop and further explored specific issues. The presentations and discussions in the second workshop focused on the use of a patient segmentation strategy to inform which care models are most appropriate for specific subpopulation of high-need patients. They also reviewed sources of data to drive segmentation strategies, efforts to build a taxonomy of high-need patients, and specific design elements of a successful care model. Sessions at this workshop also discussed specific replication strategies to spread and scale those models, the barriers to scaling new delivery models, and essential elements for a policy framework that could mitigate those barriers.

The third workshop, held in October 2016, discussed the implications of the findings of HSPH's study and the policy strategies identified by the BPC. The presentations and discussions at the third workshop examined tools to improve care delivery for high-need patients, including a taxonomy that matches patient needs to care models with the most potential to improve outcomes and lower costs of caring for high-need patients. This workshop also discussed policy-level approaches to support and accelerate the spread and scale of effective care models. An independent rapporteur prepared factual summaries of what occurred at the workshops. Statements, recommendations, and opinions expressed at the workshops were those of individual presenters and participants and have not been endorsed or validated by the NAM.

In addition to the three workshops, the planning committee initiated several important supplementary activities. A taxonomy workgroup reviewed existing approaches and developed guidance on adaptation and application of a taxonomy in practice. Chapter 3 includes the findings from the workgroup's efforts and supporting research. A review of care models examined in the literature identified promising types of care models and key attributes for success. This review informs a four-part framework described in Chapter 4, as well as how successful care models might map to different high-need patient segments. A subgroup of the planning committee also examined policy options most likely to reduce the barriers to the spread and scale of successful models. Those deliberations, together with the work of the BPC and others, provided much of the content for Chapter 5.

RECURRING THEMES

Informed by discussions, presentations, and concurrent work throughout the course of the project period, this publication reports and reflects on the following issues: (1) key characteristics of high-need patients; (2) the use of a patient categorization scheme—or a taxonomy—as a tool to inform and target care; (3) promising care models and attributes to better serve this patient population, as well as insights on "matching" these models to specific patient groups; and (4) areas of opportunity for policy-level action to support the spread and scale of evidence-based programs. Each of the main chapters begins with a fictional patient vignette highlighting a main point discussed in the chapter. The publication concludes by exploring common themes and opportunities for action in the field.

Recurring themes throughout the initiative include those related to:

- **Functional status.** Functional status is a central determinant of the nature and level of health care needs.
- **Cost.** Patients with complex needs are often high-cost patients, but some high-cost patients do not necessarily have complex needs—for example, those with conditions effectively treated by high-cost interventions.
- **Social circumstances.** Accommodation of social circumstances is key to addressing individuals with high needs.

- **Social services.** Improving care for high-need patients usually requires engaging services outside of the care system and creating patient- and care-partner-specific care plans.
- **Service linkages.** Coordination of care is critical for high-need patients, and success depends on alignment and cooperation between the health care system and services delivered through social, economic, and behavioral programs.
- **Targeting specificity and timeliness.** Health care systems with effective and efficient approaches to sustaining and improving levels of function of high-need patients are those most deliberate and active in identifying and targeting needs early on.
- **Payment alignment.** Payment models segmented according to individual services offer incentives counter to successful models of care for high-need patients, including those of certain Medicare and Medicaid payment policies.
- **Duration.** The nature and level of needs can change over time. A significant number of high-need patients are only transiently high-need.
- **Variability.** High-need patients are heterogeneous and no single care model can provide all the services required by high-need patients; relevant approaches must therefore be guided by a taxonomy that matches intervention options with the specific needs of different categories of high-need patients.

REFERENCES

Hayes, K., G. W. Hoadland, N. Lopez, M. Workman, P. Fise, K. Taylor, R. Meltzer, and S. Seong. 2016. *Delivery system reform: Improving care for individuals dually eligible for Medicare and Medicaid.* Washington, DC: Bipartisan Policy Center.

Joynt, K. E., J. F. Figueroa, N. Beaulieu, R. C. Wild, E. J. Orav, and A. K. Jha. 2017. Segmenting high-cost Medicare patients into potentially actionable cohorts. *Healthc (Amst)* 5(1-2):62-67.

Mitchell, E. M. 2016. Statistical Brief #497: Concentration of Health Expenditures in the US Civilian 298 Noninstitutionalized Population, 2014. Agency for Healthcare Research and Quality.

2

KEY CHARACTERISTICS
OF HIGH-NEED PATIENTS

Fictional Patient vignette: Mark is a 54-year-old man with rheumatoid arthritis and chronic heart disease. Many days he was reliant on a wheelchair to get around because of chronic pain. His job didn't allow him to telework, yet it was difficult to get to the handicap entrance in the back of the building and his schedule was firmly fixed at 9 to 5. As a result, Mark spent more than an hour a day commuting in his car (public transportation wasn't readily available). Everyday tasks like running errands and getting groceries were difficult. Between his pain and his heavy work schedule, he was left with little time to visit with other people, both friends and family, and it had left him feeling incredibly isolated and alone. He really missed having a pet, but he'd had to give his cat, Felix, away because Mark could no longer take care of him properly. Mark felt he wouldn't mind his disease so much if it didn't impact his life and relationships so heavily.

Who are high-need patients? A simple definition describes them as individuals with complex conditions and circumstances requiring multiple services that, for the most part, are not currently delivered easily or effectively by the health care system. This definition is impractical, however, for the task of identifying a population. In general, high-need individuals are the most costly patients, but not all high-cost individuals are also of high-need (Zodet, 2016). Many high-need patients are seniors, but younger adults with disabilities, chronic mental illness, and/or substance abuse disorders also require extensive care (Blumenthal et al., 2016b). Some individuals are of high-need for an extended time because they have multiple chronic conditions that may be stable with treatment but persist for years while other individuals, such as those treated for certain cancers or complex orthopedic surgeries, may be high-need only temporarily

(Johnson et al., 2015b). In addition to their formal diagnoses, many high-need patients have functional limitations that affect their ability to get care or engage in activities of daily living. Others may have severe, persistent behavioral health issues, or their conditions may be exacerbated by such nonmedical factors as a lack of housing, food, and supportive personal relationships (Johnson et al., 2015a; Kansagara et al., 2011).

This chapter explores candidate criteria used to identify high-need patients along with key demographic and experiential characteristics. The next chapter will consider taxonomic approaches to categorizing this heterogeneous population into subgroups with shared management characteristics as a means of developing strategies to inform planning and delivery of targeted and more effective care for specific subgroups.

IDENTIFYING HIGH-NEED PATIENT POPULATIONS

In her presentation at the first workshop, Melinda Abrams from The Commonwealth Fund noted that, to date, little has been written about the characteristics of high-need individuals using empirical data, and, as a result, there is not yet a consistent definition of need. Most studies have examined people who have a specific disease, have multiple chronic conditions, frequently use emergency department services, annually have high individual health care costs, have a disability, or have a mental illness. At some point, noted Abrams, the field will need to settle on a definition.

Health care systems and researchers have used several approaches to identifying high-need populations. One common and direct approach—which focuses on those patients who accrue the largest annual expenditures on health care—is based on the well-established observation that a small percentage of patients account for a large percentage of the nation's health care expenditures (Cohen, 2015; Cohen and Uberoi, 2013; Stanton and Rutherford, 2006; Zodet, 2016). In 2014, for example, the top 1 percent of spenders accounted for more than 20 percent of total health care expenditures, and the top 5 percent accounted for about 50 percent of the nation's health care costs (Mitchell, 2016) (see Figure 2–1).

On the other hand, focusing exclusively on cost provides an incomplete picture of high-need patients. A substantial percent of high-cost individuals incurs those costs for only a limited time (Cohen and Yu, 2012). Medical Expenditure Panel Survey (MEPS) data show, for example, that only 42 percent of individuals who accounted for the top 10 percent of medical expenditures had persistently high spending over a 2-year period. Approximately 30 percent had some reduction in spending in the second year, while 28 percent had episodic high spending, with lower spending in the second year.

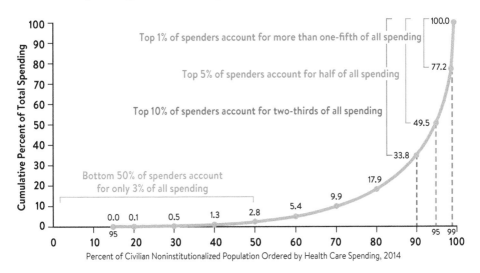

FIGURE 2–1 | Distribution of personal health care spending in the US civilian noninstitutionalized population, 2014.
SOURCE: Dzau et al., 2017

Profiling chronic or complex conditions, including behavioral health issues, offers another approach that, on the surface, seems sensible. Ashish Jha from the Harvard T.H. Chan School of Public Health and Jose Figueroa from Harvard Medical School and Brigham and Women's Hospital, together with colleagues, conducted an analysis of Medicare data to segment the high-cost patient population into clinically meaningful subgroups (Joynt et al., 2017).[4] As part of this analysis, they developed a list of complex and noncomplex chronic conditions that could be used to help determine level of patient need (see Table 2–1) from key chronic disease groups included by the Centers for Medicare & Medicaid Services in its measure for unplanned admission for patients with multiple chronic diseases (RTI International, 2015). The nine complex chronic diseases in Table 2–1 were differentiated by Jha, Figueroa, and colleagues because they account for the majority of spending and morbidity.

In fact, an analysis of MEPS data conducted by The Commonwealth Fund (Hayes et al., 2016c) identified approximately 79 million people age 18 or older

---

4   More details about the segmentation work are discussed in Chapter 3.

(i.e., 30 percent of the population) with three or more chronic conditions,[5] indicating—as was mentioned in the article—that simply counting conditions is an oversimplified approach, and additional factors must be taken into account.

TABLE 2-1 | Complex and Noncomplex Chronic Conditions

COMPLEX CHRONIC CONDITIONS	NONCOMPLEX CHRONIC CONDITIONS
Acute myocardial infarction	Amputation status
Ischemic heart disease	Arthritis and other inflammatory tissue disease
Chronic kidney disease	Artificial openings
Congestive heart failure	Benign prostatic hyperplasia
Dementia	Cancer
Diabetes	Cystic fibrosis
Chronic lung disease	Endocrine and metabolic disorders
Psychiatric disease	Eye disease
Specified heart arrhythmias	Hematological disease
Stroke	Hyperlipidemia
	Hypertension
	Immune disorders
	Inflammatory bowel disease
	Liver and biliary disease
	Neuromuscular disease
	Osteoporosis
	Paralytic diseases/conditions
	Skin ulcer
	Substance abuse
	Thyroid disease

NOTE: Complexity designation is based on spending and morbidity.
SOURCE: Reproduced from Joynt et al., 2017

The most basic identifiers of high need are functional limitations. These include limitations in activities of daily living—self-care tasks that include dressing, bathing or showering, ambulating, self-feeding, grooming, and toileting—or instrumental activities of daily living that support an independent lifestyle, such as housework, shopping, managing money, taking medications, using the telephone, or being able to use transportation (Hayes et al., 2016c). If high-need populations are defined as individuals who have three or more chronic conditions plus functional limitations, roughly 11.8 million individuals age 18 or older (i.e., approximately 5 percent of the US adult population) would be classified as high-need individuals (Hayes, 2016).

Also relevant to the consideration of functional limitations and the way they are best managed is the interplay of physical capacity and mental or emotional status.

---

5 For this study, chronic diseases were identified using an approach that assigns ICD-9 diagnosis codes (first three digits) to the Agency for Healthcare Research and Quality's Clinical Classification System (Hwang et al., 2001; Paez et al., 2009).

For example, the following six circumstances represent compelling limitations and needs:

- Recovery from acute injury or surgery
- Intensive therapeutic interventions
- Chronic addiction-related impairment
- Long-term mobility impairment
- Long-term cognitive impairment
- Needs at the end-of-life

Any of these may represent a very high degree of functional impairment or limitation at any given time, but the nature, intensity, and combination of interventions required may vary considerably.

Determining an ideal definition for a high-need patient requires a delicate balance. A highly constrained definition will risk missing people, potentially depriving them of needed resources. On the other hand, casting an overly broad definition might include people who are not high-need and do not need additional resources. Abrams noted that basing identification of high-need patients exclusively on cost will miss many people, and if the focus is exclusively on chronic conditions, a large number of people may be identified whose chronic conditions are under control.

THE OVERLAP OF HIGH-NEED AND HIGH-COST DEFINITIONS

Regardless of which definition is used to identify a high-need patient population, many of the characteristics of other definitions emerge from the analysis. For example, Jha, Figueroa, and colleagues analyzed Massachusetts claims data, looking broadly at high-cost patients in three categories: the non-Medicare population under age 65, the Medicare population, and the dual-eligible population (Joynt et al., 2017). The analyses of these data reveal that high-cost individuals have more chronic conditions than non-high-cost individuals (see Figure 2–2).

Moreover, the number of chronic conditions increases when moving from the non-Medicare under 65 to the Medicare and dual-eligible populations. High-cost patients are also more likely to have a higher number of frailty indicators (see Figure 2–3), which attempt to capture an individual's ability to engage in activities of daily living or their functional limitation status.

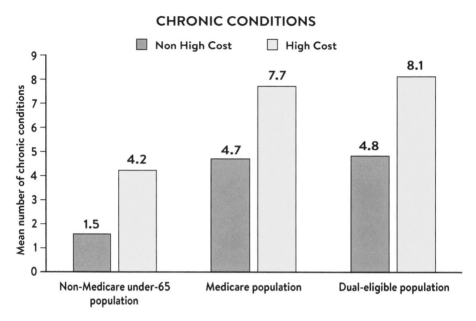

FIGURE 2–2 | Mean number of chronic conditions among three groups of Massachusetts residents.
SOURCE: Reproduced from Jha presentation, January 19, 2016

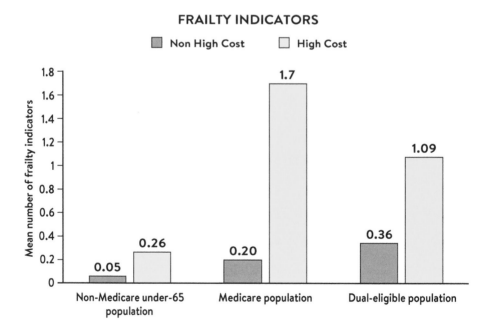

FIGURE 2–3 | Mean number of frailty indicators among three groups of Massachusetts residents.
SOURCE: Reproduced from Jha presentation, January 19, 2016

Likewise, by considering adults who have three or more chronic conditions and also have functional limitations, Hayes and colleagues at The Commonwealth Fund (2016) found that high-need adults averaged more than $21,000 a year in health care and prescription drug expenses, more than fourfold the average for all US adults, and almost three times more than for adults with three or more chronic conditions but no functional limitation. Out-of-pocket expenses for high-need adults averaged $1,669 per person per year, approximately three times higher than for the average US adult ($702) and 44 percent higher than for adults with three or more chronic conditions ($1,157). Annual spending by the top 5 percent of high-need individuals in terms of yearly expenditures exceeded $73,000 compared to nearly $27,600 by the top 5 percent of those with three or more chronic conditions and just under $21,000 by the average adult (see Figure 2–4).

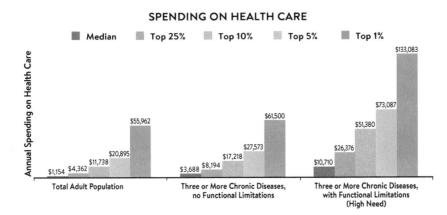

FIGURE 2–4 | High-need adults had higher spending on health care than did those with three or more chronic conditions without functional limitations.
SOURCE: Reproduced from Hayes et al., 2016c

Concordant with their higher expenditures, these high-need individuals also made greater use of the emergency department; had more hospitalizations than did either the average adult or adults with multiple chronic conditions (see Figure 2–5); had more doctor visits; and had more paid home health care days. Finally, the high-need adults were more likely to incur and maintain high health care spending over a 2-year period than were either adults with three or more chronic conditions but no functional limitations or US adults overall.

It is necessary to use major characteristics identified and validated through various studies to develop a consistent and reliable definition of high-need. For example, taken together, total accrued health care costs, intensity of care utilized for a given period of time, and functional limitations could form a basis for defining and identifying a high-need population.

EMERGENCY DEPARTMENT AND HOSPITAL USAGE

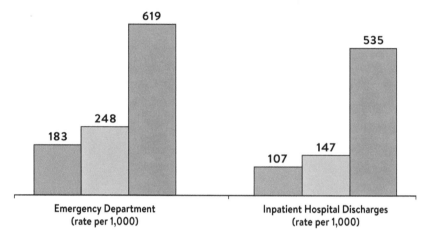

FIGURE 2-5 | High-need adults have more emergency department visits and hospital stays.
SOURCE: Reproduced from Hayes et al., 2016c

CHARACTERISTICS OF PEOPLE WITH HIGH NEEDS RELATIVE TO OTHERS

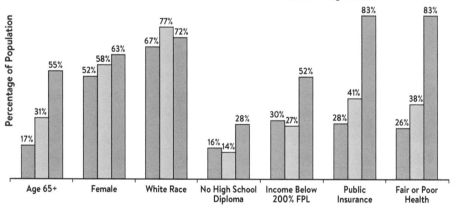

FIGURE 2-6 | Demographic characteristics of high-need adults.
NOTE: FPL = federal poverty line.
SOURCE: Reproduced from Hayes et al., 2016c

THE IMPACT OF BEING A HIGH-NEED PATIENT

A rough understanding of the demographics of the high-need patient population does emerge from the research. According to analyses by The Commonwealth Fund and by the Agency for Healthcare Research and Quality (Cohen, 2015), high-need adults are disproportionately older, female, white, and less educated. Jha, Figueroa, and colleagues found the high-cost Medicare population to be disproportionately older, female, and nearly twice as likely to be dual-eligible (Joynt et al., 2017). Hayes and colleagues (2016) reported similar findings (see Figure 2–6). As a group, high-need patients are also more likely to be publicly insured (83 percent were insured under Medicare, Medicaid, or both), have fair to poor self-reported health, and have a behavioral or substance abuse condition. The average median household income for high-need adults ($25,668) was less than half of that of the overall adult population ($52,685), which was only slightly higher than the median household income for adults with three chronic conditions but no functional limitations ($52,499).

Functional limitations are key drivers of need. Adults with functional limitations tend to have higher health care expenses than adults with no such limitations (Olin and Dougherty, 2006; Zhang et al., 2015). Studies have also shown that adults with functional limitations are more likely to require care in a nursing home or assisted living facility (Foley et al., 1992; Gaugler et al., 2007). Functional limitations are also one type of patient-reported outcome that researchers believe represents an accurate assessment of an individual's health status and need for services (Wolinsky et al., 2011).

A substantial literature shows that, for the population as a whole, medical care influences only a relatively small portion of overall health (McGinnis et al., 2002; Taylor et al., 2015b) and that social services expenditures significantly impact population health outcomes (Bradley et al., 2011). Similarly, the importance of social services to the well-being of high-need patients also has a disproportionate impact relative to medical care. Inadequate availability of social services, such as a lack of stable housing, a reliable food source, or basic transportation, can clearly worsen health outcomes in high-need patients (Taylor et al., 2015b).

A reality for high-need patients is that their needs often go beyond care for their physical ailments. For example, a study of high-need patients in Washington State who are frequent users of the emergency department for their health care needs found that a majority of these individuals had an alcohol or a substance abuse disorder and mental illness (Mancuso et al., 2004). In fact, for some high-need individuals, alcohol and substance abuse disorders can be important contributors to chronic physical and behavioral health conditions, including hypertension, congestive heart failure, depression, anxiety, and other mental and physical disorders (Mertens et al., 2003; Mertens et al., 2005). Jha, Figueroa, and colleagues also found that a mental health diagnosis and an alcohol or a substance abuse diagnosis were both predictors of high-cost status (Joynt et al., 2017).

The results of a series of The Commonwealth Fund surveys further illustrate some of the challenges high-need individuals face in receiving adequate care. A 2014 survey, in which high-need individuals were defined as those 65 years or older with three or more chronic conditions or functional limitations, found that high-need individuals are particularly susceptible to a lack of coordination within the health care system (Sarnak and Ryan, 2016). Lack of coordination was determined to be in evidence when test results or records were not available at a medical appointment; there were duplicate tests orders; conflicting information was received from different providers; or a specialist lacked a patient's medical history or the patient's primary care provider was not informed about specialist care. Some 44 percent of high-need individuals reported a care coordination problem over the preceding 2 years compared to 27 percent of other older adults (Sarnak and Ryan, 2016). Additionally, more high-need adults reported that they thought a medical mistake was made in their treatment or care (13 percent) compared to the overall population of older adults (6 percent) and, despite the high level of insurance among this population, some 22 percent reported cost-related problems accessing care compared to 16 percent of the overall population of older adults.

A subsequent study by The Commonwealth Fund (Salzberg et al., 2016), based on an analysis of the 2009–2011 MEPS data, also found that being a high-need individual had a substantial impact on the care experience. According to this analysis, high-need adults were more likely to report having an unmet medical need—defined as forgoing or delaying needed medical care or prescription medication in the prior year—and less likely to report having good patient-provider communications compared to all adults or those with multiple chronic illnesses but no functional limitations. Unmet needs were greatest among high-need adults with private insurance and Medicaid. Easy access to specialists did not differ appreciably among the three groups, with approximately 50 percent of the individuals in each group reporting they had no trouble getting referred to a specialist when they believed they needed to see one.

One troubling finding from this analysis was that, although 93 percent of high-need adults have a usual source of care, only 46 percent of high-need adults reported that they had a usual source of care meeting the definition of a medical home in providing care that is comprehensive, accessible, and responsive to the patients' needs. This finding is important, the authors wrote, because medical homes benefit all patients and may especially help high-need patients improve outcomes and reduce spending. They also noted that, while low, the proportion of high-need patients receiving care in a medical home model was greater than the 36 percent of the general adult population who have a usual source of care meeting the definition of a medical home.

The most recent survey by The Commonwealth Fund included adults with two or more major chronic conditions, with or without functional limitations; individuals under 65 with a disability; and elderly individuals with multiple functional limitations (Ryan et al., 2016). The findings reiterated many of the conclusions from previous studies, but they also provided a focus on nonmedical aspects of care. For example, Ryan and colleagues (2016) stressed the social isolation and unmet social needs expressed by high-need patients, with nearly two-thirds articulating concern about such material hardships as housing, meals, or utilities. Additionally, of those high-need patients who reported a need for assistance with activities of daily living, only slightly more than one-third (38 percent) responded that they usually or always had someone available. Emotional counseling services were also cited as difficult to access, with less than half of those who may have needed them in the past 2 years able to set up an appointment in a timely fashion.

As Blumenthal and his colleagues stated in a discussion paper for the National Academy of Medicine's *Vital Directions for Health and Health Care* Initiative (Blumenthal et al., 2016a), addressing just the health care needs—or, for that matter, the social and behavioral health needs—of high-need patients in isolation is likely to be inadequate. As the authors of this paper concluded, "Health-system leaders, payers, and providers will need to look beyond the regular slate of medical services to coordinate, integrate, and effectively manage care for behavioral-health conditions and social-service needs for functional impairments to improve outcomes and lower spending." They also noted that the heterogeneity of the high-need population speaks to the implausibility of finding one delivery model or one program that meets the needs of all high-need patients, stating, "Payers and health systems may need to divide these patients into groups that have common needs so that specific complex care-management interventions can be targeted to the people who are most likely to benefit." Addressing clinical needs alone will not improve outcomes or reduce costs. Rather, it will also be necessary to address an individual's functional, social, and behavioral needs, largely through the provision of social and community services that today are not typically the province of health care delivery systems.

REFERENCES

Blumenthal, D., G. Anderson, S. Burke, T. Fulmer, A. K. Jha, and P. Long. 2016a. *Tailoring complex-care management, coordination, and integration for high-need, high-cost patients: A vital direction for health and health care.* Discussion Paper, National Academy of Medicine, Washington, DC.

Blumenthal, D., B. Chernof, T. Fulmer, J. Lumpkin, and J. Selberg. 2016b. Caring for high-need, high-cost patients—an urgent priority. *New England Journal of Medicine* 375(10):909–911.

Bradley, E. H., B. R. Elkins, J. Herrin, and B. Elbel. 2011. Health and social services expenditures: Associations with health outcomes. *BMJ Quality & Safety* 20(10):826–831.

Cohen, S. B. 2015. *The concentration and persistence in the level of health expenditures over time: Estimates for the US Population, 2012–2013.* Rockville, MD: Agency for Healthcare Research and Quality.

Cohen, S. B., and N. Uberoi. 2013. *Differentials in the concentration in the level of health expenditures across population subgroups in the US, 2010.* Statistical Brief #421. Rockville, MD: Agency for Healthcare Research and Quality.

Cohen, S. B., and W. Yu. 2012. *The concentration and persistence in the level of health expenditures over time: Estimates for the US Population, 2008–2009.* Rockville, MD: Agency for Healthcare Research and Quality.

Dzau, V. J., M. B. McClellan, J. M. McGinnis, and et al. 2017. Vital directions for health and health care: Priorities from a national academy of medicine initiative. *JAMA* 317(14):1461–1470.

Foley, D. J., A. M. Ostfeld, L. G. Branch, R. B. Wallace, J. McGloin, and J. C. Cornoni-Huntley. 1992. The risk of nursing home admission in three communities. *Journal of Aging and Health* 4(2):155–173.

Gaugler, J. E., S. Duval, K. A. Anderson, and R. L. Kane. 2007. Predicting nursing home admission in the US: A meta-analysis. *BMC Geriatrics* 7:13.

Hayes, S. L., C. A. Salzberg, D. McCarthy, D. C. Radley, M. K. Abrams, T. Shah, and G. F. Anderson. 2016. *High-need, high-cost patients: Who are they and how do they use health care?* New York: The Commonwealth Fund.

Jha, A. 2016. *Targeting High Cost Patients and their Needs.* Presentation at the January 19th NAM Models of Care for High-Need Patients meeting, Washington, DC.

Johnson, T. L., D. J. Rinehart, J. Durfee, D. Brewer, H. Batal, J. Blum, C. I. Oronce, P. Melinkovich, and P. Gabow. 2015b. For many patients who use large amounts of health care services, the need is intense yet temporary. *Health Affairs* 34(8):1312–1319.

Joynt, K. E., J. F. Figueroa, N. Beaulieu, R. C. Wild, E. J. Orav, and A. K. Jha. 2017. Segmenting high-cost medicare patients into potentially actionable cohorts. *Healthc (Amst)* 5(1-2):62-67.

Mancuso, D., D. J. Nordlund, and B. Felver. 2004. *Frequent emergency room visits signal substance abuse and mental illness.* Olympia, WA: Washington State Department of Social and Health Services.

McGinnis, J. M., P. Williams-Russo, and J. R. Knickman. 2002. The case for more active policy attention to health promotion. *Health Affairs* 21(2):78–93.

Mertens, J. R., Y. W. Lu, S. Parthasarathy, C. Moore, and C. M. Weisner. 2003. Medical and psychiatric conditions of alcohol and drug treatment patients in an HMO: Comparison with matched controls. *Archives of Internal Medicine* 163(20):2511–2517.

Mertens, J. R., C. Weisner, G. T. Ray, B. Fireman, and K. Walsh. 2005. Hazardous drinkers and drug users in HMO primary care: Prevalence, medical conditions, and costs. *Alcoholism, Clinical and Experimental Research* 29(6):989–998.

Mitchell, E. M. 2016. *Statistical Brief #497: Concentration of Health Expenditures in the US Civilian Noninstitutionalized Population, 2014.* Agency for Healthcare Research and Quality.

Olin, G., and D. D. Dougherty. 2006. *Characteristics and medical expenses of adults 18 to 64-years old with functional limitations, combined years 1997–2002.* Rockville, MD: Agency for Healthcare Research and Quality.

RTI International. 2015. *Accountable care organization 2015 program analysis quality performance standards narrative measure specifications.* Rockville, MD: Centers for Medicare & Medicaid Services.

Ryan, J., M. K. Abrams, M. M. Doty, T. Shah, and E. C. Schneider. 2016. How High-Need Patients Experience Health Care in the United States: Findings of the 2016 Commonwealth Fund Survey of High-Need Patients. New York: The Commonwealth Fund.

Salzberg, C. A., S. L. Hayes, D. McCarthy, D. Radley, M. K. Abrams, T. Shah, and G. Anderson. 2016. *Health system performance for the high-need patient: A look at access to care and patient care experiences.* New York: The Commonwealth Fund.

Sarnak, D. O., and J. Ryan. 2016. How high-need patients experience the health care system in nine countries. *Issue Brief (The Commonwealth Fund)* 1:1–14.

Stanton, M. W., and M. K. Rutherford. 2006. *The high concentration of US Health care expenditures.* Rockville, MD: Agency for Healthcare Research and Quality.

Taylor, L. A., C. E. Coyle, C. Ndumele, E. Rogan, M. Canavan, L. Curry, and E. H. Brandley. 2015. *Leveraging the social determinants of health: What works?* Boston, MA: Blue Cross Blue Shield of Massachusetts Foundation.

Wolinsky, F. D., S. E. Bentler, J. Hockenberry, M. P. Jones, M. Obrizan, P. A. Weigel, B. Kaskie, and R. B. Wallace. 2011. Long-term declines in ADLs, IADLs, and mobility among older Medicare beneficiaries. *BMC Geriatrics* 11(1):43.

Zhang, J. X., J. U. Lee, and D. O. Meltzer. 2015. The effect of functional limitations and hospitalization on out-of-pocket medical payments in older adults. *Annals of Community Medicine and Practice* 1(1).

Zodet, M. 2016. *Characteristics of persons with high health care expenditures in the US civilian noninstitutionalized population, 2014.* Agency for Healthcare Research and Quality.

3

PATIENT TAXONOMY AND IMPLICATIONS FOR CARE DELIVERY

Fictional patient vignette: Sarah is a 26-year-old woman who was recently involved in a car accident that left her paralyzed from the waist down. She was having a lot of trouble not only adjusting to her new reality but also navigating all of her new health care needs. Sarah had been a regular runner before the accident, and she had always been in good health, so she was largely unfamiliar with the ins and outs of doctors' offices. She turned to Nora for advice because it seemed as if this family friend was always either coming from or going to one doctor or another. Nora was in her mid-sixties and had been living with diabetes and heart disease for almost 20 years. Nora talked about how her nutritionist had helped her manage her diet, and how helpful her general practitioner was. Sarah was really hoping Nora would be able to help her understand how to navigate appointments with specialists and to recommend a way to get mental health care that wasn't readily covered by insurance. Even though Nora had tried to help, Sarah left their conversation feeling more confused. It was apparent that even though she and Nora each had a severe illness, their health care needs were incredibly different.

The 12 million high-need patients in the United States are members of a diverse group of individuals affected by a range of medical, behavioral, and functional conditions and limitations (Hayes et al., 2016). Adding a layer of complexity to the effective care of high-need patients is the disproportionate impact of social circumstances—isolation, unemployment, lack of permanent or safe housing, and food insecurity, for example—on this population's health and well-being. Because of the varying needs and preferences of high-need patients, multiple tools and approaches are necessary to ensure that they receive the most appropriate care, with individual patient characteristics and preferences informing selection from among care models. Therefore, serving this heterogeneous population more effectively and efficiently requires construction of a taxonomy that has groupings based on shared characteristics and functional needs.

Drawing from discussions and common themes throughout the workshop series and the published evidence, this chapter reports on current approaches in—and evidence for—the application of taxonomies to the management of high-need patients as a means of improving their care. In particular, it provides an overview of the taxonomies used by two organizations, the Harvard T.H. Chan School of Public Health and The Commonwealth Fund, and guidance on the adoption and application of their key elements in practice. Given the profound role of social risk and behavioral health factors on the health of high-need patients, the intersection of these factors with the clinical domain receives particular attention. This chapter has been informed by two main sources: the insights gleaned from the workshop series presentations and discussions, and the assessment of an expert group of researchers, clinicians, and policy experts on the state of the evidence around the use of a patient taxonomy and their insights on how to advance its utility and adoption.

PURPOSE AND OPERATION OF PATIENT SEGMENTATION

Segmenting target populations is not a novel concept. Marketing agencies divide populations and target potential strategies based on shared characteristics. In health care, triage has long been a foundational concept for ensuring that patients with the most urgent needs are given priority for treatment (Robertson Steel, 2006), and it is an increasingly common protocol to sort cancer patients, for example, based on genomic characterization and various molecular markers to better inform therapeutic strategies (Konecny et al., 2016; Wang et al., 2014). Health system leaders can use a taxonomy to better understand their systems' patient populations and inform program planning, care team compositions and work flow, training, and infrastructure investments—leading to improved health and well-being outcomes and reduced costs.

Patient stratification strategies can take several forms. For instance, whole population risk stratification segments a health care system's entire patient population based on a projected risk of requiring care. Health systems create these risk profiles using various risk prediction algorithms that group their patients according to their utilization of services or specific health conditions, such as diabetes or high blood pressure. Health systems have developed whole population risk stratification methods to predict the anticipated costs for their specific patient populations. This approach, however, captures only a small fraction of the patients who could benefit from greater oversight or help in managing their conditions (Kansagara et al., 2011), in part because any technique based on the presumption of homogeneity is structurally limiting, and in part because it does not account for the socioeconomic characteristics and behaviors that affect health outcomes. For example, patients with diabetes have highly varied treatment requirements, and those with social challenges face still other requirements (Hostetter and Klein, 2015).

One of the earliest stratification systems was developed by Kaiser Permanente's cofounder Sidney Garfield, whose parsimonious categorization system comprised four groups for all patients: sick, well, worried well, and early sick (Garfield, 1970). These categories have since been revised: no chronic conditions, one or more chronic conditions, advanced illness, and extremely frail and near end of life (Zhou et al., 2014). The "Bridges to Health" model, first proposed by Lynn and colleagues at Centers for Medicare & Medicaid Services, divides the entire population into eight groups, from healthy to failing health near death (Lynn et al., 2007).

Patient segmentation using a taxonomy of the sort described in this chapter is driven by the goal of grouping the individuals in a health system's population by the care they need as well as how often they might need it. Segmentation involves separating the highest-risk patients (as determined using whole population risk stratification) into subgroups with common needs. A key operational concept for a useful taxonomy for patient segmentation is that it should account for the unique factors that drive an individual's health care needs.

Patient targeting goes one step further by looking within each segment to identify which patients need the highest intensity of complex care management. Both the literature and discussions with providers indicate that most successful care models, such as those discussed in Chapter 4, use targeting to refine further how they allocate resources more efficiently among their high-need patients.

DEVELOPING A TAXONOMY

The need for greater precision is a natural product of the move toward value-based care, the emphasis on patient-engaged care, and the better insights emerging on what works best under different circumstances. While a general consensus exists on the benefits of segmenting high-need patients to target care (Vuik et al., 2016), work is still in progress on the optimal definitions of patient groups. For high-need patients in particular, we know that any taxonomy must take into account social risk and behavioral health factors at play—areas that need much elaboration (Johnson et al., 2015a; Kansagara et al., 2011).

Developing and implementing any taxonomy to guide service delivery to high-need patients requires solving numerous challenges. Segmenting high-need patients into meaningful subgroups requires access to information about their physical and behavioral conditions, their care utilization, and their social challenges. Most health information technology systems, however, do not support this type of integrated and streamlined data collection. The most readily available source of information is claims-based data, but these data offer a limited, condition-based perspective of patients and are not available in real time. Electronic health records (EHRs) can serve as a key source of data, but the design of many EHR systems does not enable them to collect data on behavioral issues, social challenges, or functional limitations (Institute of Medicine, 2014a, 2014b). The burden on health systems to collect, store, and properly use data are additional practical and logistical considerations.

A patient taxonomy that is effective in driving more productive treatment strategies for the high-need patient pool requires a delicate balance between precision and generalization. It is impractical to assume that every relevant feature can be captured and characterized for each patient. Although defining patient subgroups and sub-subgroups introduces more precision into categorizing patients, a taxonomy that contains too many subgroups is not feasible to implement. On the other hand, having too few groups is an oversimplification and does not meaningfully inform care planning and management. In addition, multiple payers and varied benefits packages pose administrative and operational hurdles for the implementation of any taxonomy. Medicaid is of particular concern because a disproportionate number of high-need patients are covered—at least in part—by the program, yet coverage varies widely from state to state. Chapter 5 covers this subject in more detail.

IDENTIFYING SEGMENTS

To address the challenge of creating an actionable stratifying tool, the taxonomy workgroup developed a conceptual starter taxonomy. In the third workshop, Melinda Abrams, vice president for delivery system reform at The Commonwealth Fund and chair of the taxonomy workgroup, explained that the medical aspects of this taxonomy build largely on the work of the Harvard T.H. Chan School of Public Health group, led by Ashish Jha and Jose Figueroa.

Jha, Figueroa, and colleagues conducted a set of analyses of Massachusetts claims data to empirically derive mutually exclusive subpopulations of high-need patients in three distinct populations: the non-Medicare population under age 65, the Medicare population, and the dual-eligible population (Joynt et al.,

2017). While claims data are often maligned, said Jha in the second workshop, in his opinion they are currently the best way to draw a picture of high-need, high-cost individuals in the United States. Through a yearlong iterative process, with input from clinical leaders and working closely with a group led by Gerard Anderson at Johns Hopkins University, the Harvard team defined the subpopulations with a noniterative, hierarchical categorization that assigned patients to groups of increasing complexity. The resulting six subpopulations, in the order in which individuals are classified, are listed as follows: under-65 disabled who are not included in the non-Medicare under-65 population; frail, with two or more frailty indicators; major complex chronic, with two or more chronic conditions from a list of nine major chronic diseases that account for the majority of spending and morbidity; minor complex chronic, with one chronic condition from the list of nine major chronic diseases; simple chronic, which includes less severe conditions such as hyperlipidemia; and relatively healthy. Individuals are assigned to no more than one of these groups by first determining whether the patient is under 65 or 65 or older. Individuals under 65 are assigned to the first category. Of those individuals age 65 or older, those with two or more frailty indicators are assigned to the frail elderly group. Last, the remaining individuals are assigned to one of the final four categories based on the number of chronic conditions they have (Joynt et al., 2016).

Jha noted that this may not be the ideal way to segment the population, but he believes it is a reasonable approach. One limitation is that it does not specifically address patients with advanced illness or those patients at the end of life. Jha added that it would be important to examine other populations, particularly children, and try to understand the characteristics of providers that do better with one subpopulation as compared to another.

Building on the Harvard group's work and an analysis of Medical Expenditure Panel Survey (MEPS) data by Anderson and colleagues at Johns Hopkins (Roberts and Anderson, 2014), Abrams and collaborators at The Commonwealth Fund looked at how to characterize some of the issues and challenges facing high-need and high-cost patients. As explained by Melinda Abrams during the second workshop, the Commonwealth Fund team examined segmentation and programmatic literature, such as program evaluations and case studies, as a "reverse engineering" strategy to identify patient groups based on how existing programs identified and segmented patients. The team also conducted interviews with health system leaders, program experts, and payers, and they collaborated with an advisory group to define 11 specific patient groups, including a standalone segment for individuals with social risk and behavioral health factors. After further consideration and analysis, Abrams and colleagues merged some of these segments into six subpopulations: under-65 disabled, advancing illness, frail elderly, complex chronic conditions, multiple chronic conditions, and children with complex needs.[6] At any given time, patients are assigned to just one of these six segments and their designation is determined by their medical needs that are driving their health care costs. For example, a frail elderly individual with multiple chronic conditions would be assigned to the frail elderly segment because the frailty indicators are what is driving medical needs and ultimately costs. However, over time, as their medical needs change, patients may shift between segments.

In her presentation at the second workshop, Abrams explained some of the logic behind merging categories and settling on these six subpopulations. For example, for people with functional limitations, it did not matter whether they were under or over age 65. The two larger subcategories that made more sense practically were under-65 disabled and frail elderly. With regard to Jha's subcategories of major complex chronic, minor complex chronic, and simple chronic, Abrams said those were based on elegant work, but for practical purposes, those were too finely divided. As a result, The Commonwealth Fund team merged them into two categories: complex chronic conditions and multiple chronic conditions. Additionally, the stand-alone category of patients with social risk and behavioral health factors actually spanned all of the medical categories. Abrams noted that while the segmentation literature is small and greatly variable in terms of quality and rigor, it did suggest some additional segments beyond Anderson's and Jha's work, including advanced illness, end-of-life, and children with complex conditions (Lynn et al., 2007; Zhou et al., 2014).

Addressing some of the limitations of this work, Abrams said there are multiple plausible segmentation strategies, and the approach taken depends on the audience and the purpose. In addition, this work was based on limited data sources. "We need more information from patients, social services agencies, and interoperable systems," said Abrams during the second workshop. She noted, too, that segmentation is, at this stage, inherently imprecise, and she emphasized the need for more comprehensive data on patients that would be more informative than claims data, as was stated in a 2014 Institute of Medicine report (Institute of Medicine, 2014a).

---

6 This taxonomy was presented by Abrams at the second workshop. More information can be found at http://www.bettercareplaybook.org/resources/overview-segmentation-high-need-high-cost-patient-population (accessed on March 29, 2017).

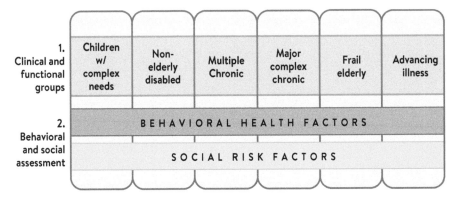

FIGURE 3–1 | A conceptual model of a starter taxonomy for high-need patients.
NOTE: For this taxonomy, functional impairments are intrinsically tied to the clinical segments.
SOURCE: Adapted from Abrams presentation, October 21, 2016

A CONCEPTUAL "STARTER" TAXONOMY

While still theoretical, taxonomies such as the ones Jha and Abrams laid out are medically oriented approaches. Given the availability of data, grouping patients according to medical characteristics is a feasible starting point for most health systems: the patient groups are clinically meaningful and carry implications for care delivery, and health systems can access information needed to identify and assign patients to groups via claims and EHR data. Assigning a patient to one of these groups tells only part of the patient story, however, and may neglect other characteristics and factors that are key drivers of functional limitations and health care spending. Here, the taxonomy workgroup offers a conceptual "starter" taxonomy for high-need patients (see Figure 3–1) that builds on the ones Jha and Abrams described to illustrate the incorporation of functional, social, and behavioral factors into a medically oriented taxonomy, not as independent segments but as factors that influence the care model or care team composition most likely to benefit a particular patient in one of the segments.

Fundamentally, this starter taxonomy aims to be actionable to inform care and workforce decisions and to reflect the reality of the data that are available to health system leaders. Table 3–1 describes the criteria for each group.

Because the segments were based largely on the work of both the Harvard and The Commonwealth Fund teams, there are limitations to clinical grouping that arise from the fact that the categorization was informed by the structure of limited datasets. For example, while children with complex needs are included, other high-risk groups worth further consideration, such as high-risk pregnancies, adolescents, and those who have suffered a traumatic event such as a brain or spinal injury, were not specifically designated as a segment. In addition, because identification of functional impairment is intrinsically tied to the clinical segments, the segments may not capture the complete diversity of functional limitations.

TABLE 3-1 | Clinical Group Features

CLINICAL GROUP	FEATURES
Children with complex needs	Have sustained severe impairment in at least four categories together with enteral/parenteral feeding or sustained severe impairment in at least two categories and requiring ventilation or continuous positive airway pressure[A]
Non-elderly disabled	Under 65 years and with end-stage renal disease or disability based on receiving Supplemental Security Income
Multiple chronic	Only one complex condition and/or between one and five noncomplex conditions[B,C]
Major complex chronic	Two or more complex conditions or at least six noncomplex conditions[B,C]
Frail elderly	Over 65 years and with two or more frailty indicators[D]
Advancing illness	Other terminal illness, or end of life

A Categories for children with complex needs are: learning and mental functions, communication, motor skills, self-care, hearing, vision.

B Complex conditions, as defined in Joynt et al., 2016, are listed in Table 2-1.

C Noncomplex conditions, as defined in Joynt et al., 2016, are listed in Table 2-1.

D Frailty indicators, as defined in Joynt et al., 2016, are gait abnormality, malnutrition, failure to thrive, cachexia, debility, difficulty walking, history of fall, muscle wasting, muscle weakness, decubitus ulcer, senility, or durable medical equipment use.

This starter taxonomy can, however, provide guidance for health system leaders and payers on how to embed social risk factors, behavioral health factors, and functional limitations in a taxonomy for high-need patients. Patients would first be assigned to one clinical segment based on what medical needs are driving their health care costs, with follow-on assessment of behavioral health issues and social services needs to determine the specific type of services an individual requires. For example, the major complex chronic conditions patient segment would include patients who simultaneously have diabetes, heart disease, and kidney disease, suggesting that a care team should include a complex care manager. If some of the patients also have severe depression, bipolar illness, or other behavioral health conditions, their care team would require someone with training in behavioral health issues. If the patient subpopulation also has unstable housing and sources of food, the care team would require personnel with expertise in addressing housing and food security. The model also assumes that the medical, behavioral, and social needs of patients will change. For example, an individual patient could move from frail elderly to advancing illness, which would suggest shifting resources from medical care to hospice care.

HIGH-IMPACT SOCIAL RISK AND BEHAVIORAL HEALTH VARIABLES

Two important components of this starter taxonomy are the social risk and behavioral health factors that affect a patient's health and influence the specific needs of each individual in a particular segment defined by medical and functional status. A review of the literature on social domains that affect care, insights from planning committee members and outside experts, and a survey of available resources (such as the National Association of Community Health Center's Protocol for Responding to and Assessing Patients' Assets, Risks, and Experiences [PRAPARE], a tool for assessing their patients' social determinants of health),[7] produced a list of four high-impact variables in the social services domain which were determined to be the most likely to affect care delivery decisions (see Table 3–2).

TABLE 3–2 | High-Impact Social Variables

VARIABLE	CRITERIA/MEASUREMENT	SOURCES
1. Low socioeconomic status	Income and/or education	Adler et al., 1994; Bengle et al., 2010; Bisgaier and Rhodes, 2011; Metallinos-Katsaras et al., 2012; Vijayaraghavan et al., 2011
2. Social isolation	Marital/relationship status and whether living alone	Ennis et al., 2014; House, 2001; Seeman, 1996
3. Community deprivation	Median household income by census tract; proximity to pharmacies and other health care services	Cutts et al., 2011; Wang et al., 2013; Bartley et al., 2003
4. Housing insecurity	Homelessness; recent eviction	Cutts et al., 2011; Schanzer et al., 2007

An analysis of MEPS data conducted by Claudia Salzberg at Johns Hopkins University for The Commonwealth Fund (Hayes et al., 2016b) shows the importance of behavioral health factors, as she found that 56 percent of high-need adults, or approximately 6.7 million people, have a behavioral health condition (such as depression, anxiety, or alcohol- or substance-related disorders) or a severe mental

---

7 For more information, see http://nachc.org/research-and-data/prapare/toolkit (accessed on March 9, 2017).

illness (such as schizophrenia) as one of their three or more chronic conditions. Salzberg also found that high-need individuals with behavioral health conditions made 27 percent more visits to hospital emergency departments, used 35 percent more home health care days, were more likely to have unmet medical needs, and were less likely to have easy access to specialists or have good patient-provider communication compared to high-need individuals who did not have a behavioral health condition. Moreover, 34 percent of high-need adults with a behavioral health condition remained in the top 10 percent of spending over a 2-year period compared to 23 percent of high-need adults without a behavioral health condition.

The subpopulation of high-need adults with a behavioral health condition is relatively younger; is more likely to be white, female, and less educated; is more likely to have lower income and fair or poor health status; and is more likely to be insured by Medicaid, either alone or in combination with Medicare. A list of four high-impact behavioral variables, which were determined to be the most likely to affect care delivery decisions (see Table 3–3), was developed by a review of the literature, insights from planning committee members and outside experts, and a survey of available resources.

TABLE 3–3 | High-Impact Behavioral Variables

VARIABLE	CRITERIA/MEASUREMENT	SOURCES
1. Substance abuse	Excessive alcohol, tobacco, prescription and/or illegal drug use	Doll et al., 2004; Eisenhauer et al., 2011; Fagerstrom, 2002; Lai and Huang, 2009; Makela et al., 1997; Ryan, 1995
2. Serious mental illness	Schizophrenia and other psychotic disorders, bipolar, major depression	De Hert et al., 2011; Katon, 2003
3. Cognitive decline	Dementia disorders (Alzheimer's, Parkinson's, vascular dementia)	Schulz and Sherwood, 2008; Zeisel et al., 2003
4. Chronic toxic stress	Functionally impairing psychological disorders or conditions (e.g., PTSD, ACE, anxiety)	Brunner, 1997; Cohen et al., 2007; King and Chassin, 2008; Kivimaki et al., 2002; Schnurr and Green, 2004; Stansfeld et al., 2002; Taft et al., 2007

NOTES: ACE = Adverse Childhood Experiences; PTSD = Post-Traumatic Stress Disorder.

For both lists of variables, social risk and behavioral health, the criteria for being "high-impact" included whether a variable had the potential for impact on both health and the type of care delivered, whether adding the variable would capture an otherwise missed patient population, and whether the variable would alter a person's status in the taxonomy in a manner that would be linked readily to clinical care. Some variables, such as race and ethnicity (Jackson et al., 2016; Larney et al., 2016; Morton et al., 2016; Segal et al., 2016) and incarceration (Wang et al., 2013), can affect health but are rooted in deeper systemic issues that are beyond the scope or purpose of this taxonomy. A variable such as health literacy can have a significant effect on health (Baker et al., 2007; Bennett et al., 2009; Institute of Medicine, 2004; Schillinger et al., 2002; Taylor et al., 2016), but the inventory of effective care models discussed in Chapter 4 does not directly address health literacy. As Abrams explained, the committee thought about the process of selecting the four social and the four behavioral health variables in terms of the taxonomy and its ability to match with the care model exemplars.

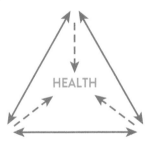

Medical System Determinants
- Children w/ complex needs
- Non-elderly disabled
- Multiple chronic
- Major complex chronic
- Frail elderly
- Advancing illness

HEALTH

Social Determinants
- Low SES
- Social isolation
- Community deprivation
- Housing insecurity

Individual Behavioral Determinants
- Substance abuse
- Serious mental illness
- Cognitive decline
- Chronic toxic stress

FIGURE 3-2 | A framework for health with all of the factors that would go into an ideal taxonomy.
NOTE: SES = Socioeconomic status.
SOURCE: Reproduced from Abrams presentation, October 21, 2016

ADVANCING THE USE OF A TAXONOMY

Categorizing high-need patients into smaller groups around which the delivery system can shape appropriate resources and strategies is sensible, given their heterogeneous medical needs, the varying impact of behavioral health issues and social factors on their functional abilities, and the high cost of caring for these individuals, as described in Chapter 2 (Boyd et al., 2010; Cohen and Uberoi, 2013; Stanton and Rutherford, 2006). In the third workshop, Abrams described an ideal patient taxonomy—one not yet achieved—that could provide a holistic assessment of how care should be targeted and delivered to improve the health of high-need individuals (see assessment of a patient's medical, behavioral, functional, and social characteristics to inform Figure 3–2). Developing such an approach for each patient segment, however, requires the integration of systems that capture physical, behavioral, and social information. Currently, this level of systems integration is only just starting to take place.

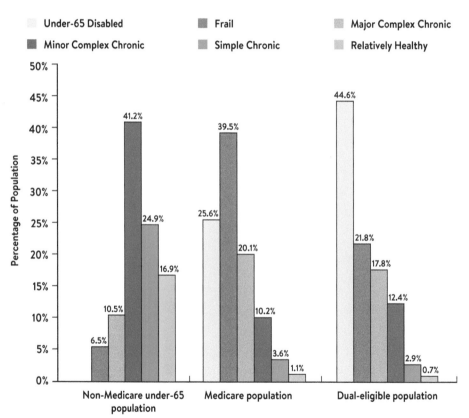

FIGURE 3–3 | Differences in the proportion of high-cost patients in six patient categories for three distinct payer groups.
SOURCE: Adapted from Jha presentation, January 19, 2016

Even with the proposed conceptual models, though, it is possible for health system leaders and payers to determine practical information about their high-need population segments. In the second workshop, Jha provided an example of the type of useful indicators a medically grounded taxonomy could produce. When Jha, Figueroa, and colleagues analyzed spending patterns among the three payer groups and six subpopulations of patients used in their taxonomy, the analysis revealed some surprises (see Figure 3–3), Jha said. For example, in the commercially insured, under-65 non-Medicare population, the majority of spending is by individuals in the minor complex chronic and simple chronic segments. Spending in the Medicare population differs greatly, he noted, with the frail and under-65 disabled accounting for the bulk of the high-cost patients. In the dual-eligible population, the under-65 disabled segment accounts for nearly half of the high-cost patients.

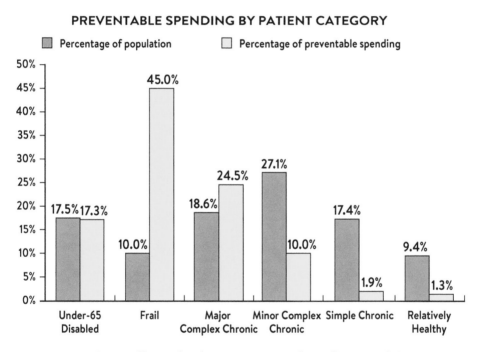

FIGURE 3–4 | Preventable spending by patient group in the Medicare population.
SOURCE: Reproduced from Jha presentation, January 19, 2016

The Harvard team also examined preventable spending among all of the Medicare patients included in the Massachusetts dataset (see Figure 3–4). For a definition of preventable, they looked at ambulatory care-sensitive conditions. For ambulatory care-sensitive conditions, most of the spending is by the frail elderly, who account for 10 percent of the total Medicare population and 45 percent of all hospitalizations for ambulatory care-sensitive conditions.

Jha discussed another analysis showing the mean distributional spending among high-cost patients (see Figure 3–5). For example, average annual inpatient spending by a high-cost under-65 disabled individual is $15,947, and outpatient spending accounts for another $13,344, but the biggest cost for these individuals is Medicare Part D spending on drugs, which is $23,003 (Joynt et al., 2016). In contrast, Part D spending by the frail elderly represents a small proportion of total spending, with inpatient care and postacute care and long-term care being the big-ticket items for this group (Joynt et al., 2016).

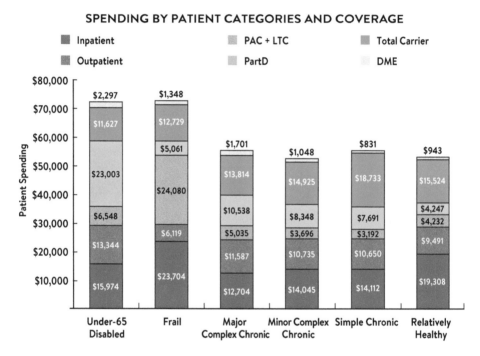

FIGURE 3-5 | High-cost Medicare patients' distributional mean spending by patient category.
NOTES: DME = Durable Medical Equipment; PAC = Post-Acute Care; LTC = Long-Term Care.
SOURCE: Adapted from Joynt et al., 2016

This sort of distributional analysis, Jha explained, highlights the different spending profiles of the subpopulations and the need for health system leaders and payers to think carefully about how to address the expense of caring for these different types of high-cost patients. Segmentation offers opportunities for payers to more effectively target finite resources and improve outcomes, which ideally will reduce the total cost of care.

In this way, a formal taxonomy can ideally inform the development of care plans and the allocation of resources to the interventions, assisting in a threefold aim to improve the care match with patient goals, improve patient outcomes, and improve the efficiency of care delivery. Highlighting the needs and use profiles of the various subpopulations, a taxonomy can help health care system leaders and payers make informed investments in a program, care team composition, work flow, training, and infrastructure. In Chapter 4, we discuss some models—many focused on specific segments of the high-need population—that health care system leaders can implement or look to for best practices. For a taxonomy to serve those purposes, however, it is necessary to align efforts across health systems and payers to ensure that payment structures incentivize, rather than hinder, effective care—a subject discussed in more detail in Chapter 5.

REFERENCES

Abrams, M. 2016. *Matching patients to tailored care models: a strategy to enhance care, improve outcomes, and curb costs.* Presentation at the October 21st NAM Models of Care for High-Need Patients meeting, Washington, DC.

Adler, N. E., T. Boyce, M. A. Chesney, S. Cohen, S. Folkman, R. L. Kahn, and S. L. Syme. 1994. Socioeconomic status and health. The challenge of the gradient. *The American Psychologist* 49(1): 15–24.

Baker, D. W., M. S. Wolf, J. Feinglass, J. A. Thompson, J. A. Gazmararian, and J. Huang. 2007. Health literacy and mortality among elderly persons. *Archives of Internal Medicine* 167(14):1503–1509.

Bartley, M., D. Blane, E. Brunner, D. Dorling, J. Ferrie, M. Jarvis, M. Marmot, M. McCarthy, M. Shaw, A. Sheiham, S. Stansfeld, M. Wadsworth, and R. Wilkinson. 2003. *Social Determinants of Health: The Solid Facts Second Edition.* The World Health Organization: Copenhagen, Denmark.

Bengle, R., S. Sinnett, T. Johnson, M. A. Johnson, A. Brown, and J. S. Lee. 2010. Food insecurity is associated with cost-related medication non-adherence in community-dwelling, low-income older adults in Georgia. *Journal of Nutrition for the Elderly* 29(2):170–191.

Bennett, I. M., J. Chen, J. S. Soroui, and S. White. 2009. The contribution of health literacy to disparities in self-rated health status and preventive health behaviors in older adults. *Annals of Family Medicine* 7(3):204–211.

Bisgaier J., and K. V. Rhodes. 2011. Cumulative adverse financial circumstances: associations with patient health status and behaviors. *Health and Social Work* 26(2) 129–137.

Boyd, C., B. Leff, C. Weiss, J. Wolff, A. Hamblin, and L. Martin. 2010. *Clarifying multimorbidity patterns to improve targeting and delivery of clinical services for Medicaid populations.* Hamilton, NJ: Center for Health Care Strategies.

Brunner E. J. 1997. Stress and the biology of inequality. *British Medical Journal* 314:1472–1476.

Cohen, S., D. Janicki-Deverts, and G. E. Miller. 2007. Psychological stress and disease. *Journal of the American Medical Association* 298(14):1685–1687

Cohen, S. B., and N. Uberoi. 2013. *Differentials in the concentration in the level of health expenditures across population subgroups in the US, 2010.* Statistical Brief #421. Rockville, MD: Agency for Healthcare Research and Quality.

Cutts, B. D., A. F. Meyers, M. M. Black, P. H. Casey, M. Chilton, J. T. Cook, J. Geppert, S. Ettinger De Cuba, T. Heeren, S. Coleman, R. Rose-Jacobs, D. A. Frank. 2011. US housing insecurity and the health of very young children. *American Journal of Public Health.* 101(8): 1508–1514.

De Hert, M., C. U. Correll, J. Bobes, M. Cetkovich-bakmas, D. Cohen, I. Asai, J. Detraux, S. Gautam, H. Moller, D. M. Ndetei, J. W. Newcomer, R. Uwakwe, and S. Leutcht. 2011. Physical illness in patients with severe mental disorders. I. Prevalence, impact of medications and disparities in health care. *World Psychiatry* 10(1): 52–57.

Doll, R., R. Peto, J. Boreham, and I. Sutherland. 2004. Mortality in relation to smoking: 50 years observations on male British doctors. *British Medical Journal* 328(7455):1519.

Eisenhauer, E., D. E. Uddin, P. Albers, S. Paton, and R. L. Stoughton. 2011. Establishment of a low birth weight registry and initial outcomes. *Maternal and Child Health Journal* 15(7):921–930.

Ennis, S. K., E. B. Larson, L. Grothaus, C. D. Helfrich, S. Balch, and E. A. Phelan. Lai, H. M. X., and Q. R. Huang. 2014. Association of living alone and hospitalization among community-dwelling elders with and without dementia. *Journal of General Internal Medicine* 29(11):1451–1459.

Fagerström, K. 2002. The epidemiology of smoking. *Drugs* 62(2):1–9.

Garfield, S. R. 1970. The delivery of medical care. *Scientific American* 222(4):15–23.

Hayes, S. L., D. McCarthy, and D. Radley. 2016. *The impact of a behavioral health condition on high-need adults.* New York: The Commonwealth Fund.

Hayes, S. L., C. A. Salzberg, D. McCarthy, D. C. Radley, M. K. Abrams, T. Shah, and G. F. Anderson. 2016. High-need, high-cost patients: Who are they and how do they use health care? New York: The Commonwealth Fund.

Hostetter, M., and S. Klein. 2015. *In focus: Segmenting populations to tailor services, improve care.* New York: The Commonwealth Fund.

House, J. S. 2001. Social isolation kills, but how and why? *Psychosomatic Medicine* 63(2):273–274.

Institute of Medicine. 2004. *Health literacy: A prescription to end confusion.* Edited by L. Nielsen-Bohlman, A. M. Panzer, and D. A. Kindig. Washington, DC: The National Academies Press.

———. 2014a. *Capturing social and behavioral domains and measures in electronic health records: Phase 2.* Washington, DC: The National Academies Press.

————. 2014b. *Capturing social and behavioral domains in electronic health records: Phase 1.* Washington, DC: The National Academies Press.

Jackson, C. S., M. Oman, A. M. Patel, and K. J. Vega. 2016. Health disparities in colorectal cancer among racial and ethnic minorities in the United States. *Journal of Gastrointestinal Oncology* 7(Suppl 1):S32-43.

Jha, A. 2016. *Targeting High Cost Patients and their Needs.* Presentation at the January 19th NAM Models of Care for High-Need Patients meeting, Washington, DC.

Johnson, T. L., D. Brewer, R. Estacio, T. Vlasimsky, M. J. Durfee, K. R. Thompson, R. M. Everhart, D. J. Rinehart, and H. Batal. 2015. Augmenting predictive modeling tools with clinical insights for care coordination program design and implementation. *eGEMs* 3(1):1181.

Joynt, K. E., J. F. Figueroa, N. Beaulieu, R. C. Wild, E. J. Orav, and A. K. Jha. 2017. Segmenting high-cost Medicare patients into potentially actionable cohorts. *Healthc (Amst)* 5(1-2):62-67.

Kansagara, D., H. Englander, A. Salanitro, D. Kagen, C. Theobald, M. Freeman, and S. Kripalani. 2011. Risk prediction models for hospital readmission: A systematic review. *JAMA* 306(15):1688–1698.

Katon, W. J. 2003. Clinical and health services relationships between major depression, depressive symptoms, and general medical illness. *Biol Psychiatry* 54(3):216–226.

King K. M., and L. Chassin. 2008. Adolescent stressors, psychopathology, and young adult substance dependence: A prospective study. *Journal of Studies on Alcohol and Drugs* 69(5): 629–638.

Kivimaki M., P. Leino-Arjas, R. Luukkonen, H. Riihimäki, J. Vahtera, and J. Kirjonen. 2002. Work stress and risk of cardiovascular mortality: prospective cohort study of industrial employees. *British Medical Journal* 325:857–860.

Konecny, G. E., B. Winterhoff, and C. Wang. 2016. Gene-expression signatures in ovarian cancer: Promise and challenges for patient stratification. *Gynecologic Oncology* 141(2):379–385.

Lai, H. M. X., and Q. R. Huang. 2009. Comorbidity of mental disorders and alcohol- and drug-use disorders: Analysis of New South Wales inpatient data. *Drug and Alcohol Review* 28(3):235–242.

Larney, S., N. D. Zaller, D. M. Dumont, A. Willcock, and L. Degenhardt. 2016. A systematic review and meta-analysis of racial and ethnic disparities in hepatitis c antibody prevalence in United States correctional populations. *Annals of Epidemiology* 26(8):570–578.

Lynn, J., B. M. Straube, K. M. Bell, S. F. Jencks, and R. T. Kambic. 2007. Using population segmentation to provide better health care for all: The "Bridges to Health" model. *Milbank Quarterly* 85(2):185–208; discussion 209–112.

Makela, P., T. Valkonen, and T. Martelin. 1997. Contribution of deaths related to alcohol use of socioeconomic variation in mortality: register based follow-up study. *British Medical Journal* 315:211–216.

Metallinos-Katsaras, E., A. Must, and K. Gorman. 2012. A longitudinal study of food insecurity on obesity in preschool children. *Journal of the Academy of Nutrition and Dietetics* (12):1949–58.

Morton, R. L., I. Schlackow, B. Mihaylova, N. D. Staplin, A. Gray, and A. Cass. 2016. The impact of social disadvantage in moderate-to-severe chronic kidney disease: An equity-focused systematic review. *Nephrology, Dialysis, Transplantation* 31(1):46–56.

Roberts, E., and G. Anderson. 2014 (unpublished). *Analysis of Medical Expenditure Panel Survey.* Johns Hopkins University.

Robertson Steel, I. 2006. Evolution of triage systems. *Emergency Medicine Journal* 23(2):154–155.

Ryan, J., M. K. Abrams, M. M. Doty, T. Shah, and E. C. Schneider. 2016. How High-Need Patients Experience Health Care in the United States: Findings of the 2016 Commonwealth Fund Survey of High-Need Patients. New York: The Commonwealth Fund.

Schanzer, B., B. Dominguez, P. E. Shrout, and C. L. M. Caton . 2007. *Homelessness, health status, and health care use.* American Journal of Public Health 97(3): 464–469.

Schillinger, D., K. Grumbach, J. Piette, F. Wang, D. Osmond, C. Daher, J. Palacios, G. D. Sullivan, and A. B. Bindman. 2002. Association of health literacy with diabetes outcomes. *JAMA* 288(4):475–482.

Schnurr, P. P., and B. L. Green. 2004. Understanding relationships among trauma, post-traumatic stress disorder, and health outcomes. *Advances in Mind-Body Medicine* 20(1):18–29.

Schulz, R., and P. R. Sherwood. 2008. Physical and mental health effects of family caregiving. *American Journal of Nursing.* 108(9): 23–27.

Seeman T. E.. 1996. Social ties and health: The benefits of social integration. *Annals of Epidemiology* 6(5):442–451.

Segal, N., D. Greenberg, R. Dagan, and S. Ben-Shimol. 2016. Disparities in PCV impact between different ethnic populations cohabiting in the same region: A systematic review of the literature. *Vaccine* 34(37):4371–4377.

Stanton, M. W., and M. K. Rutherford. 2006. *The high concentration of US Health care expenditures.* Rockville, MD: Agency for Healthcare Research and Quality.

Stansfeld S. and M. Marmot. 2002. Stress and heart disease. *BMJ Books.*

Taft, C. T., D. S. Vogt, M. B. Mechanic, and P. A. Resick. 2007. Posttraumatic stress disorder and physical health symptoms among women seeking help for relationship aggression. *Journal of Family Psychology* 21(3): 354–362.

Taylor, D. M., J. A. Bradley, C. Bradley, H. Draper, R. Johnson, W. Metcalfe, G. Oniscu, M. Robb, C. Tomson, C. Watson, R. Ravanan, and P. Roderick. 2016. Limited health literacy in advanced kidney disease. *Kidney International* 90(3):685–695.

Vijayaraghavan M., E. A. Jacobs, H. Seligman, and A. Fernandez. 2011. The association between housing instability, food insecurity, and diabetes self-efficacy in low-income adults. *Journal of Health Care for the Poor and Underserved* 22(4):1279–1291.

Vuik, S. L., E. K. Mayer, and A. Darzi. 2016. Patient Segmentation Analysis Offers Significant Benefits For Integrated Care And Support. *Health Affairs* 35(5): 769–775.

Wang, C., R. Machiraju, and K. Huang. 2014. Breast cancer patient stratification using a molecular regularized consensus clustering method. *Methods* 67(3):304–312.

Wang, E. A., Y. Wang, and H. M. Krumholz. 2013. A high risk of hospitalization following release from correctional facilities in Medicare beneficiaries: A retrospective matched cohort study, 2002 to 2010. *JAMA Internal Medicine* 173(17):1621–1628.

Zeisel, J., N. M. Silverstein, J. Hyde, S. Levkoff, M. Powell Lawton, and W. Holmes. 2002. Environmental correlates to behavioral health outcomes in Alzheimer's special care units. *The Gerontologist* 43(5): 697–711.

Zhou, Y. Y., W. Wong, and H. Li. 2014. Improving care for older adults: A model to segment the senior population. *The Permanente Journal* 18(3):18–21.

4

CARE MODELS THAT DELIVER

Fictional patient vignette: Raphael was glad that emergency surgery to fix a hip fracture in his 70-year-old mother, Gloria, had gone so well. But he was unsure of what to do afterward. Gloria had steadily advancing dementia, and she wouldn't be able to take care of herself after surgery, which meant that wound care and other recovery duties would fall on Raphael and his wife, Maria. When Gloria first returned home, Raphael and Maria struggled. Neither had any medical background beyond Maria's CPR training, and they weren't sure how to tell if Gloria's surgery site was healing correctly. Their insurance offered to pay for a visiting home nurse, however, who came twice a day to change Gloria's bandages and to check on her. When Gloria began to show signs of infection, the nurse recognized it before Raphael even knew something was wrong, and she was able to have it treated quickly. She also taught them about community resources—which their insurance would cover—that would help them handle Gloria's dementia symptoms. Raphael was incredibly thankful for the service and unsure how they would have managed without it.

For a patient taxonomy to be actionable, it needs to inform the care of high-need patients by identifying key care elements that align with the needs for specific patient populations. At the same time, providing effective and sustainable care for high-need individuals within those populations requires identifying attributes and features of care models shown to improve the experience and outcomes of the patients and reduce the cost for individual patients and the communities in which they live (Berwick et al., 2008). To examine how these two critical components relate, speakers at the first and second workshops discussed the intersection of models of care and taxonomies. Additionally, a review of evidence syntheses and other literature on care models for high-need patients identified promising models, classified areas of convergence, and produced a list of attributes holding the most potential to improve outcomes and to lower costs.

CHARACTERIZING SUCCESSFUL MODELS

Defining a successful care model starts with the goals of the stakeholders involved. In general, successful care models foster effectiveness across three domains: health and well-being, care utilization, and costs. The success of even the best care models depends on the particular needs and goals of the patient a model intends to serve, and those will vary even within segments of the high-need population. Dual-eligible patients, for example, are often considered a high-need group or segment as a whole, but as Randall Brown from Mathematica Policy Research explained at the second workshop, nearly 40 percent of this population does not need extensive services (see Figure 4–1). Even among those dual-eligible individuals who have severe chronic illnesses, only some require long-term support services that need to be integrated and coordinated. Each of these different dual-eligible subpopulations benefits from different managed care models or fee-for-service models.

Percentage of Dual-Eligible Individuals

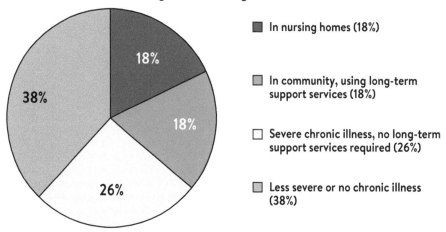

■ In nursing homes (18%)

☐ In community, using long-term support services (18%)

☐ Severe chronic illness, no long-term support services required (26%)

■ Less severe or no chronic illness (38%)

FIGURE 4–1 | Variations in the needs of dual-eligible individuals.
SOURCE: Adapted from Brown presentation, January 19, 2016

Different high-need segments will require different services and workforce competencies. A patient taxonomy may help define the competencies needed in the workforce, noted David Atkins from the Department of Veterans Affairs during workshop 2, but there are likely to be generalizable aspects that cut across the different segments. "As we look at these segments and map successful programs to the different populations, we may find [that] two segments that look different from a program perspective are actually served by similar looking programs or that there are common elements in each of the programs that address the needs of these segments."

At the third workshop, Arnold Milstein of Stanford University noted the profound changes that models of care have undergone over time. "It wasn't that long ago that there were five boxes that defined America's care models. You could either end up in the office of a surgeon, a medical doctor, or an internist, or you could end up in a hospital general surgical ward or a hospital general medical ward, and maybe an OB ward, but that was it. Over the last 100 years, as medical knowledge and health care delivery science have begun to advance, there has been a lot of evolution and customization, most of it with very good results."

Milstein's statement is borne out by the increasing abundance of care models available for high-need patients. As the number of models has grown, researchers have reviewed and classified these models and their attributes to determine how and why different models realize success (Anderson et al., 2015; Berry-Millett and Bodenheimer, 2009; Bleich et al., 2015; Brown et al., 2012; Cohen et al., 2015; Davis et al., 2015; McCarthy et al., 2015; Nelson, 2012; Salzberg et al., 2016; Taylor et al., 2015a; Zurovac et al., 2014). These reviews and syntheses span the heterogeneous populations and settings for which the models are designed.

Synthesizing areas of convergence in the evidence base for the wide variety of models, attributes, and implementation techniques in the third workshop, Milstein outlined four dimensions or areas of focus that constitute a possible analytical framework for identifying successful care models: (1) focus of service setting; (2) care and condition attributes; (3) delivery features; and (4) organizational culture. In the remainder of the chapter, a selection of the supporting research for each dimension of this framework is provided, together with a summary of a conceptual mapping exercise to illustrate how a patient taxonomy may inform care or care model selection. In addition, the chapter presents an example of implementing a population health approach to delivering primary care.

FOCUS OF SERVICE SETTING

The first dimension of the framework categorizes the service setting of models. In general, the most successful programs for managing high-need individuals focus on either a targeted age group with broad combinations of diagnoses or individuals classified as high-utilizers. Models tend to fall into several broad categories related to care settings: enhanced primary care, transitional care, and integrated care. In a synthesis review they conducted in 2009 (Berry-Millett and Bodenheimer, 2009), Berry-Millett and Bodenheimer found a similar categorization of care management by setting. Their categories included primary care, vendor-supported care, integrated multispecialty groups, hospital-to-home systems, and home-based care.

A review of evidence for successful models of comprehensive care for older adults with chronic illness identified 15 types of models, including comprehensive patient care, pharmaceutical care, and preventive home visits (Boult et al., 2009b). Each type of model had different levels of supporting evidence for measures of success such as quality of care, increased functional autonomy, and use or cost of health services. A separate study by Brown and colleagues found the strongest evidence for reductions in hospital use and cost of care from select interdisciplinary primary care models, care coordination programs focused on high-risk patients, chronic disease self-management programs, and transitional care interventions (Brown et al., 2012).

Grounded primarily in the typology of successful care models for older adults with chronic conditions (Boult et al., 2009b) and The Commonwealth Fund's evidence synthesis of care models for high-need patients (McCarthy et al., 2015), the framework presented lays out nonmutually exclusive categories of promising care models (see Box 4–1).

The primary and transitional care settings are the two key categories because of strength of the evidence base and potential for spread and scale in today's clinical practices. Additionally, interdisciplinary and enhanced primary care—two care model categories that are often distinct in the literature—are combined because overlapping and indistinguishable definitions suggest a single category for primary care models. The three subcategories of primary care—interdisciplinary primary care, care and case management, and chronic disease self-management—are highlighted but are not mutually exclusive. For example, Care Management Plus is a successful example of an interdisciplinary primary care model, but there is clear overlap with a care management approach (Brown et al., 2012).

Furthermore, there is a specifically emphasized category for models that features the integration of medical, social, and behavioral services because of the importance and impact that engaging factors outside of the medical care system has on improving care for high-need patients. Meaningful care often requires alignment, coordination, and cooperation by the care system with social and behavioral health programs and services. For example, during the first workshop Robert Master, of Commonwealth Care Alliance, explained that a challenge

BOX 4–1
Service Setting and Focus of Successful Care Models

- **Enhanced primary care**. Programs in the primary care setting defined by the use of supplemental health-related services that enhance traditional primary care and/or employ a team-based approach, with a provider and at least one other person.
  - **Interdisciplinary primary care**. A team comprising a primary care provider and one or more other health care professionals (e.g., nurse, social worker, rehabilitation therapist) who communicate frequently and provide comprehensive primary care *(e.g., Guided Care, GRACE, IMPACT, PACE, or Care Management Plus)*.
  - **Care and case management**. Collaborative models in which a nurse or social worker helps patients with multiple chronic conditions and their families assess problems, communicate with providers, and navigate the health care system *(e.g., Integrated Care Management Program at Massachusetts General Hospital)*.
  - **Chronic disease self-management**. Structured, time-limited interventions designed to provide health information to patients and engage them in actively managing their chronic conditions *(e.g., Chronic Disease Self-Management program at Stanford)*.
- **Transitional care**. Facilitate safe and efficient transitions from the hospital to the next site of care (e.g., alternative health care setting or home). Interventions are usually led by a nurse, known as a "transition coach," who provides patient education about self-care, coaches the patient and caregiver about communicating with providers, performs a home visit, and monitors the patient *(e.g., Naylor Transitional Care Model)*.
- **Integrated care**. Cross-disciplinary models which engage or focus on social risk interventions and behavioral health services in addition to medical care and functional assistance *(e.g., IMPACT or Camden Coalition)*.

NOTE: Categories are not mutually exclusive. For more information on the Integrated Care Management Program at Massachusetts General Hospital, see http://www.massgeneral.org/integrated-care-management/. For more information on Camden Coalition, see https://www.camdenhealth.org/national-center/.
SOURCES: Bleich et al., 2015; Boult et al., 2009

with the One Care population[8] is that many within it have never been nor likely ever will be bonded to a primary care practice, given the large number of people in this population with persistent mental illness, intermittent homelessness, and

8 One Care is a program started in October 2013 by Commonwealth Care Alliance. At the time of the first workshop, 10,300 dual-eligible individuals under age 65 with disabilities were enrolled. Some 42 percent, most of whom enrolled voluntarily, have serious physical, developmental, or mental-illness–related disabilities. Additional information about this program is available at: http://www.commonwealthfund.org/publications/case-studies/2016/dec/commonwealth-care-alliance.

concurrent substance abuse. For many segments of high-need patients, these highly integrated models can be the most effective, especially for populations with high levels of social or behavioral health needs.

CARE AND CONDITION ATTRIBUTES

While the details of any given model will be guided by specific conditions, successful care models share many common care attributes—the second dimension of the framework. Research has identified attributes that lead to successful models. For example, in their evidence synthesis McCarthy and colleagues (McCarthy et al., 2015) found several attributes to be widespread in successful models, including targeting patients likely to benefit from the intervention; coordinating care and communication among patients and providers; promoting patient and family engagement in self-care; comprehensively assessing patients' risks and needs; providing appropriate care in accordance with patients' preferences; relying on evidence-based care planning and patient monitoring; and facilitating transitions from the hospital and referrals to community resources.

Targeting patients who are most likely to benefit from an intervention, based on a comprehensive patient assessment and subsequent segmentation, is a key common attribute of successful programs (Boult et al., 2009b). Reviews of existing care models have indicated that comprehensive assessments should include multiple dimensions such as medical diagnoses, physical functioning, social risk factors, and behavioral health concerns (Boult and Wieland, 2010; Hong et al., 2014b). The factors that determine who is most likely to benefit include both the conditions that cause them to need a high level of care (Brown et al., 2012) and the patient's amenability to complying with treatment protocols and change behaviors (Hibbard et al., 2016; Hibbard et al., 2015). With a more complete understanding of the full spectrum of needs of the patient, care providers can select a suitable care plan.

Another common attribute among successful models is that a dedicated care coordinator—usually a social worker or registered nurse—located in the physician's office coordinates care for patients. One important role for the care coordinator is to develop an ongoing working relationship with the patient, family members, and other informal caregivers, as well as with the physicians caring for that patient (Berry-Millett and Bodenheimer, 2009; Bodenheimer and Berry-Millett, 2009; Brown et al., 2012; Hong et al., 2014b). An analysis of program design in Medicare's demonstration projects on disease management, care coordination, and value-based payment found that the nature of interactions among care managers, patients, and physicians was the strongest predictor of success in reducing hospital use (Nelson, 2012). These interactions occurred in a variety of ways, such as meeting patients in the hospital or occasionally accompanying patients on visits to their physician.

Effective care communication, through coaching and education, can play an important role in engaging the patient and family in sharing decision making, actively managing care, and developing a care plan that best reflects a given patient's goals and desires—all common attributes of successful care models. When describing Minnesota's Health Care Home (HCH) program at the first workshop, Bonnie LaPlante, HCH interim director and capacity building and certification supervisor in the Health Policy Division at the Minnesota Department of Health, explained that care coordinators develop relationships with the patients while physicians identify their panel of patients and commit to helping each one understand that better care results from choosing a primary care provider.

Patient monitoring, strategic use of data to provide timely feedback to the care team, and facilitating transitions between inpatient and outpatient or nursing home care are other important attributes of successful programs. Transitional care interventions have been shown, for example, to reduce hospital readmissions by as much as one-third (Englander et al., 2014; Feltner et al., 2014; Kansagara et al., 2015).

On the whole, there is convergence in the literature around many common care attributes. The eight attributes highlighted in the framework (see Box 4–2) are based on McCarthy and colleagues' (2015) synthesis, as well as other pertinent literature.

BOX 4–2
Care and Condition Attributes of Successful Care Models

- **Assessment**. Multidimensional (medical, functional, and social) patient assessment
- **Targeting**. Targeting those most likely to benefit
- **Planning**. Evidence-based care planning
- **Alignment**. Care matched with patient goals and functional needs
- **Training**. Patient and care partner engagement, education, and coaching
- **Communication**. Coordination and communication among and between the patient and care team
- **Monitoring**. Proactive tracking of the health status and adherence to care plans
- **Continuity**. Seamless transitions across time and settings

SOURCES: Anderson et al., 2015; Bodenheimer and Berry-Millett, 2009; Boult and Wieland, 2010; Brown et al., 2012; McCarthy et al., 2015; Nelson, 2012

DELIVERY FEATURES

The third dimension of the framework addresses delivery features. As with the evidence supporting common care attributes, there is substantial overlap in the indications supporting specific features. In the second workshop, for example, Brown highlighted two managed care plan models that show some evidence for improvement and that share many of the same features. The first model, Geisinger Health System's Patient-Centered Medical Home (ProvenHealth Navigator) (Maeng et al., 2015), embeds care managers with primary care providers to identify and work with the truly high-risk cases that are identified on a list the case managers receive. The care managers have links to physicians at other care sites and serve as the communication hub. The second model Brown discussed, the Comprehensive Care Physician model (Meltzer and Ruhnke, 2014), has eliminated hospitalists to improve the continuity of care for all of its high-risk patients and instead allocates these patients to specific physicians who have limits to their panel size to increase their interaction with their patients. This model uses interdisciplinary teams and data-driven meetings to improve care and care coordination. Both of these programs achieve meaningful shared savings.

Brown and colleagues' analysis of the Medicare Care Coordination Demonstration identified six practices of care coordinators that were common among the more successful programs for high-need individuals (Brown et al., 2012): Care coordinators had monthly face-to-face contact with patients; they built a strong rapport with physicians through face-to-face contact at the hospital or the office; and they acted as a communications hub for the many providers involved in the care of these patients and between the patient and those providers. In addition, the care coordinators used behavior-change techniques, not just patient education, to help patients adhere to medication and self-care plans; they also had reliable information about patients' prescriptions and access to pharmacists or medical directors. Finally, the care coordinators knew when patients were hospitalized and provided support for the transition home.

In his presentation at the second workshop, Rahul Rajkumar, deputy director at the Center for Medicare & Medicaid Innovation (CMMI), noted that after 5 years of studying various approaches for change, CMMI has developed an abstract understanding of some of the common delivery features of successful models. Among those features are using team-based approaches, providing enhanced access to providers, proactively using continuous data to improve care, working across the medical neighborhood with a very select group of medical subspecialists, engaging patients in shared decision making, and stratifying patients based on risk.

The common delivery features highlighted in the framework (see Box 4–3) represent these more granular activities that are required to realize the common attributes.

BOX 4–3

Delivery Features of Successful Care Models

- **Teamwork**. Multidisciplinary care teams with a single, trained care coordinator as the communication hub and leader
- **Coordination**. Extensive outreach and interaction among patient, care coordinator, and care team, with an emphasis on face-to-face encounters among all parties and collocation of teams
- **Responsiveness**. Speedy provider responsiveness to patients and 24/7 availability
- **Feedback**. Timely clinician feedback and data for remote patient monitoring
- **Medication management**. Careful medication management and reconciliation, particularly in the home setting
- **Outreach**. The extension of care to the community and home
- **Integration**. Linkage to social services
- **Follow-up**. Prompt outpatient follow-up after hospital stays and the implementation of standard discharge protocols

SOURCES: Anderson et al., 2015; Bodenheimer and Berry-Millett, 2009; Brown et al., 2012; Hasselman, 2013; McCarthy et al., 2015; Nelson, 2012; Rodriguez et al., 2014

ORGANIZATIONAL CULTURE

McCarthy and colleagues' (2015) synthesis of common attributes, in which they separate the feature content (i.e., the what) and the method (i.e., the how), inspired the fourth dimension of the framework: the incorporation of organizational culture.

A study of 18 successful complex care management programs for high-need, high-cost patients with multiple or complex conditions—often combined with behavioral health problems or socioeconomic challenges—recommended a number of operational approaches (Hong et al., 2014b). In particular, this study highlighted the success of programs that adapted and customized their approaches and teams to the local context and caseload. Success often involved structuring the size of the program to better facilitate communication and adapting the program as local circumstances changed or evolved (Anderson et al., 2015).

During the first workshop, LaPlante described an example of a clinic in Minnesota's HCH that might start with a care plan in which a registered nurse serves as the care coordinator, but over time the plan adapts to changing circumstances and adds a social worker or a community health worker as a care coordinator and involves other health care team members to contribute their talents to care coordination. She noted that some of the state's small, rural, solo-practice clinics do not have the resources to hire a care coordinator and have just started assessing their population and identifying what would be best for that population.

In addition, because care management programs are highly specialized, customized training for team members enhances success. This may involve offering specialized education and training for providers and team members (American Geriatrics Society Expert Panel on the Care of Older Adults with Multimorbidity, 2012; Hong et al., 2014b) or using care managers who have already received specialized training (Bodenheimer and Berry-Millett, 2009; McCarthy et al., 2015).

The Health Resilience Program (HRP) in Oregon, which was a 4-year-old program at the time of the first workshop, is a care program for high-need, high-cost patients that marries a nontraditional workforce with a safety net of primary care practices. The program's primary workforce, explained Rebecca Ramsay, director of community care at CareOregon, consists of master's degree–level community outreach specialists paired with culturally specific peer-support specialists and addiction recovery mentors to work intensively with CareOregon's highest-risk and highest-need patients. These specialists focus primarily on the social determinants of health, but they are embedded in practices and function as part of a primary care team. "We have hired skilled behaviorists and peers with community outreach capacity and excellent engagement skills who spend 60 to 70 percent of their time in the community going to shelters, hospitals, park benches, and single-room occupancy housing, the places where our clients are living their lives," said Ramsay during the first workshop. She continued, "They are trained in trauma-informed care, and they are learning evidence-based trauma-recovery interventions." Those interventions include seeking-safety methods (Najavits, 2001) and eye-movement desensitization and reprocessing (EMDR), both of which have proven effective in treating posttraumatic stress disorder (PTSD) and substance abuse. Behavioral health clinicians provide clinical supervision, with dotted-line supervision provided by a primary care champion.

Ramsay also discussed the strong operational relationships that have developed among HRP program staff, and McCarthy and colleagues' (2015) synthesis of care models cites effective interdisciplinary teamwork as of one of the execution methods of successful models. Boult and Wieland, however, noted that, for many primary doctors, the inability to effectively treat complex chronic patients was exacerbated by not having the proper training or experience to work in a team setting (Boult and Wieland, 2010). Molly Coye, social entrepreneur in residence at the Network for Excellence in Health Innovation, explained in the second workshop that some programs have seen substantial changes in workforce roles, highlighted by the inclusion of social workers, licensed professional counselors, behavioral health specialists, and pastoral professionals as principal members of the integrative care teams who serve to coordinate a broad range of behavioral health and social services, including help with housing and financing. Embedding case managers in the practice to facilitate access and build trusting relationships with both patients and primary care providers can help solidify complex networks (Hong et al., 2014b; Nelson, 2012).

The workforce is not the only adaptive feature of successful care models. Effective use of data access, sources, and application can vary considerably and have a significant impact on the construction and responsiveness of a program (Hong et al., 2014b; McCarthy et al., 2015). Data sources themselves range from qualitative in-person assessments to such sophisticated health information technologies as interoperative electronic health records and patient-generated outcomes data from wearables and trackers—all of which care programs could use to assess outcomes or attribute value. Health systems can also use metrics gathered by the care team to evaluate and improve care models and their performance (American Geriatrics Society Expert Panel on the Care of Older Adults with Multimorbidity, 2012; McCarthy et al., 2015).

As an example of how metrics can inform care, John O'Brien, vice president of public policy at CareFirst BlueCross BlueShield, explained how CareFirst gives providers access to a suite of data and analytic reports, called SearchLight, that uses clinical claims and other information to help them hot-spot across their population. If these analytic tools identify a patient who needs additional services, SearchLight provides a link to the iCentric service request hub for referrals or requests for additional services, such as a medication consult with a pharmacist. To help the providers use and make sense of the SearchLight data, CareFirst employs 22 program consultants. In addition, CareFirst uses 300 nurse care coordinators as the interface between the patient, the provider, the care plan, and the community at large. O'Brien said a care coordinator who senses something is missing from someone's care can request a consult from a registered nurse, who will go into the home to look for fall risks, gaps in care, lack of medication adherence, and lack of a caregiver. The information from that consult then feeds back to the care team.

Informed by these practices, and with grounding in recommendations from Hong et al., 2014, Anderson et al., 2015, and others, the six elements of organizational culture included in the framework reflect the strong convergence of common operational approaches to successful care models (see Box 4–4).

BOX 4–4

Organizational Culture of Successful Care Models

- Leadership across levels
- Customization to context
- Strong team relationships, including patients and care partners
- Training appropriate to circumstances
- Continuous assessment with effective metrics
- Use of multiple sources of data

SOURCES: Anderson et al., 2015; Hong et al., 2014; McCarthy et al., 2015

CARE MODELS THAT DELIVER AND THE PATIENT TAXONOMY

A Conceptual "Crosswalk" Exercise

Examples of health care systems that use validated care models to successfully address the high-need and high-cost patients abound (see Appendix A for examples). Indeed, the lack of models is not a significant barrier for any delivery system that truly wants to improve care delivery for this population (Anderson et al., 2015; Boult et al., 2009; Brown et al., 2012; McCarthy et al., 2015). Specific characteristics of a given system's patient population will influence the requirements, as Brown discussed during the second workshop: a patient in the community is going to have different care delivery requirements than is a patient in an institution, while individuals with a fee-for-service Medicare plan may have different needs than are individuals who are in a managed care plan.

To demonstrate the utility of the starter taxonomy described in Chapter 3 for selecting appropriate care models, the committee performed the following conceptual mapping exercise on a sample of 14 successful care models that highlight many of the attributes, delivery features, and operational practices described in the framework Milstein proposed. Selected programs span the range of potential models, including interdisciplinary primary care (e.g., Guided Care, Centers for Medicare & Medicaid Services' Program of All-Inclusive Care for the Elderly [PACE]); care and case management (e.g., Integrated Care Management Program at Massachusetts General Hospital); transitional care (e.g., Naylor Transitional Care Model); and programs with strong integration of medical, social, and behavioral services (e.g., Improving Mood: Promoting Access to Collaborative

Treatment [IMPACT]). The sample programs were chosen in part due to the available evidence to support effectiveness across three domains: health and well-being, care utilization, and costs.[9]

Using the targeted populations described by the selected models, the committee determined which segment or segments proposed in the taxonomy would be served by that care model. The committee also determined whether the selected models were designed to specifically target individuals with complex behavioral or social factors.

An illustration of the resulting "crosswalk" is shown in Figure 4–2. This diagram shows that there are successful care models that apply to each of the

PROGRAM \ SEGMENT	Children w/ complex needs	Non-elderly disabled	Multiple chronic	Major complex chronic	Frail elderly	Advancing illness
Care Management Plus				*		*
Commonwealth Care Alliance		*				
Complex Care Program at Children's National Health System						
GRACE				*		
Guided Care						
Health Quality Partners						
Health Services for Children with Special Needs	*					
Hospital at Home						
H-PACT		*				
IMPACT			*		*	
Partners HealthCare Integrated Care Management Program						
MIND at home					*	
Naylor Transitional Care Model (Penn)						
PACE					*	

FIGURE 4–2 | A sample of 14 care models which have evidence of success, matched to the six population segments identified in the taxonomy showing that each segment has been matched to at least one program. A subset of these care models also targets social and/or behavioral risk factors faced by high-need patients and is marked with an (*).

NOTE: Many of these programs could be matched and/or adapted to other patient segments.

SOURCE: Models of Care for High-Need Patients Planning Committee, National Academy of Medicine

---

9 An exception was made for pediatric-specific programs because of a dearth of evidence.

different segments defined by the taxonomy. Additionally, the diagram shows that there are areas of overlap, with some programs being applicable to multiple segments in the taxonomy and some segments being served by multiple programs. Even with this limited selection of care models, the range of available options enables targeting of individual care models to specific patient groups based on characteristics and needs. Consequently, this crosswalk demonstrates that, with a patient taxonomy and "menu" of evidence-based care models that incorporate many of the care attributes, delivery features, and operational practices identified in the framework laid out in this chapter, health systems would be better equipped to plan for and deliver targeted care based on patient characteristics, needs, and challenges.

This crosswalk was performed solely as a conceptual mapping exercise to illustrate how a patient taxonomy can inform care: it is not an exhaustive crosswalk of all evidence-based care models. The intent of this exercise was to demonstrate the practicality of matching specific care models (e.g., GRACE or Hospital at Home) to identified patient groups (major complex chronic with social risk and/or behavioral health factors or advancing illness, respectively) to guide practical translation of this knowledge. In addition, many models could be matched or adapted to multiple patient groups, which Figure 4–2 suggests but may not fully reflect. Similar to the taxonomy, this is one approach—a starting approach—and is intended only to be illustrative. Theoretically, such a mapping exercise could also identify programs that are needed to meet the needs of specific segments otherwise lacking in targeted care models.

An Example from the Crosswalk

As a specific example of a well-served segment, Milstein highlighted two populations during his presentation at the second workshop: the frail elderly, and the frail elderly with social risk and/or behavioral health. He then discussed those programs that he and his colleagues identified as favorably impacting health and well-being, measures of utilization, or cost (net of the cost of the program itself). He noted that although a range of interventions improved the health and well-being and cost domains, much of the research used to evaluate the programs was completed before the field recognized the growing importance of patient experience. He expressed confidence, however, that "some of these programs would have also moved the needle on patient experience."

For the frail elderly population,[10] Milstein described two potential programs as appropriate matches. The two programs were the Transitional Care Model, developed by Naylor and colleagues at the University of Pennsylvania (Bradway et al., 2012; Hirschman et al., 2015; Naylor, 2000), and CMS's PACE (Boult and Wieland, 2010; Hirth et al., 2009; Lynch et al., 2008), which was developed to serve elderly in San Francisco's Chinatown-North Beach neighborhood (Ansak and Zawadski, 1983; Zawadski and Ansak, 1983). In reviewing the two programs, Milstein explained that the Transitional Care Model has a target population of hospitalized, high-risk older adults with chronic conditions. Key components of this intervention include multidisciplinary provider teams, led by advanced practice nurses that engage in comprehensive discharge planning; 3-month post-discharge follow-up that includes frequent home visits and telephone availability; and active involvement of patients and family members in identifying patient and family goals and building self-management skills. Research has demonstrated that this program is effective at reducing rehospitalizations and patient health care expenditures (Coalition for Evidence-Based Policy, 2017).

The target population for PACE includes adults age 55 and older who are publicly insured, have chronic conditions and functional and/or cognitive impairments, and live in the service area of a local PACE organization. Many PACE participants are dual-eligible individuals. Each PACE site provides comprehensive preventive, primary, acute, and long-term care and social services, including adult day care, meals, and transportation. An interdisciplinary team of health professionals provides PACE participants with coordinated care that for most participants enables them to remain in the community rather than receive care in a nursing home. Patients receive all covered Medicare and Medicaid services through the local PACE organization and at a local PACE center, thereby enhancing care coordination. Clinical staff are employed or contracted by the local PACE organization, which is paid on a per-capita basis and not based on volume of services provided.

Several research groups have evaluated PACE programs around the country (Boult et al., 2009b; Eleazer, 2000; Gross et al., 2004; Hirth et al., 2009; Lynch et al., 2008; Meret-Hanke, 2011; Pacala et al., 2000; Weaver et al., 2008). These evaluations have found that participants in PACE programs are hospitalized less frequently but make more frequent use of nursing homes; Milstein noted, however, there is also evidence that PACE programs may be more effective than

---

10 Frail elderly is defined as over 65 and with two or more frailty indicators, as defined in (Joynt et al., 2016) (gait abnormality, malnutrition, failure to thrive, cachexia, debility, difficulty walking, history of fall, muscle wasting, muscle weakness, decubitus ulcer, senility, or durable medical equipment use). For more information, see Chapter 3.

home- and community-based waiver programs in reducing long-term nursing home use, especially for those individuals with cognitive impairments. PACE program enrollees have lower mortality rates and experience better quality care on some measures, such as pain management. The program appears to be cost neutral to Medicare and may have increased costs for Medicaid, though Milstein said more research is needed on this facet of the program.

Another subcategory, frail elderly with social risk and/or behavioral health problems,[11] benefited from a different set of programs, including the IMPACT program developed at the University of Washington (Callahan et al., 2005; Lin et al., 2003; Unutzer et al., 2002; Unutzer et al., 2008; Van Leeuwen Williams et al., 2009), and the Maximizing Independence at Home (MIND at Home) program developed at Johns Hopkins University (Black et al., 2013; Johnston et al., 2011). The IMPACT program targets older adults with depression and includes collaborative care and a care manager. Each individual's primary care physician works with a consulting psychiatrist and a depression care manager—who can be a nurse, social worker, or psychologist supported by a medical assistant or some other paraprofessional—to develop and implement a treatment plan, including antidepressant medication and/or short-term counseling. The care manager also educates the patient about depression and coaches the patient on self-care techniques. Providers use ongoing measurement and track outcomes validated through use of a depression screening tool, such as the Patient Health Questionnaire-9, and adapt care to changing symptoms. Once a patient improves, the care manager and patient jointly develop a plan to prevent relapse.

A randomized, controlled trial of 1,801 adults over age 60 with depression or dysthmic disorder or both revealed that half of patients had a greater than 50 percent reduction in depressive symptoms compared to 19 percent of patients in the control group (Unutzer et al., 2002). Net of intervention costs, the total cost of health care was $3,363 less per patient than for patients in the control group (Unutzer et al., 2008).

The MIND at Home program targets elderly patients with memory disorders. It is a home-based program that links individuals with dementia and their caregivers to community-based agencies, medical and mental health care providers, and community resources. An interdisciplinary team, comprising trained nonclinical community workers and mental health clinicians, delivers individualized care planning, implementation, and monitoring for both patient and caregiver based on comprehensive in-home dementia-related needs assessments the clinicians

---

11   High-impact social risk variables are low socioeconomic status, social isolation, community deprivation, and housing insecurity. High-impact behavioral health variables are substance abuse, serious mental illness, cognitive decline, and chronic toxic stress. For more information, see Chapter 3.

conduct. In addition to ongoing monitoring, assessment, and planning for emergent needs, the team uses six basic care strategies: resource referrals, attention to environmental safety, dementia care education, behavior management skills training, informal counseling, and problem solving. Each component of the intervention is based on best practice recommendations and evidence from prior research, and the components are combined for maximum impact. The team also provides education, skills training, and self-management support for patients and families.

An 18-month trial of MIND at Home, involving 303 people age 70 and older with memory disorders—primarily dementia—and mild cognitive impairment, found that those individuals in the MIND at Home program were able to stay in their homes an average of 288 extra days over the subsequent 2 years compared to individuals who received no special care. Participants who met regularly with care coordinators were less likely to leave their homes or die than were those in the control group, and they had fewer unmet care needs, particularly with regard to safety and legal and advance care issues (Samus et al., 2014). The researchers reported that the caregivers of individuals in the MIND at Home program also seemed to benefit in terms of reducing the amount of time they needed to spend with the individuals in their care (Tanner et al., 2015).

While these care models share many of the care attributes, delivery features, and organizational characteristics outlined in the framework presented in this chapter and include a variety of different service settings, in order to be successful, they need to be tailored to the health system, the community, and the unique patient characteristics that drive health care need. For example, in the case of the frail elderly segment, the characteristics that drive the need for health care relate to the frailty indicators that must be managed by interdisciplinary teams, often with social supports including family members and community social services, where available. When these individuals also have mental health issues, specialized coordination with appropriate mental health care providers becomes important.

DENVER HEALTH: A "REAL-WORLD" APPLICATION

Denver Health represents one example that pulls together the use of whole population risk stratification, the practical use of a patient taxonomy, targeted care, and many of the care attribute and delivery features of successful care models. Simon Hambidge, chief ambulatory officer at Denver Health and professor of pediatrics at the University of Colorado, spoke about the program at the second workshop. Referring to Denver Health as "unusual," Hambidge explained that it combines a safety net hospital, a large federally qualified health center (FQHC), a public health department, an emergency 9-1-1 call center, and several school-based health centers. Though the work he discussed in his presentation took place in Denver Health's FQHC, it impacted the rest of the organization. The goal of this CMMI-funded project was to improve the experience of care, improve the health of populations, and reduce per capita costs of health care. To meet that goal, however, a fourth goal should be added: improving provider engagement and creating healthier and happier providers. Some $9 million of the $19.8 million CMMI award was spent on redesigning health teams; another $9 million was spent on health information technology to enable population segmentation and patient risk stratification; and the remaining funds were spent on rapid-cycle evaluation to enable design iteration.

Patient Risk Stratification

Denver Health's risk stratification approach uses clinical risk groups (CRGs), a clinically based classification system originally developed by 3M to measure a population's burden of illness (Hughes et al., 2004). This approach uses input from clinicians and data analysts to assign every CRG-classified patient to one of four tiers of increasing complexity and risk (see Figure 4–3), with additional criteria used to override a CRG designation.[12] As an example, Hambidge explained that a child on Denver Health's special health needs registry or individuals with certain mental health diagnoses would receive increased care coordination regardless of what their CRGs would normally warrant. Similarly, a family history of premature birth would result in a pregnant woman being targeted for more intensive interventions no matter where she fell on the CRG stratification scale. He also noted that different stratification algorithms are used for adults and children.

Matching Care Delivery to Tier Level

For healthy adults (i.e., those assigned to Tier 1), standard panel management techniques, including a heavy reliance on Denver Health's eTouch text messaging program, have produced good clinical outcomes, Hambidge said. These outcomes include decreased no-show rates, higher immunization rates, and higher well-child appointment rates. Individuals in Tier 2 start to get increased care management for chronic diseases. For children, Tier 2 care management involves lay patient navigators, some nurse care coordination, and some home visits and environmental scans for children with asthma. For adults, Tier 2 care

---

12   This risk stratification does not directly map on to the taxonomy described in Chapter 3. However, it is an example of a system that could be used to assist in care delivery.

includes more pharmacotherapy management and emphasizes transitions of care to reduce readmissions.

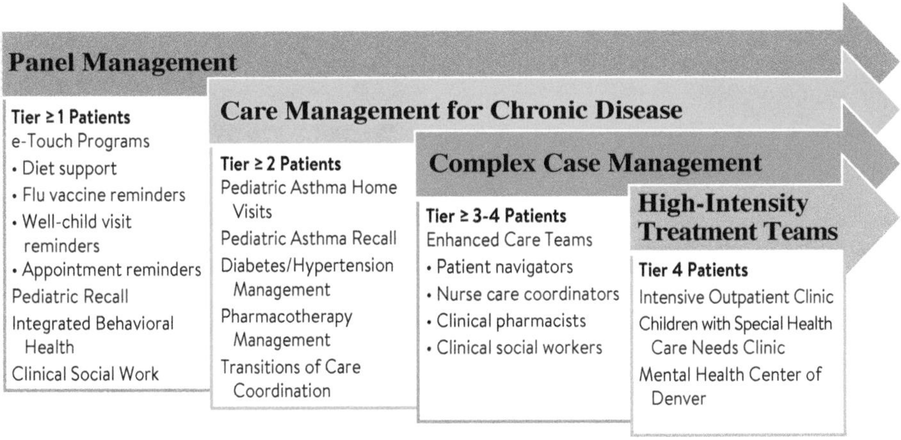

Panel Management

Tier ≥ 1 Patients
e-Touch Programs
• Diet support
• Flu vaccine reminders
• Well-child visit
  reminders
• Appointment reminders
Pediatric Recall
Integrated Behavioral
  Health
Clinical Social Work

Care Management for Chronic Disease

Tier ≥ 2 Patients
Pediatric Asthma Home
  Visits
Pediatric Asthma Recall
Diabetes/Hypertension
  Management
Pharmacotherapy
  Management
Transitions of Care
  Coordination

Complex Case Management

Tier ≥ 3-4 Patients
Enhanced Care Teams
• Patient navigators
• Nurse care coordinators
• Clinical pharmacists
• Clinical social workers

High-Intensity Treatment Teams

Tier 4 Patients
Intensive Outpatient Clinic
Children with Special Health
  Care Needs Clinic
Mental Health Center of
  Denver

FIGURE 4–3 | Denver Health's use of Clinical Risk Groups to assign patients to care programs.
NOTE: This is an example of risk stratification. It does not map directly on to the taxonomy proposed in Chapter 3.
SOURCE: Hambidge presentation, January 19, 2016

Complex case management strategies using enhanced care teams come into play for Tier 3 and Tier 4 patients. Integrated behavioral health assessments and care are standard for patients in these two tiers, as is the involvement of nurse care coordinators, clinical pharmacists, and clinical social workers. For Tier 4 patients, which Hambidge said is where the biggest cost savings and clinical benefits are realized, Denver Health relies on specialized intensive outpatient clinics for adults and multidisciplinary special needs clinics, similar to those prevalent in children's hospitals, for its highest-risk pediatric patients. The intensive outpatient clinic is targeted to adults with multiple, potentially avoidable, inpatient admissions within 1 year, and it serves as the patient's medical home. Panel sizes in this clinic are smaller, and the care teams include a dedicated social worker and navigator. This clinic also works closely with the Mental Health Center of Denver.

Outcomes

Hambidge said the total number of "super-utilizers" is stable, but individual turnover is high, which creates a dynamic population (Johnson et al., 2015b). A population- and individual-level analysis of Denver Health's data showed that over a 2-year period only a small number of superutilizers continuously met the criteria to be considered a superutilizer, and a slightly larger number went back and forth between meeting and not meeting those criteria. This analysis, he said, shows the importance of developing a population-based stratification system even though individuals are getting care. "You have to step back and look across the population to see who is coming into and going out of your system."

These data also show the importance of taking a population-based, actuarial approach when conducting financial analyses. As Hambidge explained, the natural tendency for high-utilizing patients to become less so over time would lead to an overestimation of cost savings based on individual results. Denver Health's data at the individual patient level, for example, showed that charges were reduced by 44 percent and admissions fell by 53 percent without any clinical intervention simply because of this natural tendency for individuals to move out of the high-utilization group. When the financial analysis was conducted using population-based cost avoidance as the metric, however, the true savings were approximately 2 percent, or $6.7 million, over a 1-year period, which Hambidge characterized as significant and important. "Even though programs such as this have significant clinical impact and significant impact on family and provider satisfaction, they are going to be sustainable based on financial performance." Most of the savings, he added, came from Denver Health's adult population, but some 15 to 20 percent of the savings were realized from its Tier 4 pediatric population.

The demonstrated success of models of care such as those being implemented by Denver Health and other forward-thinking health systems to improve the care of high-need patients and perhaps reduce the cost of care raises an obvious question: why are more health systems not adopting these models of care? Chapter 5 discusses some of the barriers to the wider spread and scale of successful models of care and raises some possible policy solutions to address those barriers.

REFERENCES

American Geriatrics Society Expert Panel on the Care of Older Adults with Multimorbidity. 2012. Patient-centered care for older adults with multiple chronic conditions: A stepwise approach from the American Geriatrics Society: American Geriatrics Society expert panel on the care of older adults with multimorbidity. *Journal of the American Geriatrics Society* 60(10):1957–1968.

Anderson, G. F., J. Ballreich, S. Bleich, C. Boyd, E. DuGoff, B. Leff, C. Salzberg, and J. Wolff. 2015. Attributes common to programs that successfully treat high-need, high-cost individuals. *American Journal of Managed Care* 21(11):e597-600.

Ansak, M. L., and R. T. Zawadski. 1983. On Lok CCODA: A consolidated model. *Home Health Care Services Quarterly* 4(3–4):147–170.

Berry-Millett, R., and T. S. Bodenheimer. 2009. Care management of patients with complex health care needs. *Synth Proj Res Synth Rep.*(19).

Berwick, D. M., T. W. Nolan, and J. Whittington. 2008. The triple aim: Care, health, and cost. *Health Affairs* 27(3):759–769.

Black, B. S., D. Johnston, P. V. Rabins, A. Morrison, C. Lyketsos, and Q. M. Samus. 2013. Unmet needs of community-residing persons with dementia and their informal caregivers: Findings from the maximizing independence at home study. *Journal of the American Geriatrics Society* 61(12):2087–2095.

Bleich, S. N., C. Sherrod, A. Chiang, C. Boyd, J. Wolff, E. Chang, C. Salzberg, K. Anderson, B. Leff, and G. Anderson. 2015. Systematic review of programs treating high-need and high-cost people with multiple chronic diseases or disabilities in the United States, 2008–2014. *Preventing Chronic Disease* 12:e197.

Bodenheimer, T., and R. Berry-Millett. 2009. Follow the money—controlling expenditures by improving care for patients needing costly services. *New England Journal of Medicine* 361(16):1521–1523.

Boult, C., A. F. Green, L. B. Boult, J. T. Pacala, C. Snyder, and B. Leff. 2009. Successful models of comprehensive care for older adults with chronic conditions: Evidence for the Institute of Medicine's "retooling for an aging America" report. *Journal of the American Geriatrics Society* 57(12):2328–2337.

Boult, C., and G. D. Wieland. 2010. Comprehensive primary care for older patients with multiple chronic conditions: "Nobody rushes you through." *JAMA* 304(17):1936–1943.

Bradway, C., R. Trotta, M. B. Bixby, E. McPartland, M. C. Wollman, H. Kapustka, K. McCauley, and M. D. Naylor. 2012. A qualitative analysis of an advanced practice nurse-directed transitional care model intervention. *Gerontologist* 52(3):394–407.

Brown, R. S., D. Peikes, G. Peterson, J. Schore, and C. M. Razafindrakoto. 2012. Six features of Medicare-coordinated care demonstration programs that cut hospital admissions of high-risk patients. *Health Affairs* 31(6):1156–1166.

Callahan, C. M., K. Kroenke, S. R. Counsell, H. C. Hendrie, A. J. Perkins, W. Katon, P. H. Noel, L. Harpole, E. M. Hunkeler, and J. Unutzer. 2005. Treatment of depression improves physical functioning in older adults. *Journal of the American Geriatrics Society* 53(3):367–373.

Coalition for Evidence-Based Policy. 2017. *Top Tier Evidence Initiative: Evidence Summary for the Transitional Care Model.* Washington, DC.

Cohen, D. J., M. M. Davis, J. D. Hall, E. C. Gilchrist, and B. F. Miller. 2015. *A guidebook of professional practices for behavioral health and primary care integration: Observations from exemplary sites.* Rockville, MD: Agency for Healthcare Research and Quality.

Davis, K., C. Buttorff, B. Leff, Q. M. Samus, S. Szanton, J. L. Wolff, and F. Bandeali. 2015. Innovative care models for high-cost Medicare beneficiaries: Delivery system and payment reform to accelerate adoption. *American Journal of Managed Care* 21(5):e349-356.

Eleazer, G. P. 2000. The challenge of measuring quality of care in PACE. Program of All-Inclusive Care for the Elderly. *Journal of the American Geriatrics Society* 48(8):1019–1020.

Englander, H., L. Michaels, B. Chan, and D. Kansagara. 2014. The care transitions innovation (C-TRAIN) for socioeconomically disadvantaged adults: Results of a cluster randomized controlled trial. *Journal of General Internal Medicine* 29(11):1460–1467.

Feltner, C., C. D. Jones, C. W. Cene, Z. J. Zheng, C. A. Sueta, E. J. Coker-Schwimmer, M. Arvanitis, K. N. Lohr, J. C. Middleton, and D. E. Jonas. 2014. Transitional care interventions to prevent readmissions for persons with heart failure: A systematic review and meta-analysis. *Annals of Internal Medicine* 160(11):774–784.

Gross, D. L., H. Temkin-Greener, S. Kunitz, and D. B. Mukamel. 2004. The growing pains of integrated health care for the elderly: Lessons from the expansion of pace. *Milbank Quarterly* 82(2):257–282.

Hambidge, S. 2016. *21st Century Care: Redesigning Care at Denver Health.* Presentation at the January 19th NAM Models of Care for High-Need Patients meeting. Washington, DC.

Hibbard, J. H., J. Greene, Y. Shi, J. Mittler, and D. Scanlon. 2015. Taking the long view: How well do patient activation scores predict outcomes four years later? *Medical Care Research Review* 72(3):324–337.

Hibbard, J. H., J. Greene, R. Sacks, V. Overton, and C. D. Parrotta. 2016. Adding a measure of patient self-management capability to risk assessment can improve prediction of high costs. *Health Affairs* 35(3):489–494.

Hirschman, K. B., E. Shaid, K. McCauley, M. V. Pauly, and M. D. Naylor. 2015. Continuity of care: The transitional care model. *Online Journal of Issues in Nursing* 20(3):1.

Hirth, V., J. Baskins, and M. Dever-Bumba. 2009. Program of all-inclusive care (PACE): Past, present, and future. *Journal of the American Medical Directors Association* 10(3):155–160.

Hong, C. S., A. L. Siegel, and T. G. Ferris. 2014. *Caring for high-need, high-cost patients: What makes for a successful care management program?* New York: The Commonwealth Fund.

Hughes, J. S., R. F. Averill, J. Eisenhandler, N. I. Goldfield, J. Muldoon, J. M. Neff, and J. C. Gay. 2004. Clinical risk groups (CRGs): A classification system for risk-adjusted capitation-based payment and health care management. *Medical Care* 42(1):81–90.

Johnson, T. L., D. J. Rinehart, J. Durfee, D. Brewer, H. Batal, J. Blum, C. I. Oronce, P. Melinkovich, and P. Gabow. 2015. For many patients who use large amounts of health care services, the need is intense yet temporary. *Health Affairs* 34(8):1312–1319.

Johnston, D., Q. M. Samus, A. Morrison, J. S. Leoutsakos, K. Hicks, S. Handel, R. Rye, B. Robbins, P. V. Rabins, C. G. Lyketsos, and B. S. Black. 2011. Identification of community-residing individuals with dementia and their unmet needs for care. *International Journal of Geriatric Psychiatry* 26(3):292–298.

Kansagara, D., J. C. Chiovaro, D. Kagen, S. Jencks, K. Rhyne, M. O'Neil, K. Kondo, R. Relevo, M. Motu'apuaka, M. Freeman, and H. Englander. 2015. VA evidence-based synthesis program reports. In *Transitions of care from hospital to home: An overview of systematic reviews and recommendations for improving transitional care in the Veterans Health Administration.* Washington, DC: US Department of Veterans Affairs.

Lin, E. H., W. Katon, M. Von Korff, L. Tang, J. W. Williams, Jr., K. Kroenke, E. Hunkeler, L. Harpole, M. Hegel, P. Arean, M. Hoffing, R. Della Penna, C. Langston, and J. Unutzer. 2003. Effect of improving depression care on pain and functional outcomes among older adults with arthritis: A randomized controlled trial. *JAMA* 290(18):2428–2429.

Lynch, M., M. Hernandez, and C. Estes. 2008. PACE: Has it changed the chronic care paradigm? *Social Work in Public Health* 23(4):3–24.

Maeng, D. D., N. Khan, J. Tomcavage, T. R. Graf, D. E. Davis, and G. D. Steele. 2015. Reduced acute inpatient care was largest savings component of Geisinger Health System's patient-centered medical home. *Health Affairs* 34(4):636–644.

McCarthy, D., J. Ryan, and S. Klein. 2015. Models of care for high-need, high-cost patients: An evidence synthesis. *Issue Brief (The Commonwealth Fund)* 31:1–19.

Meltzer, D. O., and G. W. Ruhnke. 2014. Redesigning care for patients at increased hospitalization risk: The comprehensive care physician model. *Health Affairs* 33(5):770–777.

Meret-Hanke, L. A. 2011. Effects of the Program of All-Inclusive Care for the elderly on hospital use. *Gerontologist* 51(6):774–785.

Najavits, L. M. 2001. *Seeking safety: A treatment manual for PTSD and substance abuse.* The Guilford Press.

Naylor, M. D. 2000. A decade of transitional care research with vulnerable elders. *Journal of Cardiovascular Nursing* 14(3):1–14; quiz 88–19.

Nelson, L. 2012. *Lessons from Medicare's demonstration projects on disease management, care coordination, and value-based payment.* Washington, DC: Congressional Budget Office.

Pacala, J. T., R. L. Kane, A. J. Atherly, and M. A. Smith. 2000. Using structured implicit review to assess quality of care in the Program of All-Inclusive Care for the Elderly (PACE). *Journal of the American Geriatrics Society* 48(8):903–910.

Salzberg, C. A., S. L. Hayes, D. McCarthy, D. Radley, M. K. Abrams, T. Shah, and G. Anderson. 2016. *Health system performance for the high-need patient: A look at access to care and patient care experiences.* New York: The Commonwealth Fund.

Samus, Q. M., D. Johnston, B. S. Black, E. Hess, C. Lyman, A. Vavilikolanu, J. Pollutra, J. M. Leoutsakos, L. N. Gitlin, P. V. Rabins, and C. G. Lyketsos. 2014. A multidimensional home-based care coordination intervention for elders with memory disorders: The Maximizing Independence at Home (MIND) pilot randomized trial. *American Journal of Geriatric Psychiatry* 22(4):398–414.

Tanner, J. A., B. S. Black, D. Johnston, E. Hess, J. M. Leoutsakos, L. N. Gitlin, P. V. Rabins, C. G. Lyketsos, and Q. M. Samus. 2015. A randomized controlled trial of a community-based dementia care coordination intervention: Effects of mind at home on caregiver outcomes. *American Journal of Geriatric Psychiatry* 23(4):391–402.

Taylor, E. F., S. Dale, D. Peikes, R. S. Brown, and G. Arkadipta. 2015. *Evaluation of the comprehensive primary care initiative: First annual report.* Princeton, NJ: Mathematica Policy Research.

Unutzer, J., W. Katon, C. M. Callahan, J. W. Williams, Jr., E. Hunkeler, L. Harpole, M. Hoffing, R. D. Della Penna, P. H. Noel, E. H. Lin, P. A. Arean, M. T. Hegel, L. Tang, T. R. Belin, S. Oishi, and C. Langston. 2002. Collaborative care management of late-life depression in the primary care setting: A randomized controlled trial. *JAMA* 288(22):2836–2845.

Unutzer, J., W. J. Katon, M. Y. Fan, M. C. Schoenbaum, E. H. Lin, R. D. Della Penna, and D. Powers. 2008. Long-term cost effects of collaborative care for late-life depression. *American Journal of Managed Care* 14(2):95–100.

Van Leeuwen Williams, E., J. Unutzer, S. Lee, and P. H. Noel. 2009. Collaborative depression care for the old-old: Findings from the impact trial. *American Journal of Geriatric Psychiatry* 17(12):1040–1049.

Weaver, F. M., E. C. Hickey, S. L. Hughes, V. Parker, D. Fortunato, J. Rose, S. Cohen, L. Robbins, W. Orr, B. Priefer, D. Wieland, and J. Baskins. 2008. Providing all-inclusive care for frail elderly veterans: Evaluation of three models of care. *Journal of the American Geriatrics Society* 56(2):345–353.

Zawadski, R. T., and M. L. Ansak. 1983. Consolidating community-based long-term care: Early returns from the On Lok demonstration. *Gerontologist* 23(4):364–369.

Zurovac, J., R. Brown, B. Schmitz, and R. Chapman. 2014. *The effectiveness of alternative ways of implementing care management components in Medicare D-SNPS: The Care Wisconsin and Gateway study.* Princeton, NJ: Mathematica Policy Research.

5

POLICY TO SUPPORT THE SPREAD AND SCALE OF CARE MODELS

Fictional patient vignette: Andy is a 75-year-old man whose arthritis, anxiety, and heart disease make it difficult for him to be on his feet and out of the house for long periods of time. He has frequent doctor appointments, and he feels lucky that between his Medicare and Medicaid benefits, most of his costs—for his general practitioner, pain management specialist, psychiatrist, and cardiologist—are covered. Often, the most difficult part of his health care routine is trying to figure out what is covered under Medicare and Medicaid, and by whom. Even though the staff at his various doctors' offices are willing to help him, Andy still spends hours trying to figure out what he is eligible for, and whether Medicare or Medicaid or both will pay for it. Andy doesn't understand why his Medicare and Medicaid coverage are so separate. They're both part of the federal government, aren't they?

While a range of programs have been shown to improve care for high-need patients, a variety of barriers have prevented successful programs from expanding beyond a single site or led them to be discontinued after an initial trial. These barriers are complex and span a range of factors: health system fragmentation, high implementation start-up costs with uncertain returns on investment; the challenge of integrating (and paying for) social and other nonmedical services with medical care; the difficulty of replicating care models developed in one setting across disparate settings; workforce training issues; and the need for appropriate quality measures and a data infrastructure to inform those measures. A number of barriers, however, have actionable solutions, with the key foundational issue often being federal-, state-, and health-system-level policies that exacerbate the challenges of caring for high-need patients. This chapter explores areas in which policy initiatives could accelerate the spread and scale of care models for high-need patients—particularly the programmatic integration of social supports and medical care—through developing a workforce to deliver comprehensive health care, expanding and realigning payment policies, reexamining quality measurement, and improving the data infrastructure.

Although the committee recognizes that prevention of the chronic conditions associated with high-need patients—through both public health and medical interventions—is a critical pursuit, this publication does not address policies that focus on population health and prevention. Many elements central to population health strategies (e.g., integration of social services and medical care) are relevant to the issues in this publication, however, and considering steps to increase prevention efforts could perhaps be the focus for future work by those concerned with improving the lives of high-need patients.

SPREADING AND SCALING SUCCESSFUL CARE MODELS

In his presentation at the second workshop, Arnold Milstein from the Clinical Excellence Research Center at Stanford University noted that an important barrier to spreading and scaling care models is the complexity of health care delivery systems. In Milstein's experience, system leaders are interested in adopting a new care model if the model would affect only one area of operations, such as primary care or neurology. Any idea for lowering the cost of providing better care that required cooperation among and across multiple departments, however, was typically rejected by system executives. "We are still in a situation where systems are challenged by the complexity of the job they face simply in delivering care, let alone improving it," he said. He also noted the challenge and cost of adapting a model developed to serve one particular subpopulation of high-need patients in one specific setting to another subpopulation in a different health care setting.

One approach Milstein suggested to dealing with these challenges would be to create a network of improvement communities that would bring together parties interested in scaling models of care to chart what does and does not work for various settings. Creating a network of improvement communities could accelerate the transfer of insights about better care methods and scaling approaches, and he credited organizations such as the Institute for Healthcare Improvement for starting to engage in these types of learning activities. Milstein also suggested that spreading and scaling efforts might benefit from a research effort to apply simulation modeling, using continuously generated patient data, to identify actions to improve care and lower cost. The resulting simulation models would then be available as a national asset.

Though the challenges to spreading and scaling models of care are significant, research has identified helpful tactics for spread and scale. During the first workshop, Deborah Peikes from Mathematica Policy Research discussed some of the factors for successful scaling that she and her colleagues found in studies conducted for the Centers for Medicare & Medicaid Services (CMS). The identified success factors included substantial financial incentives; support from multiple payers, such as coordination and aligning spending, technical assistance, data feedback, staff support, and reporting requirements; adapting data and technical assistance to reflect the considerable diversity of practices, health systems, markets, and patients; and monitoring or auditing, particularly if the funder bears risk, to ensure that programs are implemented as intended (Dale et al., 2016; Taylor et al., 2015a).

Despite Milstein's observation that health system leaders are reluctant to adopt models that require widespread changes in a health system, Peikes and colleagues found that practices that spread a model broadly throughout the practice were the most successful at implementing the model. Strong and consistent leadership is also critical for successful model adoption, and technical assistance on leadership and teamwork may help spread interventions. She noted that implementing a care model piecemeal in an organization puts too much burden on clinician champions, leads to unclear roles and responsibilities, and does not encourage the development of a learning health system.

At the first workshop Lisa Mangiante from the Pacific Business Group on Health (PBGH) discussed lessons learned from efforts to spread the Intensive Outpatient Care Program (IOCP) model that Milstein and Alan Glaseroff developed for high-need patients in California's Health Homes program. Between May 2012 and July 2015, this high-touch, care-coordinated, patient-involved, and team-based care model (see Appendix A) has been spread to 23 delivery system partners in Arizona, California, Idaho, Nevada, and Washington, and it encompasses some 500 practices and 15,000 patients. Of the 23 health system partners who participated in this CMS-funded scaling project, 20 are sustaining this model in their operations by integrating the model into their overall population health strategies. Mangiante explained that there is a great deal of payment and organizational variation among the partners, including the Medicare Shared Savings Program, Pioneer accountable care organizations (ACOs), Medicare Advantage Plans, and fee-for-service operations. Partners included independent practice associations, medical foundations, and both integrated and nonintegrated systems.

When discussing what was involved in scaling the IOCP model, Mangiante said PBGH started with what it called the A List of medical groups in California: those that already had track records of innovation, did well with innovation, had an infrastructure in place to implement this model, and had supportive leadership. Those A List groups had IOCP operational within 10 months. Once Mangiante and her colleagues had successful experiences working with the A List groups, they added less aligned and less sophisticated providers who required ongoing support.

Mangiante noted the following key characteristics that enable this model to scale and launch successfully at new sites, many of which overlap with the framework of attributes for successful care models described in Chapter 4: provider-hospital integration and integration into a larger population health strategy; adapting to the local environment after meeting core requirements; a strong analytical capability enabling aggressive patient monitoring with regular feedback; hiring effective care coordinators; identifying physicians and nurses who welcome disruptive innovation; training staff in didactic, interactive, and peer-to-peer learning; giving physicians a role in patient selection; developing intensive local patient outreach with close contact between physician and patient; ensuring strong support from senior leadership; having dedicated physician champions; and targeting those most likely to benefit from this program. With regard to sustaining the model once it is operational, she said it is critical for the programs to involve multiple payers as a means of creating a solid revenue stream.

Given these types of lessons, an important consideration for spreading and scaling successful models of care for high-need patients could be having payers and health systems work both separately and in tandem to more aggressively implement these models. Gerard Anderson from Johns Hopkins Bloomberg School of Public Health reported at the third workshop that payers could help foster success by tying payments to improving the patient experience, improving the health of populations, and reducing per capita cost of care; they could also target resources to populations most likely to benefit from these models as well as in a manner consistent with best practice. Health systems, meanwhile, could work with peers to identify promising models and work with payers to develop alternative contracts that pay for services not covered by fee-for-service arrangements (see page 86 for more on payment policies). Health systems could also commit to adequate investments in training, practice redesign, and information technologies. Working together, payers and health systems could explore the use of the patient taxonomy as a tool to match patient groups to tailored care models that better meet individual characteristics, needs, and challenges.

Anderson also pointed to the need for more research on developing programs that can be adopted widely in a variety of settings. To help inform efforts to spread and scale effective models of care, he suggested more research in areas such as identifying people at high need in actual practice settings, identifying individuals who are likely to be high-need patients in the future, identifying the best methods of care coordination, developing cost-effective implementation practices, and developing methods for effectively integrating medical and social services. As he noted, the importance of integrating social services and medical care is embedded in the other four policy areas—workforce development, payment policy, quality measures, and data infrastructure.

INTEGRATION OF SOCIAL SUPPORTS AND MEDICAL CARE

A recent analysis by McCarthy and colleagues found that comprehensive transitional care and case management involving patients and their caregivers after hospitalization is an important integrative feature of successful care models for high-need patients (McCarthy et al., 2015). As part of an effort to provide a framework for understanding the nature and extent of integration in programs that integrate long-term services and supports (LTSS) with medical care and behavioral health, the Long-Term Quality Alliance concluded that a critical element of a fully integrated model includes having a plan for health systems to accept responsibility for integrating medical care, postacute care, behavioral health care, pharmaceutical care, transitional care, and LTSS, including transportation and housing (Long-Term Quality Alliance, 2016).

As noted in Chapter 2, functional limitations are an important contributor to the disproportionate share of health care spending in the United States associated with high-need patients. In his presentation at the first workshop, Bruce Chernof from The SCAN Foundation noted that addressing a person's medical needs without also addressing functional limitations will have little impact on the cost or quality of care for these high-need patients. He also pointed out that social determinants of health,[13] which have been largely considered beyond the purview of the medical system, can have the biggest effect on ameliorating functional limitations. This is why successful models for improving care for high-need patients, such as those described in Chapter 4, often include the integration and delivery of social services in addition to better coordinated medical care. Enacting policies to facilitate the integration of social services and medical care is crucial for obtaining better outcomes for high-need individuals.

---

13   The Department of Health and Human Services' Office of Disease Prevention and Health Promotion defines social determinants of health to be social, economic, and physical conditions of an individual's life and surrounding environment, such as income, house, and nutritional factors, that impact the health outcomes of individuals (Secretary's Advisory Committee on Health Promotion and Disease Prevention Objectives for 2020, 2010).

A report prepared by Taylor and colleagues for Blue Cross Blue Shield of Massachusetts Foundation (Taylor et al., 2015b) points to the extensive scientific literature showing that nonmedical factors can play a substantially larger role than medical factors in health and health outcomes. On page 3, the report states there is "strong evidence that increased investment in selected social services as well as various models of partnership between health care and social services can confer substantial health benefits and reduce health care costs for targeted populations." Hayes and colleagues at the Bipartisan Policy Center (BPC) recently made a similar observation with regard to high-need Medicare patients and dual-eligible patients who receive care from both Medicare and Medicaid programs (Hayes et al., 2016). As an example, Hayes and colleagues (2016) noted that a recent evaluation of the Minnesota Senior Health Options program, which coordinates care for dual-eligible patients, found that this program increased the use of home- and community-based LTSS while decreasing hospitalizations for treatment of chronic illnesses and days spent in nursing homes (Anderson et al., 2016).

Two studies from Bradley and colleagues at the Yale School of Public Health further emphasize the importance of providing social services to improve health outcomes. The first study compared national spending on health services and social services among Organisation for Economic Co-operation and Development (OECD) countries and found that a larger ratio of social expenditures to health expenditures was significantly associated with better health outcomes (Bradley et al., 2011). OECD data used in this study (OECD, 2009) show that, compared to the United States, most highly developed countries spend a greater percentage of gross domestic product on social support and a smaller percentage on health care. In the second study, a state-to-state comparison of spending on social services and health care between 2000 and 2009 found that states with higher ratios of social service spending to health care spending[14] had better health outcomes and fewer days with functional limitations (Bradley et al., 2016). This team's analysis of 74 studies examining the impact of various health outcomes and health care costs found that three types of services were particularly important: supportive housing, nutritional support such as in-home meals for older adults, and case management and outreach programs.

While these and other studies reveal the important role social supports play in achieving the best health outcomes for high-need patients, it can be difficult to integrate social service and medical care programs into a seamless system, often because there are separate funding streams that hinder integration. For

---

14 This ratio was calculated as the sum of social service spending and public health spending divided by the sum of Medicare spending and Medicaid spending.

example, for the 10.3 million dual-eligible beneficiaries—many of whom are also high-need patients—Medicare is the primary payer for acute and postacute care services, while Medicaid covers services not included in Medicare benefits, such as case management services, transportation to medical appointments, personal-care services to help patients with functional limitations, and other LTSS. Too often, according to the work from Hayes and colleagues (2016), the separation of Medicare and Medicaid benefits and the "carving out" of certain Medicaid benefits from managed care contracts can lead to a fragmented care model in which the beneficiaries and their family caregivers must navigate multiple plans or payers depending on the type of service provided (Hayes et al., 2016a).

While this chapter addresses the negative effect that current payment policies have on integration in more detail below, one step the federal government, states, and payers could consider taking would be to revise financial incentives and organizational systems in a manner that recognizes the importance of providing social supports in conjunction with medical care. Currently, said Anderson, health systems and payers invest money for social services primarily when doing so saves money for the medical care system, even though providing social services for high-need patients has importance aside from cost savings. Moreover, savings accrued from social service investment are often not reinvested in social services, missing an opportunity to provide even better care. One caution to exercise when integrating social services and medical care is to not "medicalize" social services by making them the responsibility of health care systems. Doing so would create the risk that all services aimed at improving outcomes for high-need patients become "health care" and therefore subject to the administrative and payment rules that govern health systems.

While there are many system constraints to integration, there are opportunities nonetheless to better link medical and social services. For example, the Office of the Assistant Secretary for Planning and Evaluation could take the lead in overseeing integration efforts, perhaps in conjunction with an interagency task force involving the Departments of Agriculture, Health and Human Services, Transportation, and Urban Development that would work to embed health in all policies.[15] The federal government will likely need to engage in a strategy coordinated with state leadership to incentivize provision of evidence-based social support services in conjunction with the delivery of medical services. In addition, the nation would be well-served if the federal government studied the

---

15   Health in all policies is a strategy for addressing the complex factors that influence health and equity, including educational attainment, housing, transportation options, and neighborhood safety. Additional information is available at: http://www.naccho.org/uploads/downloadable-resources/Programs/Community-Health/HiAP-FAQ-Final-12-04-24.pdf.

impact of providing social services on health outcomes for high-need patients and encouraged states to support integration of social support services through "no wrong door" approaches that link patients to needed services regardless of how or where they enter health care or social services systems.

State governments, which control Medicaid spending, can also play a role in fostering the integration of health and social services. McGinnis and colleagues at The Commonwealth Fund developed a policy framework to help states move beyond isolated pilot efforts and establish the infrastructure necessary to support ongoing integration of health and social services, particularly for Medicaid beneficiaries (McGinnis et al., 2014). Their framework focuses on creating a statewide integrator to assume responsibility for ensuring coordination and communication across state-level services, establishing a robust set of tools to measure health outcomes and costs and share data among health systems, and developing long-term financing sources and payment models with incentives to encourage ongoing integration.

EXPAND AND ALIGN PAYMENT POLICIES

As multiple speakers at the first two workshops noted, payment policies that misalign financial incentives—particularly those that reimburse providers on a fee-for-service basis and that fail to pay for social services benefiting high-need patients—are perhaps the most prominent barrier to the widespread adoption of successful models of care for high-need patients. Many workshop participants stated the need for new payment policies that incentivize integration of social services and medical care and improved outcomes for high-need patients: Melissa Abrams from The Commonwealth Fund; Alan Glaseroff from Stanford Coordinated Care and Stanford School of Medicine; Bruce Chernof from The SCAN Foundation; Lisa Iezzoni from Harvard Medical School and the Mongan Institute for Health Policy at Massachusetts General Hospital; Robert Master from Commonwealth Care Alliance; John O'Brien from CareFirst Blue Cross Blue Shield; Peter Long from the Blue Shield of California Foundation; and Rahul Rajkumar from the Center for Medicare & Medicaid Innovation. A research synthesis compiled by The Commonwealth Fund also concluded that a lack of reimbursement under fee-for-service payment policies for providing care coordination and social supports is a major obstacle to spreading and scaling patient-focused care models for high-need patients (McCarthy et al., 2015).

Significant improvements have been made in paying for care coordination, and there is an increasing recognition that social supports are important components of effective care plans for high-need patients. Many insurers, including states and the federal government, are starting to embrace value-based purchasing that includes paying for care delivered outside of the traditional medical silo (Bachrach et al., 2014; Hamblin et al., 2011). In a recent perspective on the urgency of caring for high-need, high-cost patients, Blumenthal and colleagues point out, for example, that the Affordable Care Act catalyzed the formation of 838 ACOs covering more than 28 million people (Blumenthal et al., 2016b). At least some of these ACOs have allocated independent resources—not reimbursed by Medicare—toward providing short-term housing upon hospital discharge as a means of reducing hospital readmissions for vulnerable patients and keeping Medicare per-member spending below predetermined spending benchmarks (Viveiros, 2015). They also note that under the Medicare Access and Children's Health Insurance Program Reauthorization Act (MACRA), physicians will face strong incentives to participate in alternative, value-based payment models.

Fee-for-service Medicare Advantage Plans now pay for care coordination, and Medicare managed care plans have recognized the importance of care coordinators for high-need patients. In addition, CMS has granted an increasing number of Medicaid demonstration waivers for states that want to provide greater flexibility in covering community-based services as a means of reducing health care costs. Anderson noted that state and local public agencies are developing programs and task forces to support integration of social service and medical care programs. Examples include housing-related interventions such as the National Governors Association's Housing as Health Care program[16] and state-led Balancing Incentives Program and no wrong door approaches to provide access to LTSS for all populations and payers.[17]

The analysis conducted by Hayes and colleagues at the BPC and the recommendations they developed were intended to accelerate delivery system reform (Hayes et al., 2016a). Their analysis focused on the 10.3 million dual-eligible patients. Though only 20 percent of Medicare beneficiaries and 14 percent of Medicaid beneficiaries are dual-eligible individuals, they account for 35 percent of Medicare spending and 33 percent of combined federal and state spending on Medicaid. According to BPC's analysis, some 87 percent of dual-eligible beneficiaries have multiple chronic conditions, 54 percent have at least one behavioral health condition or cognitive impairment, and 29 percent have two or more limitations affecting activities of daily living. BPC's team noted that provider organizations seeking to improve care integration for high-need patients

---

16 For more information, see https://www.nga.org/cms/home/nga-center-for-best-practices/center-publications/page-health-publications/col2-content/main-content-list/housing-as-health-care-road-map.html (accessed on July 31, 2017).

17 For more information, see http://www.balancingincentiveprogram.org (accessed on July 31, 2017).

frequently run into the complex maze of federal and state reimbursement rules that preclude payment for, and in some cases coverage of, services that health providers believe could avert costlier emergency or hospital inpatient visits, which are major driving forces for the high costs associated with high-need patients.

To best appreciate the challenges arising from dual-eligible status, it is necessary to understand how dual-eligible patients receive their benefits from these two distinct programs. Although both Medicare and Medicaid are authorized under the Social Security Act, the federal government administers Medicare, while federal and state governments jointly finance Medicaid. States cover certain mandatory benefits under Medicaid, while other services are optional and coverage is determined on a state-by-state basis. As Hayes explained in her presentation at the third workshop, Medicaid covers LTSS, including many services that deal with functional limitations. As of June 2015, only some 20 percent of dual-eligible individuals were enrolled in the type of organized systems of care that blend social services and medical care, such as Medicare managed care plans, Program of All-Inclusive Care for the Elderly (PACE), and Dual Eligible Special Needs Plans (D-SNPs).

In their report, Hayes and colleagues (2016) state that the specific care delivery model and state implementation of the model will likely determine whether full integration of Medicare and Medicaid services will improve quality and lower the total cost of care for dual-eligible beneficiaries. There is mounting evidence, however, that integration does improve quality and value. As noted earlier in this chapter, for example, dual-eligible patients enrolled in Minnesota's Senior Health Options program had fewer hospitalizations and emergency department visits and increased use of home- and community-based LTSS compared to individuals receiving benefits through Medicare fee-for-service plans (Anderson et al., 2016).

BPC's team pointed out that there is much to learn about integrating care for dual-eligible beneficiaries. Hayes and colleagues (2016) explained that only a relatively small number of states have more than a few years of experience fully integrating Medicare and Medicaid services for dual-eligible beneficiaries over age 65. Even fewer states have experience with the under-65 population, which has higher-than-average rates of untreated behavioral health issues and/ or prevalence of homelessness according to Medicare managed care sponsors. Summarizing BPC's recommendations, Hayes explained that they include changing existing reimbursement structures, consolidating regulatory authority for dual-eligible programs within the Medicare-Medicaid Coordination Office at CMS, and building on lessons learned through implementation of existing programs and demonstrations to develop a consolidated framework for programs serving dual-eligible beneficiaries. Critical to that framework is the ability to combine Medicare and Medicaid financing streams into an integrated benefit structure that allows flexibility in benefit design to address patient needs. See Box 5–1 for selected excerpts of BPC's recommendations.

While BPC's recommendations aim to harmonize Medicare and Medicaid benefits to improve care of dual-eligible individuals, other efforts are under way to take advantage of Medicare and Medicaid programs that enable providers, payers, and state agencies with opportunities to test delivery system innovations that improve outcomes and patient experiences while increasing the value of care. Health Homes, Patient-Centered Medical Homes, Community Health Teams, and Transition Care Models are among the many programs using value-based strategies to replace traditional fee-for-service payment models. Recently, the Center for Health Care Strategies outlined approaches to value-based payments (Houston, 2016), some of which supplement fee-for-service payments, and others that replace them. Foundational payments, for example, are a flat or per-member per-month (PMPM) fee to reimburse providers for upfront investments they make to better coordinate care. Meaningful-use payments from the Office of the National Coordinator for Health Information Technology, which aim to reimburse practices for installing electronic health record systems, are an example of a foundational payment. Pay-for-performance models supplement fee-for-service payments by rewarding providers with performance incentive payments linked to outcomes and patient satisfaction metrics. The Medicare Physician Group Practice Demonstration is an example of this type of value-based payment model. Other approaches include bundled payments for a set of services for a specific care intervention, a common mechanism that state Medicaid programs use; shared savings programs that manage the total cost of care based on risk, such as the Medicare Shared Savings Program and state Medicaid ACOs; and capitation and global payments that pay a single PMPM fee to a provider to cover all of an individual's care, a model used by Oregon's Coordinated Care Organizations.

These types of payment methodologies can incentivize care investments in evidence-based best practices for high-need individuals and reduce the incentives that lead to ineffective and uncoordinated care. To increase their effectiveness, however, such payment models could be constructed to account for the increased financial risk associated with caring for high-need patients (Barnett et al., 2015). Health systems that focus exclusively on high-need patients can be at a market disadvantage and may be financially unstable.

They may be further disadvantaged by value-based purchasing arrangements that do not recognize the unique requirements of the high-need population. It may also be the case that capital markets would be less likely to finance organizations to better serve high-need patients because of the potential for competitive

BOX 5–1

Selected Excerpts from the Bipartisan Policy Center's Recommendations to Align Programs and Integrate Care for Dual-Eligible Beneficiaries

Special-Needs Plans (SNPs): Permanently authorize Medicare Advantage Dual-Eligible SNPs. However, all plans fully integrate clinical health services, behavioral health, and LTSS by January 1, 2020. [Additionally], the combined Medicare and Medicaid benefits offered through all SNPs [should be] seamless to the beneficiary and to providers.

Streamlining and aligning of SNPs: For ongoing demonstrations, CMS should revise contracts to ensure that rates reflect unanticipated costs of infrastructure investment or significant differences in cost associated with serving certain special-needs populations, such as those with previously untreated mental illnesses or homeless individuals. [CMS should also] work with states to develop unique state-specific quality and access measures, and permit states to share in a greater percentage of [applicable] savings or permit added flexibility in the scope of covered benefits [as appropriate]. [Moreover,] CMS should establish additional demonstrations to integrate Medicare and Medicaid for dual-eligible beneficiaries based on findings from the evaluations of the first-round demonstrations.

Expanded PACE eligibility: CMS should test [variations of the Program of All-Inclusive Care for the Elderly (PACE) including] an expansion to individuals, regardless of age, who meet all other PACE criteria and who do not require a nursing home level of care; an option that permits individuals to enroll in PACE, but opt out of adult day services; and an option that includes both Medicare-covered services and a beneficiary "buy-in" of a limited LTSS benefit.

Streamlined dual-eligible beneficiary services: Regulatory authority for reimbursement structures serving dual-eligible beneficiaries should be consolidated into a single office or center within CMS, such as the Medicare-Medicaid Coordination Office.

CMS, states, plans alignment: Policymakers should build on lessons learned from existing programs and demonstrations to develop a contractual model similar to the innovative "three-way" contract between CMS, states, and plans under the financial alignment demonstration. A new model three-way contract should be uniform with respect to basic structure, beneficiary protections, quality requirements, care coordination, and continuity of care requirements. At the same time, it should be flexible enough to permit variation in delivery, provider, and reimbursement models, as well as state-level decisions, such as eligibility for optional populations.

SOURCE: Adapted from Hayes et al., 2016a

disadvantage compared to organizations that do not serve large numbers of high-need patients.

One issue, addressed by Blumenthal and colleagues in a discussion paper from the National Academy of Medicine's series of discussion papers *Vital Directions for Health and Health Care* (Blumenthal et al., 2016a), is that most ACOs and performance- and risk-based plans still pay clinicians on a fee-for-service basis (Bailit et al., 2015). The authors of this discussion paper note that if individual providers or practice sites do not feel accountable for health outcomes, population health, and value, the diffusion of promising practices and models of care will be slow. Another concern the authors of this paper noted is the misalignment between investment and savings: too often, the savings realized by a successful care model accrue to payers, even though it is the providers who are expected to cover the up-front costs of staff training and other investments a program requires (Hong et al., 2014). Even if savings are shared with providers, the time for these complex delivery system reforms to produce savings can be several years (Jones et al., 2016), which can discourage providers from making the necessary initial investments. Ashish Jha from the Harvard T.H. Chan School of Public Health noted at the third workshop that realizing a return on investment with even good models is a long process. Google, he pointed out, took 8 or so years to become profitable, and to expect these models to yield large returns in 2 to 3 years will lead to disappointment. Similarly, Peikes and colleagues stated, "The providers we speak to report that it takes a year and a half or longer for interventions to really click." In the third workshop, David Atkins of the Department of Veterans Affairs underscored the need for support for the long-term experiments to demonstrate meaningful returns on investments, particularly given the reluctance of health system administrators to maintain programs that are not yielding short-term benefits.

When discussing payment policies, Anderson said in the third workshop, it is important to remember that just as there is not one kind of high-need patient, corresponding flexibility will be needed when it comes to payment models that incentivize high-value care for high-need patients. In particular, reimbursements for care coordination will have to reflect the different levels of patient need that require different levels of care coordination and that entail different degrees of risk. One issue that a breakout group in the second workshop raised was the need to allow organizations to have some flexibility in the benefits they offer as long as they can demonstrate that they are providing high-quality care for all of the high-need individuals in their care, not just a selected few. Flexibility could allow providers and health care organizations to target individuals who are most likely to benefit from particular delivery models if the focus is on improving quality of care rather than squeezing cost savings out of the system. In that regard, said John O'Brien from CareFirst Blue Cross Blue Shield, payment models should incentivize targeting patients who are most likely to benefit from the right interventions.

WORKFORCE FOR COMPREHENSIVE HEALTH CARE

Both Peikes and Mangiante noted the importance of education and training in successful scaling efforts and the integration of services. Many clinicians, however, are not well trained to address the needs of high-need patients. Anderson commented that medical schools tend to emphasize "body parts" instead of the whole person and that nurses, who are often the care coordinators in these model programs, have little training in care coordination. In fact, he pointed out, care providers of all types—physicians and nurses, medical paraprofessionals, social workers, and housing and employment professionals—need to receive training on caring for and interacting with high-need individuals.

Thomas-Henkel and colleagues, in a study commissioned by the Robert Wood Johnson Foundation (Thomas-Henkel et al., 2015), noted that barriers to the spread and scale of care models for high-need patients include gaps in the training of current and newly graduated clinicians, a lack of interprofessional education among team members, low reimbursement rates that may limit recruitment efforts, and the need to develop more effective models for preventing and managing staff burnout given the professional and emotional challenges this work can entail. They highlighted the opportunity for academic health centers and professional societies to collaborate on developing new training and certification opportunities, particularly those that encompass team-based approaches and training in behavioral health, substance use disorders, and complex psychosocial factors. They also raised the point that there are new models of supervision involving the entire spectrum of traditional and nontraditional health care team members that care models are drawing upon to better serve high-need patients.

There is, therefore, a need and an opportunity for education and training to be integrated into the process of spreading and scaling any given model. Many models that have proven successful at improving care for high-need patients already put an emphasis on social supports, a trend noted by Molly Coye from the Network for Excellence in Health Innovation. As mentioned in Chapter 4, adoption of these models can lead to substantial changes in workforce roles as evidenced by assigning important roles in the care teams that integrate the broad range of social and behavioral health services high-need patients require to professionals who are often not considered key members of a health care team.

Credentialing programs, particularly for nontraditional health workers such as community health workers and peer support providers, could be developed to encourage workforce development to support high-need patients. Research has shown that properly trained community health workers can play a unique role in helping high-need patients navigate the health system, obtain necessary supportive resources, and build self-efficacy and health literacy; by doing so, they can improve patient experiences and outcomes and reduce hospital readmissions (Adair et al., 2012; Adair et al., 2013; Davis, 2013; Kangovi et al., 2014). For example, an Oregon program for high-need Medicaid patients, in which care teams were led by a nurse and two community health workers, reduced emergency department utilization from 78 percent in 2011 to 59 percent in 2013 (Takach and Yalowich, 2015).

Academic institutions, health systems, and other educators could develop curricula on the treatment and social support needs of high-need patients, including training on team-based care, patient engagement, care coordination across health and social sectors, and the social determinants of health. Key workforce sectors in need of training would include clinicians, nurses, physician assistants and other medical paraprofessionals, mental health professionals, social workers, pharmacologists, substance abuse providers, community health workers, peer providers, law enforcement officers, and housing and employment service providers. In particular, anyone involved in case management would benefit from special training that would include field training to observe delivery of evidence-based practices. Rajesh Davda from Cigna noted that physicians and nurses participating in Cigna's model program for high-need patients were generally poorly informed about care coordination when the program started. Once staff members were trained on matters of care coordination, they became the most effective instructors for training additional team members. This result prompted Cigna to develop learning collaboratives to foster workforce training. Anderson commented that high-need patients would also benefit from improved training for students in health care fields, which he believes would reduce the stigma associated with people with complex illnesses among clinical trainees, active professionals, and health system administrators, and produce a culture shift in the world of health care.

REEXAMINE QUALITY MEASUREMENT

As value-based purchasing becomes more common, it will be essential to use quality measures—and the data that inform those measures—to improve care and offer incentives for providers to treat high-need patients. As Shari Ling from

CMS noted in her presentation at the third workshop, the proper use of measures creates transparency on cost and quality of care. Most quality measures currently in use, however, focus on specific conditions and whether methods of care for those conditions are effective. Ling pointed out that meaningful quality measures are too often setting-specific rather than being aligned with patient-centered outcomes that span various settings (Conway et al., 2013). Discussion during the second workshop noted that the current system of metrics is not designed in a way that encourages providers to organize care in the most effective manner.

While condition-specific measures are important, high-need patients are more than the sum of their individual diseases, and they have additional concerns beyond the appropriate care for each specific condition. To better reflect this reality, measures for assessing the performance of care models for high-need patients could indicate the degree of care coordination, quality of life, independence, and overall mental and physical health status. In her presentation at the third workshop, Helen Burstin from the National Quality Forum highlighted the need for measures based on patient-reported outcomes, patient involvement in the decision-making process regarding their care, and the quality of home and community-based services. In his remarks at the third workshop, Rick Kronick from the University of California, San Diego, added that measures should assess whether systems are stinting on some aspects of care, whether patient preferences are elicited and respected, and whether the communication between clinician and patient is of adequate quality. During the same workshop, Richard Frank from Anthem Blue Cross Blue Shield wondered if it would be possible to measure patient behavior in some manner that would provide a better understanding of engagement and motivation to change.

The Health and Medicine Division of the National Academies of Sciences, Engineering, and Medicine has undertaken a study of the relationships between social risk factors and performance measurement (National Academies of Sciences and Medicine, 2016a, 2016b), which will also inform metrics focused on the social determinants of health for the high-need population. According to Burstin, the availability of more appropriate measures of care relevant to high-need patients will enable health care financing to move beyond reliance on claims-based risk adjustment and instead enable differentiation of risk within clinical conditions and risk-based grouping of multiple chronic conditions. Such measures could also better account for unmeasured clinical complexity, such as patient frailty, disability, poor functional status, and multiple chronic conditions. Among existing measures, recent evidence suggests that because reliable case mix accommodation approaches are still evolving, hospitals caring for a higher proportion of patients with complex medical problems tend to fare worse on certain quality measures, such as readmissions (Joynt, 2013, 2017), and may experience high penalties under value-based purchasing programs, potentially creating a disincentive to caring for these individuals.

Burstin and other participants at the third workshop voiced their concern that the proliferation of measures and "measurement for measurement's sake" has become a burden to providers. A 2016 National Academy of Medicine Perspective, *Observations from the Field: Reporting Quality Metrics in Health Care* (Dunlap et al., 2016), offered the same concern. As David Dorr from the Oregon Health & Science University noted, it takes discipline to be parsimonious with measures. It is important for payers and health systems to choose measures that reflect realistic quality and accountability goals and to understand that programs may not demonstrate marked improvements for several years. Kronick remarked that measures should not be the only means used to improve quality of care. In his opinion, public policies related to quality improvement should emphasize methods of enhancing professional intrinsic motivation while recognizing the role of organizations to promote and facilitate that motivation by providing systematic feedback to physicians, technical assistance, and opportunities for providers to collaborate on projects to improve care.

IMPROVE DATA INFRASTRUCTURE

Research shows that high-quality data and analytics are an essential component of effective models of care for high-need patients in that they are used to match high-need individuals with specific interventions (Bates et al., 2014; Bradley et al., 2016; Dale et al., 2016; Rajkumar et al., 2015). High-quality data are also needed to inform the types of measures discussed in the previous section. One major challenge Anderson noted is that there are many disparate systems that cannot easily share information, making it difficult to assess the requirements of high-need individuals and whether they are getting appropriate medical and social care. During the first workshop, Lisa Iezzoni from Harvard Medical School and the Mongan Institute for Health Policy at Massachusetts General Hospital said that reliable data are needed when identifying high-need patients to overcome the limitations of the diagnostic data by which chronic conditions are identified. International Classification of Diseases-Clinical Modification diagnostic codes may not fully capture disability, functional limitations, or frailty, while other measures of frailty and disability can carry biases, including cultural ones, or have gaming potential once reimbursements start being based on a particular measure. In addition, diagnostic claim codes may fail to capture the health of persons who have not received adequate care.

Iezzoni illustrated the problem of trying to use diagnostic claim codes to capture the health of persons who have not yet received adequate care by recounting the experience of the One Care program in Massachusetts, a dually capitated program begun on October 1, 2013, for Medicare and Medicaid enrollees ages 21 to 64. Capitation for Medicaid payments was set using rating categories that were initially assigned based on prior year MassHealth Medicaid claims for the program's participants. As soon as the One Care program started, it became obvious that many enrollees had higher needs than were indicated in their assigned rating category, in large part because they had not had Medicaid claims from a prior year since they had not received services in that prior year. Program administrators went to MassHealth and explained that they were not able to provide needed services because the capitated payments were too low because of the improper ratings. The solution was to conduct a functional status assessment once a person was enrolled in the One Care program and upgrade the rating based on that assessment. Before the upgrade, 59 percent of the enrollees had the lowest rating—a minimal care level for this high-need population—while after the upgrade only 40 percent of the enrollees fell into that category. At the same time, the percentage of independently living individuals in the highest-need categories rose from 19 percent to 35 percent. At the time of the second workshop, reimbursements were matched closely to costs, allowing One Care to provide the services its clients required.

Electronic health record (EHR) data, combined with claims data, can provide some additional insights about high-need patients that can help with managing complex patient populations. At the second workshop, Paul Bleicher from OptumLabs, a division of UnitedHealth Group, described how his organization uses these combined data sources to characterize the natural history of disease and identify specific issues and conditions associated with the biggest costs. Researchers at OptumLabs have also been using these data to examine patient clustering. They created a model that identifies patients who are at the highest risk of hospitalization and uses machine-learning clustering technologies to segment the top 10 percent of these patients. This analysis, he said, can support efforts to personalize care based on specific patient profiles.

Data from EHRs can provide a finer-grained picture of different groups of patients. For example, EHR data analysis reveals a substantial difference between prescriptions written and prescriptions filled. In the case of patients with hypertension who are not following established guidelines, this type of analysis can show whether the problem rests with the patient or the physician. Natural language processing of EHR data can create structured variables that provide detailed pictures of laboratory test results as they relate to care management, leading to the identification of possible drivers of hospital readmission, said Bleicher. He noted that significant amounts of granular information can be extracted from the EHR with natural language processing and used to gain a better understanding of patient outcomes. This value-added information includes clinical findings that are not available in claims data, such as preadjusted diagnostic and procedure information and temporal data about a patient's stay in the hospital. In addition, clinical notes can be mined for details, such as the risk of falling, that are not available in the EHR's structured data.

OptumLabs has been using this type of data analysis and mining to create predictive models that can help reduce hospitalizations. For example, a congestive heart failure predictive model uses a patient's prior health care use and clinical findings such as blood oxygenation, laboratory results, and vital signs to predict the risk of future hospitalization over the following 6 months. Individuals in the 95th percentile of risk were contacted and brought into the clinic for further assessment and treatment, with the result that hospital admissions for all patients with congestive heart failure were reduced by 60 percent from a year earlier. Bleicher explained that with claims data alone, the model was inadequate.

There are policy impediments—particularly with regard to sharing behavioral health and substance abuse information—that act as barriers to coordinating care for high-need individuals. Bleicher noted that standardizing EHR data across different systems is a major challenge, as is the fact that individual physicians capture and record data differently, and coders will code records and turn them into claims differently. For example, Bleicher stated that his team found from mining EHR data that between 11 and 31 percent of patients who had no billing code for diabetes over a 3-year period were in fact being treated for diabetes based on EHR-recorded laboratory results and prescriptions for diabetes medications. Jha added that claims data are limited when it comes to identifying which individuals either use or have used long-term care. Medicare data, for example, do not include long-term care; there is not a good national dataset with any granularity on long-term care services and supports and social services for the Medicare population. Federal, state, and local governments could identify barriers that currently inhibit data flow among the clinicians and organizations treating high-need populations and work to minimize those barriers while respecting patient privacy and data security.

In her presentation at the second workshop, Sandra Wilkniss from the National Governors Association said that access to data is one of the main challenges that states face in crafting effective policies to support better care for high-need, high-cost patients. In fact, some states have difficulty accessing even their own claims data to conduct necessary analyses, in part because state laws are barriers to effective data sharing. For the most part, explained Wilkniss, governors are taking a data-driven strategy to identify target populations primarily using Medicaid claims data, pharmacy data, and other types of high-level data to segment patient populations. A significant piece of this strategy involves what Wilkniss called "geospatial hot-spotting," or identifying communities with a disproportionate share of high-need, high-cost patients. She noted that high-value health care systems with which she has interacted are using data to conduct rapid-cycle evaluations of their programs' performance to continuously improve care and reduce costs.

In their work toward defining a state policy framework for integrating health and social services, McGinnis and colleagues at The Commonwealth Fund suggest that state- and community-level data-sharing tools could include integrated claims databases that link and share information across payers, service sectors, and provider networks (McGinnis et al., 2014). One example of such a tool is the Predictive Risk Intelligence System (PRISM) that Washington State developed to support care management for high-risk Medicaid patients (Court et al., 2011).

Integration of medical, behavioral, and social data, along with improved data sharing, is paramount to improving care for high-need patients. Integration and data sharing, however—whether across health and social services systems or within different components of the health care system—is a challenge that federal, state, and local partners could work together to address. One possible first step would be to identify the barriers to data flow among and within agencies and providers and then invest in activities to optimize information exchange. As noted at the third workshop, some of those barriers include federal confidentiality regulations (42 CFR Part II) that restrict sharing information about patients' history of alcohol and substance abuse; misinterpretation of data sharing rules in the Health Insurance Portability and Accountability Act of 1996 (HIPAA); and integration of EHRs and Prescription Drug Monitoring Program data.

Data could inform the strategic deployment of health care and social services resources. Toward that end, public and commercial payers could lead efforts to identify and share information about target populations and the potential for different models to positively affect the care of those populations. Incorporating screening tools for social risk and behavioral health variables into EHRs could serve as a source of data on patients that could be used to inform program targeting. Other sources of data could include claims, administrative data, data from patient encounters with health and social services systems, and patient-related geographical information. Medicare data, collected by CMS, could serve as a rich source of information about patients and program effectiveness. If these disparate sources of data could be integrated, they could be used to align targeting strategies across payers and to inform benefits, care delivery, and payment models.

As multiple speakers over the course of the three workshops noted, achieving the type of policy changes discussed here will not happen without the involvement of all stakeholders—federal, state, and local governments; providers; payers; and patients and caregivers. Moreover, changing policies and allowing organizations to adapt to those changes will not happen quickly. As Mary Anne Sterling from Connected Health Resources said at the conclusion of the third workshop: "I think what we are doing is culture change on a grand scale, probably [on a scale] that has never been done before in this country. I think we all need to encourage our peers that it is going to take some patience, maybe one or two do-overs, maybe a left or right turn along the way, but it is definitely doable."

REFERENCES

Adair, R., J. Christianson, D. R. Wholey, K. White, R. Town, S. Lee, H. Britt, P. Lund, A. Lukasewycz, and D. Elumba. 2012. Care guides: Employing non-clinical laypersons to help primary care teams manage chronic disease. *Journal of Ambulatory Care Management* 35(1):27–37.

Adair, R., D. R. Wholey, J. Christianson, K. M. White, H. Britt, and S. Lee. 2013. Improving chronic disease care by adding laypersons to the primary care team: A parallel randomized trial. *Annals of Internal Medicine* 159(3):176–184.

Anderson, W. L., F. Zhanlian, and S. K. Long. 2016. *Minnesota managed care longitudinal data analysis.* Washington, DC: HHS Office of the Assistant Secretary for Planning and Evaluation.

Bachrach, D., S. Anthony, and A. Detty. 2014. *State strategies for integrating physical and behavioral health services in a changing medicaid environment.* New York, NY: The Commonwealth Fund.

Bailit, M. H., M. E. Burns, and M. B. Dyer. 2015. Implementing value-based physician compensation: Advice from early adopters. *Healthcare Financial Management* 69(7):40–47.

Barnett, M. L., J. Hsu, and J. M. McWilliams. 2015. Patient characteristics and differences in hospital readmission rates. *JAMA Intern Med* 175(11):1803–1812.

Bates, D. W., S. Saria, L. Ohno-Machado, A. Shah, and G. Escobar. 2014. Big data in health care: Using analytics to identify and manage high-risk and high-cost patients. *Health Affairs* 33(7):1123–1131.

Bennett, I. M., J. Chen, J. S. Soroui, and S. White. 2009. The contribution of health literacy to disparities in self-rated health status and preventive health behaviors in older adults. *Annals of Family Medicine* 7(3):204–211.

Blumenthal, D., G. Anderson, S. Burke, T. Fulmer, A. K. Jha, and P. Long. 2016a. *Tailoring complex-care management, coordination, and integration for high-need, high-cost patients.* Vital Directions for Health and Health Care Series. Discussion Paper, National Academy of Medicine, Washington, DC.

Blumenthal, D., B. Chernof, T. Fulmer, J. Lumpkin, and J. Selberg. 2016b. Caring for high-need, high-cost patients - an urgent priority. *New England Journal of Medicine* 375(10):909–911.

Bradley, E. H., M. Canavan, E. Rogan, K. Talbert-Slagle, C. Ndumele, L. Taylor, and L. A. Curry. 2016. Variation in health outcomes: The role of spending on social services, public health, and health care, 2000–09. *Health Affairs* 35(5):760–768.

Bradley, E. H., B. R. Elkins, J. Herrin, and B. Elbel. 2011. Health and social services expenditures: Associations with health outcomes. *BMJ Qual Saf* 20(10):826–831.

Conway, P. H., F. Mostashari, and C. Clancy. 2013. The future of quality measurement for improvement and accountability. *JAMA* 309(21):2215–2216.

Court, B. J., D. Mancuso, C. Zhu, and A. Krupski. 2011. Predictive risk intelligence system (prism): A decision-support tool for coordinating care for complex medicaid clients. In *Comprehensive care coordination for chronically ill adults*: John Wiley & Sons, Inc. Pp. 349–359.

Dale, S. B., A. Ghosh, D. N. Peikes, T. J. Day, F. B. Yoon, E. F. Taylor, K. Swankoski, A. S. O'Malley, P. H. Conway, R. Rajkumar, M. J. Press, L. Sessums, and R. Brown. 2016. Two-year costs and quality in the comprehensive primary care initiative. *New England Journal of Medicine* 374(24):2345–2356.

Davis, A. C. 2013. *Leveraging community health workers within california's state innovation model: Background, options and considerations.* Sacramento, CA: California Health and Human Services Agency.

Dunlap, N. E., D. J. Ballard, R. A. Cherry, W. C. Dunagan, W. Ferniany, A. C. Hamilton, T. A. Owens, T. Rusconi, S. M. Safyer, P. J. Santrach, A. Sears, M. R. Waldrum, and K. E. Walsh. 2016. *Observations from the field: Reporting quality metrics in health care.* Discussion Paper, National Academy of Medicine, Washington, DC.

Hamblin, A., J. Verdier, and M. Au. 2011. *State options for integrating physical and behavioral health care.* Washington, DC: Center for Health Care Strategies, Inc.

Hayes, K., G. W. Hoadland, N. Lopez, M. Workman, P. Fise, K. Taylor, R. Meltzer, and S. Seong. 2016. *Delivery system reform: Improving care for individuals dually eligible for medicare and medicaid.* Washington, DC: Bipartisan Policy Center.

Hong, C. S., M. K. Abrams, and T. G. Ferris. 2014. Toward increased adoption of complex care management. *New England Journal of Medicine* 371(6):491–493.

Houston, R. 2016. *Maintaining the momentum: Using value-based payments to sustain provider innovations.* http://www.chcs.org/maintaining-the-momentum-using-value-based-payments-to-sustain-provider-innovations/ (accessed November 2, 2016).

Jones, C., K. Finison, K. McGraves-Lloyd, T. Tremblay, M. K. Mohlman, B. Tanzman, M. Hazard, S. Maier, and J. Samuelson. 2016. Vermont's community-oriented all-payer medical home model reduces expenditures and utilization while delivering high-quality care. *Popul Health Manag* 19(3):196–205.

Joynt, K. E., A. A. Gawande, E. J. Orav, and A. K. Jha. 2013. Contribution of preventable acute care spending to total spending for high-cost medicare patients. *JAMA* 309(24):2572–2578.

Joynt, K. E., J. F. Figueroa, E. J. Orav, and A. K. Jha. 2016. Opinions on the Hospital Readmission Reduction Program: Results of a National Survey of Hospital Leaders.*The American Journal of Managed Care 22(8): 287–294.*

Kangovi, S., N. Mitra, D. Grande, M. L. White, S. McCollum, J. Sellman, R. P. Shannon, and J. A. Long. 2014. Patient-centered community health worker intervention to improve posthospital outcomes: A randomized clinical trial. *JAMA Intern Med* 174(4):535–543.

Long-Term Quality Alliance. 2016. *Taxonomy of long-term services and supports integration.* Washington, DC: Long-Term Quality Alliance.

McCarthy, D., J. Ryan, and S. Klein. 2015. Models of care for high-need, high-cost patients: An evidence synthesis. *Issue Brief (Commonw Fund)* 31:1–19.

McGinnis, T., M. Crawford, and S. A. Somers. 2014. *A state policy framework for integrating health and social services.* New York, NY: The Commonwealth Fund.

National Academies of Sciences, Engineering, and Medicine. 2016a. *Accounting for social risk factors in medicare payment: Criteria, factors, and methods.* Washington, DC: The National Academies Press.

National Academies of Sciences, Engineering, and Medicine. 2016b. *Accounting for social risk factors in medicare payment: Identifying social risk factors.* Washington, DC: The National Academies Press.

OECD. 2009. *Health at a glance 2009.* Geneva: OECD Publishing.

Olin, G., and D. D. Dougherty. 2006. *Characteristics and medical expenses of adults 18 to 64-years old with functional limitations, combined years 1997–2002.* Rockville, MD: Agency for Healthcare Research and Quality.

Rajkumar, R., M. J. Press, and P. H. Conway. 2015. The cms innovation center—a five-year self-assessment. *New England Journal of Medicine* 372(21):1981–1983.

Secretary's Advisory Committee on Health Promotion and Disease Prevention Objectives for 2020. 2010. *Healthy people 2020: An opportunity to address the societal determinants of health in the United States.* Washington, DC: US Department of Health and Human Services.

Takach, M., and R. Yalowich. 2015. *Transforming the workforce to provide better chronic care: The role of a community health nurse in a high-utilizer program in Oregon.* Washington, DC: AARP Public Policy Institute.

Taylor, E. F., S. Dale, D. Peikes, R. S. Brown, and G. Arkadipta. 2015a. *Evaluation of the comprehensive primary care initiative: First annual report.* Princeton, NJ: Mathematica Policy Research.

Taylor, L. A., C. E. Coyle, C. Ndumele, E. Rogan, M. Canavan, L. Curry, and E. H. Brandley. 2015b. *Leveraging the social determinants of health: What works?* Boston, MA: Blue Cross Blue Shield of Massachusetts Foundation.

Thomas-Henkel, C., A. Hamblin, and T. Hendricks. 2015. *Opportunities to improve models of care for people with complex needs.* Princeton, NJ: Robert Wood Johnson Foundation & Center for Health Care Strategies.

Viveiros, J. 2015. *Addressing housing as a health care treatment.* Washington, DC: Center for Housing Policy and the National Housing Conference.

6

COMMON THEMES AND OPPORTUNITIES FOR ACTION

At the outset of this collaborative initiative in February 2015, the goal established by the participants—the Peterson Center on Healthcare, the National Academy of Medicine, the Harvard T.H. Chan School of Public Health (HSPH), the Bipartisan Policy Center (BPC), and The Commonwealth Fund—was to advance our understanding about how to better manage the health of high-need patients through the exploration of patient characteristics and groupings, of promising care models and attributes, and of policy solutions to spread and scale models of care. Since the launch of this project, the pace of change in the field—from the demonstration of new models of care for high-need patients to state and federal governments launching initiatives aimed at better coordinating care for this patient population—has created an encouraging new dynamic that offers promise for addressing the challenge of caring for high-need patients and reducing the outsized cost of providing that care.

The key themes and lessons from the workshops, the workgroups, and the committee as a whole are summarized below, along with areas of opportunity for various stakeholders. Given that high-need patients often face challenges in receiving adequate care, including a lack of care coordination within the health care system, and that caring for these individuals is currently a key driver of health care spending, a notable theme voiced throughout the discussions was the call for bold policy action and system and payment reform efforts. The comprehensive team-oriented services required are not currently available in most settings, yet the potential gains to health care systems are considerable. Over the past 2 years, a number of promising innovations in care delivery have emerged, but there are systemic barriers to replicating and sustaining the key practices. The research and activities of this partnership have shown how essential it is to create a policy and regulatory environment built around payment models that incentivize coordinated care and support the integration of clinical care and social services. In addition, health systems would benefit from a "taxonomy" to segment high-need patients and match the appropriate interventions as well as from a set of key measures to support value-based payment.

MAIN THEMES AND LESSONS

The first important lessons from this initiative are that the high-need patient population is diverse, complex, expensive, and often transient, and the heterogeneity of this population suggests that a similar diversity of care models will be needed to address the range of problems these individuals experience. At the same time, there is a need to strike a balance between standardized and customized approaches to care. In that regard, segmenting patients can be a useful tool for targeting care, but there is need for more real-world testing and refinement of approaches for segmenting patients in conjunction with care models demonstrated to work with certain subpopulations of high-need patients.

Another key lesson from this initiative is that just improving medical care for high-need patients will not address all of the challenges they face, nor will it lower the cost of care. To be successful, as the examples cited in Chapter 4 and in Appendix A demonstrate, care models for high-need patients will often need to address the social risk and behavioral health factors that play an outsized role in the lives of these individuals. Going forward, care models, policies, and assessment tools need to address social services and behavioral health needs in addition to those services normally considered the purview of health care systems. The final overarching lesson is that to be actionable, policy solutions must account for existing constraints and complexities arising from the lack of integration of medical, social, and behavioral services and with the way the United States finances care models.

In addition to those overarching lessons, a number of important themes emerged from the presentations and discussions in the three workshops and deliberations among the committee members. These included:

Segmentation and Taxonomy

The high-need patient population comprises a heterogeneous group of individuals that have a diverse array of conditions, making segmentation of this population into a finite number of subpopulations an important consideration when attempting to match patients with appropriate models of care. With a patient taxonomy and menu of evidence-based care models, health systems would be better equipped to plan for and deliver targeted care based on patient characteristics, needs, and challenges and to identify gaps in their ability to deliver care for specific subgroups within their patient populations. Models of care for high-need patients must balance the need for standardized approaches for diverse populations with the need for personalization around individual patients' conditions, needs, and characterization. In that regard, having too many segment groups becomes too complex and impractical for broad implementation, but having too few segments makes groupings less meaningful and undermines the objective to be able to target care effectively.

The purpose and utility of segmentation must guide the development of a taxonomy for high-need patients and reflect the fact that a taxonomy will be a dynamic and interactive tool and that a single individual can move between taxonomic segments as their health—and therefore their care needs—change over time. Starting a taxonomy from a medical perspective has limitations, but it is a feasible starting point for most health systems, given the availability of data. Additionally, functional status can be "baked in" to the various medical segments in a taxonomy, with social risk factors and behavioral health considerations spanning all clinical/functional segments.

Barriers around data collection and use, particularly among smaller clinics and providers who lack a sophisticated and interoperable health information technology infrastructure, limit the use of patient segmentation. There is a need to improve our understanding of the transient nature of the high-need patient population and how health systems need to account for it when developing care delivery models.

Tailored Care and Care Coordination

In the 2 years since the germination of this collaborative project, understanding and approaches to care delivery for high-need patients have evolved, with the demonstration that multiple care models can improve care. A successful care model is designed to respond to the goals and needs of patients, and an essential tool for standardizing and centering care around patient needs and goals—as well as for assessing patient needs across disease groups—is measuring functional status. Understanding patient needs and goals also requires better measurement of patient priorities, and meeting these goals will require flexible models of care.

Care coordination is critical for high-need patients, and improving care coordination will require the development of new workforce and training efforts. Such efforts are often costly, so special consideration should be given to potential care coordination approaches that help control costs. Additionally, improving care for high-need patients requires aligning the care system with social, economic, and behavioral programs and services, a task that will be difficult because of the fragmentation that exists in these fields.

While more research is needed to bolster the evidence base for care models and care model attributes that work for specific subpopulations of high-need patients, there is a broad consensus on universal attributes common to successful care models. There is broad agreement that the predominant location for delivering care for high-need patients should be in the home and community rather than in the hospital or nursing home whenever possible. Health systems can work with payers to better identify and target high-need patients and to test new practices, including the use of a taxonomy. A matching exercise demonstrated that individual care models can be targeted to specific groups based on characteristics and needs.

Payment Models

Current economic and payment models oriented to individual conditions lead to inefficiencies and deficiencies in care processes that have particular impact on high-need patients, who often have a diverse array of conditions. Moreover, care models for high-need patients incur high, ongoing costs, and the long-term financing of these models must be considered when identifying policy solutions. Payers can actively support the adoption of care models or specific elements of care models that research has shown are effective at improving care for high-need patients and/or reducing the cost of care. Policy makers and payers can continue progress toward a value-based system using alternative payment models, including those that work within fee-for-service structures, to support more effective care for high-need patients.

Policy Opportunities to Encourage the Spread and Scale of Care Models

Policy solutions must engage all aspects of care delivery, such as providing mental health support for home health aides and family caregivers, as well as accounting for existing system constraints and complexities (e.g., integration of medical and social financing of care models). Although having supportive policies in place can enable models to spread and scale, many care models do not scale because specifics of the models are not considered, such as the adaptations away from ideal conceptualizations to meet the on-the-ground realities or interpersonal dynamics and the role of leadership in success. Areas where policy changes could accelerate their widespread adoption and sustainability include the programmatic integration of social supports; care delivery and workforce; payment policy; quality measurement; and data infrastructure.

Furthermore, policies need to consider both state and federal perspectives to be broadly adopted. Federal structures such as the Federal Coordinated Health Care Office—also known as the Medicare-Medicaid Coordination Office or Office of the Dual—can serve an important role in bridging many different health care and social services sectors and populations.

Quality measures have proliferated and are often burdensome; a reevaluation of which limited set of measures is necessary to determine quality in specific circumstances would greatly benefit program administrators, regulators, health systems, payers, and providers. Tying payment incentives to particular measures simply because they can be measured can give too much weight to the importance of those aspects of care compared to elements that are less easily quantified.

OPPORTUNITIES FOR STAKEHOLDER ACTION

A goal of this initiative has been to identify a path forward to produce the bold actions needed to improve the lives of the nation's 12 million high-need patients, and to reduce the unsustainably high cost of providing them with effective care and support (Hayes et al., 2016). Major stakeholders—health systems, payers, providers, patients and family or unpaid caregivers, researchers, and policy makers—have opportunities to address several key challenges to improving care for high-need patients. The following list highlights stakeholder opportunities discussed throughout the workshops:

- Refine the starter taxonomy based on real-world use and experience to facilitate the matching of individual need and functional capacity to specific care programs.
- Integrate and coordinate the delivery of medical, social, and behavioral services in a way that reduces the burdens on patients and caregivers.
- Develop approaches for spreading and scaling successful programs and for training a workforce capable of making these models successful.
- Promote payment reform efforts that further incentivize adoption of successful care models.
- Establish a small set of proven quality measures appropriate for assessing outcomes, including return on investment, and continuously improving programs for high-need individuals.
- Create road maps and tools to help organizations adopt models of care suitable for their particular patient populations.

In particular, action is needed by certain key stakeholders: health systems, payers, providers, patients and their care partners, researchers, and policy makers.

Health Systems

- Engage patients and caregivers in design, implementation, and evaluation of care models.
- Work with payers to better identify and target high-need patients and to test new practices and tools, such as a taxonomy.

- Work with payers to develop interoperable electronic health records that can include functional and behavioral status and social needs.
- Identify the threshold for targeting programs to those elderly who are frail, since not all elderly need the intensive, coordinated care these programs provide.
- Use established metrics and quality improvement approaches to create an environment of continuous assessment and improvement for these models.
- Partner with community organizations, including schools and even prisons, as well as with patients, caregivers, and social and behavioral health service providers outside of the health care system to create patient-centered care plans.
- Assess established culture and promote changes needed to institute new and successful care models, blending medical, social, and behavioral approaches.

Payers

- Actively support the adoption of care models or specific elements of models that research has shown to be effective at improving care for high-need patients.
- Work with policy makers to continue progress toward a value-based system, using alternative payment models, including those that work within a fee-for-service structure, to support more effective care for high-need patients.
- Expect that return on investment for most models of care for high-need patients will take time and that a return in 2 to 3 years is unlikely.
- Develop financing models to provide social and behavioral health services that will both improve care and lower the total cost of care for high-need patients, recognizing that even cost-neutral programs are worth supporting if the outcome is positive for patients.
- Support recognition, training, and education for patients and caregivers as part of care teams.
- Lead efforts to identify and share information about high-need patients and the potential for different models to positively affect the care of those populations.

Providers

- Meet patients in their communities or connect patients to community and other social resources and accept that much of the care they need will be delivered by family and unpaid caregivers or professionals outside of the health care system.
- Learn to work collaboratively in teams, and understand that many successful care models work best when everyone works at the top of their licenses.
- Engage with patients, care partners, and their caregivers in the design and delivery of care.

- Fully adopt the proven practices of health literacy to improve patients' and caregivers' ability to follow care plans developed with their input.
- Identify and work to change cultural norms that may hinder adoption of successful care models.
- Identify and engage patients' care partners as integrated team participants.

Patients and Their Care Partners

- Seek out formal training and education experiences to enhance care, understand complex medical situations, limit injuries and other errors, and identify problems earlier.
- Explore with your care team the potential benefits of home-based care, including improved financial, social, and psychosocial outcomes.
- Request formal recognition as part of the care team.
- Participate in active communication with providers regarding quality of care, needs, and services.
- Work with a care coordinator or care coordination team to amplify self-advocacy efforts and fully utilize care models.
- Contribute to the development of quality measures to assist in better decision making around care and care delivery.

Research community

- With the involvement of patients, caregivers, and other key stakeholders, continue research on approaches for identifying and segmenting high-need patients in practice settings and matching those individuals with successful care models.
- Gather better data for care models that work, including the effective integration of social and behavioral health services.
- Develop and test a parsimonious set of metrics for measuring outcomes and return on investment for models of care.
- Identify the best methods of care coordination, workforce training, and education for caregivers.
- Study effective culture change implementation techniques to promote spread and scale of successful care models.

Policy Makers

- Increase and expand efforts to engage patient and caregiver involvement in discussions around policy options for improving care and reducing costs for high-need patients.
- Harmonize and coordinate Medicare and Medicaid programs to increase access to needed services and to reduce the burden on patients and caregivers.

- Continue payment policy reforms and alignment initiatives to incentivize pay-for-performance instead of fee-for-service.
- Incentivize adoption and use of interoperable electronic health records that include functional, behavioral health, and social factors.
- Create state- and community-level data-sharing tools which include integrated claims databases that link and share information across payers, service sectors, and provider networks, such as the Predictive Risk Intelligence System (PRISM) that Washington State developed to support care management for high-risk Medicaid patients.
- Explore the expansion of programs to mitigate financial strain of caregiving, like Medicaid's Cash & Counseling.
- Modify existing regulations, such as 42 CFR Part II and data-sharing rules in the Health Insurance Portability and Accountability Act of 1996 (HIPAA), to improve data flow among and within agencies and providers.

CONCLUSION

Common to the presentations and discussions among participants was the notion that improving the care management of high-need patients will require engagement and coordination of a broad range of stakeholders at multiple levels. While each stakeholder sector individually may impact a patient's life, a community, or even a regional health delivery system, one of the most expensive and challenging populations for the current health care system will remain underserved until there is a unified effort—rather than small, incremental steps—to improve care for the nation's high-need patients and to reduce the cost of delivering that care. It is important that different stakeholder groups convene to discuss opportunities for actions and improvement, using the potential activities identified here to guide discussion and action. The taxonomy to guide care team and care model design needs further discussion, refinement, testing, and validation, as do the implementation tactics and practices to determine elements of successful care models. Policies to accelerate the spread and scale of proven models, new workforce development initiatives, suitable quality measures, and expanded data infrastructure are all at the forefront of the national health care goals of balancing quality and associated costs. Sustained attention to these areas, too, is needed.

REFERENCES

Hayes, S. L., C. A. Salzberg, D. McCarthy, D. C. Radley, M. K. Abrams, T. Shah, and G. F. Anderson. 2016. *High-need, high-cost patients: Who are they and how do they use health care?* New York: The Commonwealth Fund.

APPENDIXES

APPENDIX A

CARE MODEL CASE STUDIES

The care models described here were presented or discussed as part of one of the workshop proceedings or came up during the deliberations of the planning committee or taxonomy workgroup.

ALIGNMENT HEALTHCARE	
Target population	**Matched Segment**
The 20 percent of a health system's members who are frail, or have complex conditions or several chronic illnesses, and who account for 80 percent of health care spending. (Furman, 2015; Kao, 2016)	Not used in matching exercise

Intervention Components

- Alignment Healthcare's program is built around a new type of clinician, the extensivist, a highly trained physician who cares for five or six patients in the hospital, instead of the 30 that a hospitalist would see, and who not only treats the patient but also speaks to the patient's family and primary care physician every day. (Furman, 2015)
- Any member of a participating health care system who was frail, whether posthospitalization or for any other reason, can be seen at a care center by a team that included the extensivist, nurse practitioners, social workers, and case workers functioning at the top of their licenses. These care centers also have teams of psychiatrists, psychologists, and psychiatric nurses who integrate mental health care and extend that care into nursing homes, skilled nursing facilities, and the patient's home. (Furman, 2015)
- Care centers incorporate nutritional counseling, podiatry services, and other key components for seniors. (Furman, 2015)
- Technology and advanced analytics play a key role in supporting the care model, with the goal being to use analytical tools to develop earlier predictive patterns that inform preventive interventions before high-cost interventions are needed. (Furman, 2015)

Outcomes

Well-being	Utilization	Cost
	X	X

Notes

- The program eliminates copayments for mental health care, which decreased costs and improved outcomes. (Furman, 2015)

SOURCES: Furman, 2015; Kao, 2016

CARE MANAGEMENT PLUS

Target population	Matched Segment
Generally adults 65 years and older, who have multiple comorbidities, diabetes, frailty, dementia, depression and other mental health needs; physician referral. (Care Management Plus, 2017; McCarthy, 2015)	Advancing illness with social risk and behavioral health factors Major complex chronic with social risk and behavioral health factors

Intervention Components

- "Specially trained care managers (usually RNs or social workers) located in primary care clinics perform person-centered assessment and work with families and providers to formulate and implement a care plan." (McCarthy, 2015)
- "Care manager ensures continuity of care and regular follow-up in office, in the home, or by phone." (McCarthy, 2015)
- "Continuity of care enhanced by specialized information technology system." (McCarthy, 2015)
- "Care manager provides coaching and self-care education for patients and families." (McCarthy, 2015)

Outcomes

Well-being	Utilization	Cost
X	X	

Notes

- Utilization results only significant among patients with diabetes. (Dorr, 2008)

SOURCES: Care Management Plus, 2017; Dorr, 2008; McCarthy, 2015

CAREFIRST'S PATIENT-CENTERED MEDICAL HOME PROGRAM

Target population	Matched Segment
The 12 percent of CareFirst BlueCross Blue Shield members with advanced or critical illness and multiple chronic illnesses who account for 72 percent of the system's hospital admissions and 63 percent of the total medical costs. (O'Brien, 2015)	Not used in matching exercise

Intervention Components

- An incentive-based program for primary care physicians that rewards them for managing patients and influencing the whole medical dollar, including the 94 percent of the plan's expenditures on specialists, inpatient care, outpatient care, and prescription drugs. (O'Brien, 2015).
- Credible data and analytic support provided through a dedicated informational portal and high-touch, superior technical support promote collaboration among physicians, local nurses, and other health professionals to manage members' care. These analytics provide primary care physicians with information to help them spot potential hot-spot individuals within their panels and then provide links to additional services for those patients. (O'Brien, 2015)
- Primary care physicians collaborate with the specialists and other medical professionals of their choice, informed by analytics that provide the primary care physician with cost and quality metrics for those other professionals, to more closely coordinate and track care for the sickest patients or those at highest risk for future illness. (CareFirst, 2017; O'Brien, 2015)
- Care plans are supported by local community-based care teams headed by a registered nurse. (O'Brien, 2015)

Outcomes

Well-being	Utilization	Cost
	X	X

Notes

- "Participating providers receive a 12 percentage point increase in their fee schedule, agreeing to higher compensation in exchange for increased effort and time devoted to improved coordination of care. They also receive additional new fees for developing care plans for select patients with certain chronic or multiple conditions and additional fees for keeping the care plans up to date." (CareFirst, 2017)
- Incentives (paid as fee increases) can be earned tied to better outcomes for the patients under the care of each panel of primary care physicians in the program. (O'Brien, 2015)
- "Of the 291 PCMH panels participating in 2013, 69 percent earned an outcome incentive award averaging 36 percent, and of the panels participating in 2011-2013, 37 percent earned the award in all three years." (O'Brien, 2015)

SOURCES: CareFirst, 2014; CareFirst, 2017; O'Brien, 2015

CAREOREGON'S HEALTH RESILIENCE PROGRAM

Target population	Matched Segment
The 10 percent of CareOregon's Medicaid members who incur 50 percent of the plan's medical expenses. Members enrolled in the Health Resilience program were more likely to experience high disease burden and psychosocial challenges. The majority of those who enrolled have experienced significant trauma in their lives. (Ramsay, 2015)	Not used in matching exercise

Intervention Components

- Health Resilience Specialists are paired with primary health homes and specialty practices to provide individualized high touch and trauma-informed support to patients with exceptional utilization with the primary emphasis of mitigating social determinants of health. (CareOregon, 2014)
- Staff are supported by clinically licensed supervisors who provide daily and weekly guidance, mentoring, and clinical supervision. (CareOregon, 2014)
- The Health Resilience Specialists, who have mental health and addictions training, an in-depth understanding of trauma dynamics, and extensive outreach experience with the Medicaid population, are paid and administered by CareOregon but operate as part of a primary care team. (CareOregon, 2014)
- The program also subcontracts with regional and culturally specific peer mentors to build longer-term sustainability into the program. (CareOregon, 2014)

Outcomes

Well-being	Utilization	Cost
X	X	X

Notes

- CareOregon's six programmatic principles of trauma-informed care include: reducing barriers; providing client-centered care; increasing transparency; taking time and building trust; avoiding judgment and labels; and providing care in a community-based setting. (CareOregon, 2014)
- Measures of access and quality increased significantly, as did member access to help with food, housing, and transportation. (Ramsay, 2015)
- Clinical staff rated the program highly on measures of care coordination, effectiveness at caring for high-need Medicaid patients, and care team satisfaction. (Ramsay, 2015)

SOURCES: CareOregon, 2014; Ramsay, 2015

CHENMED

Target population	Matched Segment
Program serves 60,000 moderate- to low-income Medicare members in more than 40 locations in six states. More than 30 percent of the members are dual-eligibles. (Klein, 2016)	Not used in matching exercise

Intervention Components

- For-profit model offers a one-stop-shop approach for delivering multispecialty services in the community utilizing a smaller physician panel size of 350 to 450 patients, allowing for intensive health coaching and preventive care. (Coye, 2016)
- Collaborative peer review, powered by customized information technology, is a central feature of this system. (Tanio, 2013)
- ChenMed practices offer a broad set of additional services on site, including dental care, digital x-ray, ultrasound, and acupuncture, as well as five to 15 high-volume specialists. (Tanio, 2013)
- Because access to care is a major issue with seniors, the practice provides door-to-door van transportation at no charge. (Tanio, 2013)
- To boost medication adherence, each practice has on-site physician pharmacy dispensing, which encourages patients to discuss side effects and other issues that interfere with medication adherence. (Tanio, 2013)

Outcomes

Well-being	Utilization	Cost
X	X	

Notes

- For-profit Medicare Advantage model of managed care that accepts capitated payments and is at full risk for patients' total health care costs. (Tanio, 2013)
- ChenMed's customized electronic health record and decision support software requires less documentation than most off-the-shelf electronic health records, allowing physicians to make concise notes and enhance productivity. (Hostetter, 2016)
- Ninety percent of ChenMed's diabetic patients reported they had an improved understanding of their medications and 80 percent reported improved communication with their physician. New Promoter Scores, a measure of how likely a member would be to refer a practice to a friend or colleague, was 90 percent compared to a national average for health insurance companies of 12 percent. (Klein, 2016)

SOURCES: Coye, 2016; Hostetter, 2016; Klein, 2016; Tanio, 2013

CIGNA COLLABORATIVE CARE MODEL

Target population	Matched Segment
High-risk, high-cost patients identified based on having multiple comorbidities and through Cigna's proprietary predictive modeling. (Davda, 2015)	Not used in matching exercise

Intervention Components

- Cigna Collaborative Care, modeled after accountable care organizations, embeds a care coordinator, typically a registered nurse, in a physician group with a substantial primary care component. (Davda, 2015)
- Care coordinators work closely with Cigna's case managers to ensure that high-need individuals receive the screenings, follow-up care, educational materials, and access to Cigna's clinical support programs, such as those for chronic condition management and lifestyle management, to help them manage their health better. (Davda, 2015)
- Cigna uses proprietary predictive modeling and analytics to provide the embedded care coordinator with a daily list of which members of a practice are in the hospital and will require a transition of care call at the time of discharge, and a monthly list of high-risk patients with multiple gaps in care, such as medication compliance issues and multiple emergency department visits. (Davda, 2015)

Outcomes

Well-being	Utilization	Cost
X		X

Notes

- Cigna offers ongoing training and best practice sharing for the care coordinators and connects them with other Cigna resources such as case managers, wellness coaches, and pharmacists to expand the clinical resources available to their patients. (Davda, 2015)
- The medical group is rewarded through a pay for value structure if it meets targets for improving quality and lowering medical costs. (Cigna, 2014)
- Large physician groups active two or more years have shown 3 percent better total medical cost and a 2 percent increase in quality performance. The return on investment for these "mature" practices is 2:1. (Davda, 2015) "Three of the highest-performing arrangements have each removed more than $3 million from the health care system." (Cigna, 2017)

SOURCES: Cigna, 2014, 2017; Davda, 2015

COMMONWEALTH CARE ALLIANCE

Target population	Matched Segment
Dual-eligible individuals 65+ in Senior Care Options program or dual-eligible individuals age 64 and younger in Disability Care Program, part of the Massachusetts One Care financial alignment demonstration. (McCarthy, 2015)	Non-elderly disabled

Intervention Components

- "Provides enhanced primary care and care coordination through multidisciplinary clinical teams led by nurse practitioners." (McCarthy, 2015)
- "After a comprehensive assessment, individualized care plans are developed to promote independence and functioning." (McCarthy, 2015)
- "Integration of behavioral health care for those who need it." (McCarthy, 2015)
- "Care team available 24/7 in the home, in the hospital, or at the doctor's office." (McCarthy, 2015)
- "Patients' records available 24/7 in proprietary electronic health record system." (McCarthy, 2015)

Outcomes

Well-being	Utilization	Cost
	X	

SOURCE: McCarthy, 2015

COMPLEX CARE PROGRAM AT CHILDREN'S NATIONAL HEALTH SYSTEM

Target population	Matched Segment
Medically complex children with 2 or more chronic conditions. (Children's National, 2017)	Children with complex needs

Intervention Components

- "Provides ongoing care coordination between visits including communication with family, primary care providers, and specialists." (Children's National, 2017)
- "Helps families negotiate the health care system and provide a link to community resources." (Children's National, 2017)
- "Creates written care plans with the family to share with the primary care provider." (Children's National, 2017)
- "Provides comprehensive care coordination through a team approach that includes nurse case management, parent navigators, and social work." (Children's National, 2017)

Outcomes

Well-being	Utilization	Cost
	X	

Notes

- Outcomes unavailable.

SOURCE: Children's National, 2017

COMPREHENSIVE CARE PHYSICIAN (CCP) MODEL (UNIVERSITY OF CHICAGO)

Target population	Matched Segment
Patients with multiple chronic illnesses who had at least one hospitalization in the previous year. (The University of Chicago, 2017)	Not used in matching exercise

Intervention Components

- Five dedicated CCPs lead teams of advanced practice registered nurses, social workers, care coordinators, and other specialists best suited to address the needs of patients who are expected to average 10 hospital days per year. (Meltzer, 2014)
- Each CCP has a panel of approximately 200 patients and serves as both primary care physician and supervisor for each panel member's care while hospitalized. (Meltzer, 2014)
- The five CCPs visit hospitalized patients each morning while the other members of the care team provide care at the physicians' clinics. One CCP is assigned afternoon rounds and weekend duties. "Providing these physicians with a high volume of inpatients and locating their clinics in or near the hospital allows them to offer many of the same benefits that hospitalists provide while offering the additional benefit of continuity across settings and over time." (Meltzer, 2014)
- "The CCP or other care team member makes postdischarge calls to the patient and both telephone and text messages are used to keep the care team and patient connected." (Meltzer, 2014)

Outcomes

Well-being	Utilization	Cost
(study not yet completed)	(study not yet completed)	(study not yet completed)

Notes

- Shared saving based on risk-adjusted estimates of predicted costs.

SOURCES: Meltzer, 2014; The University of Chicago, 2017

COMPREHENSIVE PATIENT-CENTERED MEDICAL HOME INITIATIVE

Target population	Matched Segment
This model is being tested in seven states encompassing 31 payers, nearly 500 practices, and approximately 300,000 Medicare beneficiaries (Taylor, 2015)	Not used in matching exercise

Intervention Components

- A medical home model in which practices first risk-stratify their patients within physician panels. (Taylor, 2015)
- Practices use care management methods, including care planning, registries, proactive care monitoring, and enhanced access that include home-based and team-based care. (Taylor, 2015)
- While the program is not prescriptive per se, care management activities must include at least one of the following: behavioral health integration, self-management or support for beneficiaries, or medication management. (Taylor, 2015)

Outcomes

Well-being	Utilization	Cost
(study not yet completed)	(study not yet completed)	(study not yet completed)

Notes

- Practices receive monthly case management payments of $20 per month per patient over the first two years of the program and $15 per month for years three and four. They also have an opportunity to earn shared savings on reductions in total Part A and B Medicare expenditures. (Taylor, 2015)

SOURCE: Taylor, 2015

GEISINGER'S PROVENHEALTH NAVIGATOR PATIENT-CENTERED MEDICAL HOME

Target population	Matched Segment
Elderly Medicare patients.	Not used in matching exercise

Intervention Components

- "Patient-centered primary care." (Maeng, 2012)
- "Integrated population management." (Maeng, 2012)
- "A medical 'neighborhood' that aligns key community partners, such as home health agencies, skilled nursing facilities, outpatient and ancillary services, hospital facilities, and community pharmacies. Comprehensive quality improvement. Value-based reimbursement redesign that includes a quality, outcome-based pay-for-performance program." (Maeng, 2012)

Outcomes

Well-being	Utilization	Cost
	X	X

Notes

- "The program aims to move resources further upstream in the primary care settings to reduce downstream costs from the highest acuity settings resulting from uncontrolled exacerbations of chronic disease, hospital readmissions, and unnecessary duplication of services." (Maeng, 2012)

SOURCES: Maeng, 2012; xG Health Solutions, 2017

GRACE

Target population	Matched Segment
Low-income seniors with medical complexity.	Major complex chronic with social risk and behavioral health factors

Intervention Components

- "Support team consisting of advanced practice nurse and social worker work with elderly in the home and community." (McCarthy, 2015)
- "In-home assessment and specific care protocols inform individualized care plan." (McCarthy, 2015)
- "Support team works closely with larger interdisciplinary care team." (McCarthy, 2015)
- "Patient education and self-management plans include tools for low-literacy seniors." (McCarthy, 2015)

Outcomes

Well-being	Utilization	Cost
	X	X

Notes

- "Program was cost-neutral in the first two years among high-risk patients, and cost-saving in the third year (postintervention)." (McCarthy, 2015)

SOURCES: Counsell, 2009; Indiana University, 2017; McCarthy, 2015

GUIDED CARE

Target population	Matched Segment
"Older adults with multiple chronic conditions." (McCarthy, 2015)	Major complex chronic

Intervention Components

- "Predictive modeling and 12 months of claims data used to identify the 20 to 25 percent of patients most at risk of needing complex care in the near future." (McCarthy, 2015)
- "RNs trained in complex care management perform in-home assessments and develop care plans to coordinate care with multidisciplinary providers." (McCarthy, 2015)
- "Patient education and self-management strategies focus on addressing issues before hospitalization becomes necessary." (McCarthy, 2015)

Outcomes

Well-being	Utilization	Cost
X	X	

SOURCE: McCarthy, 2015

HEALTH CARE HOME (HCH) PROGRAM (OF MINNESOTA)

Target population	Matched Segment
Medicare and Medicaid recipients who have two or more chronic illnesses. (Minnesota Department of Health, 2017)	Not used in matching exercise

Intervention Components

- Three strategic components of the HCH program are its certification process, a quality improvement process, and a learning collaborative. (LaPlante, 2015)
- At the time of certification, each clinic is evaluated by a team that includes a regional nurse planner, a consumer or patient under contract with her agency, and a community nurse or other community health professional. The purpose of the site visit is to ensure that clinics have enacted processes to redesign primary care. (LaPlante, 2015)

Outcomes

Well-being	Utilization	Cost
X	X	X

Notes

- Racial disparities were significantly smaller for Medicaid, Medicare, and dual-eligible beneficiaries served by HCH versus non-HCH clinics for most measures. (Wholey et al., 2015)
- HCH organizations report being better able to capture care coordination payments from Medicaid than from Medicare, private managed care, or commercial insurers. (Wholey et al., 2015)
- Financial incentives were not a primary driver of a clinic or organization participating in the HCH initiative. (Wholey et al., 2015)
- Minnesota did develop a care coordination tier assignment tool to support care coordination billing. (Wholey et al., 2015)

SOURCES: LaPlante, 2015; Minnesota Department of Health, 2017; Wholey et al., 2015

HEALTH QUALITY PARTNERS

Target population	Matched Segment
"Medicare beneficiaries with chronic conditions." (McCarthy, 2015)	Major complex chronic Multiple chronic

Intervention Components

- "Registered nurse care coordinators focus on changing patient behavior." (McCarthy, 2015)
- "Focus on frequent in-person contact with both patients and physicians." (McCarthy, 2015)
- "Evidence-based patient education including condition-specific self-monitoring training." (McCarthy, 2015)

Outcomes

Well-being	Utilization	Cost
	X	X

Notes

- Reduced average monthly Medicare Part A and B expenditures by 21 percent. (Brown, 2017)

SOURCES: Brown et al., 2017; McCarthy et al., 2015

HEALTH SERVICES FOR CHILDREN WITH SPECIAL NEEDS

Target population	Matched Segment
High-need, high-cost pediatric patients.	Under 65 disabled
	Children with complex needs with social risk and behavioral health factors

Intervention Components

- Provides a care manager to coordinate appointments, to assist with arranging transportation, and to connect patients with community resources and organizations. (HSCSN, 2016)
- Care Manager works with providers and patients to create a care coordination plan that's updated at least twice per year. (HSCSN, 2016)

Outcomes

Well-being	Utilization	Cost

Notes

- Outcomes unavailable.

SOURCE: Health Services for Children with Special Needs, Inc., 2016

HOMELESS PATIENT ALIGNED CARE TEAM (H-PACT)

Target population	Matched Segment
Homeless veterans coming to the emergency department with complex medical and social problems.	Non-elderly disabled with social risk and behavioral health factors

Intervention Components

- "Located on the campuses of Veterans Affairs medical centers, community-based outpatient clinics, and Community Resource and Referral Centers, H-PACT clinics colocate medical staff, social workers, mental health and substance use counselors, nurses, and homeless program staff. These professionals form a team that provides Veterans with comprehensive, individualized care, including services that lead to permanent housing." (US VA, 2017)

Outcomes

Well-being	Utilization	Cost
	X	

Notes

- Launched in 2012, so limited data are available but evidence exists to support decreased utilization.

SOURCE: US Department of Veterans Affairs, 2017

HOSPITAL AT HOME

Target population	Matched Segment
Older patients who are acutely ill and require hospital-level care. (Johns Hopkins, 2013)	Advancing illness

Intervention Components

- "Potentially eligible patients are identified in the hospital emergency department or ambulatory care site. If they meet the validated criteria and consent to participate, they are evaluated by a physician and transported home, usually via ambulance." (McCarthy, 2015)
- "One-on-one nursing for initial stage and at least daily nurse and physician visits thereafter." (McCarthy, 2015)
- "Both nurses and physicians on call around-the-clock for urgent or emergent visits." (McCarthy, 2015)
- "Some diagnostic services and treatments performed in home setting." (McCarthy, 2015)
- "Same criteria and guidelines are used to judge patient readiness for transition to skilled nursing facility, or discharge from Hospital at Home as from hospital." (McCarthy, 2015)

Outcomes

Well-being	Utilization	Cost
X	X	X

Notes

- Utilization outcomes were based on a prospective quasi-experiment. (McCarthy, 2015)
- Per patient average costs were 19 percent lower than similar inpatient per-patient average costs but excluded physician costs. (McCarthy, 2015)
  - Cost savings were due to lower average length of stay and few diagnostic and lab tests. (McCarthy, 2015)
  - Cost savings did not factor in physician costs. (McCarthy, 2015)

SOURCES: Johns Hopkins School of Medicine, 2013; McCarthy, 2015

IMPACT	
Target population	**Matched Segment**
"Older adults suffering from depression." (McCarthy, 2015)	Frail elderly with social risk and behavioral health factors
	Multiple chronic with social risk and behavioral health factors

Intervention Components

- "Collaborative care: Primary care physician works with depression care manager (e.g., nurse, social worker, or psychologist supported by medical assistant or other paraprofessional) to develop and implement treatment plan including antidepressant medication and/or short-term counseling. Team includes consulting psychiatrist." (McCarthy, 2015)
- "Care manager also educates patient about depression and coaches in self-care." (McCarthy, 2015)
- "Providers utilize ongoing measurement and tracking of outcomes with validated depression screening tool, such as Patient Health Questionnaire-9, and adapt care to changing symptoms." (McCarthy, 2015)
- "Once a patient improves, case manager and patient jointly develop a plan to prevent relapse." (McCarthy, 2015)

Outcomes

Well-being	Utilization	Cost
X		X

Notes

- "Total health care costs for IMPACT patients were $3,300 lower per patient on average than those of patients receiving usual primary care, net of program cost." (McCarthy, 2015)

SOURCE: McCarthy, 2015

INDEPENDENCE AT HOME DEMONSTRATION

Target population	Matched Segment
"Medicare beneficiaries with multiple chronic conditions." (CMS, 2016)	Not used in matching exercise

Intervention Components

- Model that uses home-based primary care teams directed by physicians and nurse practitioners designed to improve health outcomes and reduce expenditures for Medicare beneficiaries with multiple chronic conditions. (CMS, 2016)
- "Selected participants, including primary care practices, will provide home-based primary care to targeted chronically ill beneficiaries for a five-year period. Participating practices will make in-home visits tailored to an individual patient's needs and preferences." (CMS, 2016)
- "This focus on timely and appropriate care is designed to improve overall quality of care and quality of life for patients served, while lowering health care costs by forestalling the need for care in institutional settings." (CMS, 2016)

Outcomes

Well-being	Utilization	Cost
(study not yet completed)	(study not yet completed)	(study not yet completed)

Notes

- "The Independence at Home Demonstration will award incentive payments to health care providers who succeed in reducing Medicare expenditures and meet designated quality measures." (CMS, 2016)

SOURCE: CMS, 2016

MIND AT HOME (JOHNS HOPKINS UNIVERSITY)

Target population	Matched Segment
Elderly with memory disorders.	Frail elderly with social risk and behavioral health factors

Intervention Components

- "Links people with dementia and their caregivers to community-based agencies, medical and mental health care providers, and community resources." (JHU, 2014)
- "Delivered by an interdisciplinary team comprised of trained nonclinical community workers and mental health clinicians, who conduct comprehensive in-home dementia-related needs assessments and provide individualized care planning and implementation." (JHU, 2014)
- "The team uses six basic care strategies: resource referrals, attention to environmental safety, dementia care education, behavior management skills training, informal counseling, problem-solving, as well as ongoing monitoring, assessment, and planning for emergent needs." (JHU, 2014)
- "Each component of the intervention is based on best practice recommendations and evidence from prior research, and is combined for maximum impact." (JHU, 2014)
- Provides individualized needs assessments, care planning, and monitoring for both patient and caregiver. (JHU, 2014)
- Provides education, skills training, and self-management support for patients and families. (JHU, 2014)
- Model is home-based, linking medical and community-based care services delivered by nonclinical staff with support from mental health practitioners. (JHU, 2014)

Outcomes

Well-being	Utilization	Cost
X	X	

Notes

- "Primary outcomes were time to transfer from home and percent of unmet needs" (both significant effects). (Samus, 2014)

SOURCES: Johns Hopkins University, 2014; Samus et al., 2014

MISSIONPOINT HEALTH PARTNERS

Target population	Matched Segment
Serving 250,000 members in seven states. (MissionPoint, 2017b)	Not used in matching exercise

Intervention Components

- MissionPoint Health Partners is a population health management organization that uses a global financing model to provide a clear picture of the resources needed for this patient population and enable personalized responses to patient needs and iterative learning and resource shifting. This iterative approach, supported by a clear leadership commitment, is a major feature of the program's profit-and-loss strategy. (Coye, 2016)
- "Central to the MissionPoint model is [its] wraparound clinical management framework, a skilled team of Health Partners who help members solve problems and connect their medical care with everyday life. . . . [The Health Partners, who] are experienced health care professionals and social workers, are provided at no cost to members and help support members when they most need it, such as after an emergency department visit, hospital stay, or diagnosis of a chronic disease." (MissionPoint 2017a)
- Advanced analytics notify Health Partners "of members' health events within the network and provide them with relevant medical data so that the Health Partners can work hand-in-hand with members and caregivers to . . . navigate the health care system, problem-solve complex issues, and remove barriers to self-care." (MissionPoint, 22017a)

Outcomes

Well-being	Utilization	Cost
X	X	X

Notes

- Medicare shared savings plan and additional incentives for expanding member access with extended hours or email support.
- A key component of MissionPoint's success in improving the health status of its members while lowering overall health care costs is its ability to create clinically integrated networks in the communities it serves.

SOURCES: Coye, 2016; MissionPoint, 2017a, 2017b

NAYLOR TRANSITIONAL CARE MODEL (UNIVERSITY OF PENNSYLVANIA)

Target population	Matched Segment
"Hospitalized, high-risk older adults with chronic conditions." (McCarthy, 2015)	Frail elderly

Intervention Components

- "Multidisciplinary provider team led by advanced practice nurses engages in comprehensive discharge planning." (McCarthy, 2015)
- "Three-month postdischarge follow-up includes frequent home visits and telephone availability." (McCarthy, 2015)
- "Involve patients and family members in identifying goals and building self-management skills." (McCarthy, 2015)

Outcomes

Well-being	Utilization	Cost
X	X	X

Notes

- "38 percent reduction in total costs." (McCarthy, 2015)
- "36 percent fewer readmissions." (McCarthy, 2015)
- "Short-term improvements in overall quality of life and patient satisfaction." (McCarthy, 2015)

SOURCE: McCarthy, 2015

PACIFIC BUSINESS GROUP ON HEALTH'S INTENSIVE OUTPATIENT CARE PROGRAM

Target population	Matched Segment
Individuals having two or more chronic conditions and behavioral and psychosocial needs that are not being met by the current health care system. (Mangiante, 2015)	Not used in matching exercise

Intervention Components

- This high-touch, care-coordinated, patient-involved program uses team-based care with both licensed and unlicensed care coordinators to ensure seamless transitions and links to needed services. (Mangiante, 2015)
- Individuals in 23 participating delivery systems and 500 practices are identified using a predictive risk model plus cognitive assessment, as well as through physician referrals. (Mangiante, 2015)
- Interdisciplinary care teams developed longitudinal relationships with clients and provide warm handoffs to support services outside of the health care system. (Stremikis, 2016)
- Care coordinators complete a face-to-face "supervisit" within 1 month of a member's enrollment in the program. Because medically complex patients can be anxious and depressed, coordinators are particularly attentive to their patients' social and psychological needs, providing or supplying referrals for behavioral, psychosocial, and community services. (Mangiante, 2015)
- Coordinators proactively provide patients with tools for effective self-management, helping them to develop action plans and to recognize signs of exacerbations of illness, and engage in two-way communication with members at least once per month, with intensity decreasing as patients become stable. (Mangiante, 2015)

Outcomes

Well-being	Utilization	Cost
X	X	X

Notes

- Being tested in Pioneer and Medicare Shared Savings Program accountable care organizations as well as Medicare Advantage plans. (Mangiante, 2015)
- After CMS grant ended, "90 percent of participating delivery systems continued the core elements of the program for Medicare patients and 15 of the 23 expanded programs into their commercial populations." (Stremikis, 2016)
- 3.3 percent improvement in physical health functioning, 4.2 percent improvement in mental health functioning, and 31 percent improvement on depression score. Patient Activation Measure (PAM) scores increased in 37 percent of participants, and 30 percent increase in graduation from program among participants with increased PAM scores. (Mangiante, 2015)

SOURCES: Mangiante, 2015; Stremikis et al., 2016

PARTNERS HEALTHCARE INTEGRATED CARE MANAGEMENT PROGRAM

Target population	Matched Segment
"Medicare beneficiaries who are high cost and/or have complex conditions" (McCarthy, 2015) (also expanded to children) (Partners Healthcare, 2016).	Major complex chronic Children w/ complex needs

Intervention Components

- "Care managers are integrated into primary care practices." (McCarthy, 2015)
- "Care managers provide patient education and address both medical and psychosocial needs." (McCarthy, 2015)
- "Focus on preventing exacerbations that lead to emergency department visits and inpatient admissions." (McCarthy, 2015)
- "Case managers also support end-of-life decision making." (McCarthy, 2015)

Outcomes

Well-being	Utilization	Cost
	X	X

Notes

- "7 percent annual savings after accounting for intervention costs." (McCarthy, 2015)
- "20 percent reduction in hospital admissions." (McCarthy, 2015)
- "13 percent reduction in emergency department visits." (McCarthy, 2015)

SOURCES: McCarthy, 2015; Partners Healthcare, 2016

PROGRAM OF ALL-INCLUSIVE CARE FOR THE ELDERLY (PACE) PROGRAM

Target population	Matched Segment
Frail elderly, dual-eligible individuals, functional and/or cognitive impairments.	Frail elderly

Intervention Components

- "Each PACE site provides comprehensive preventive, primary, acute, and long-term care and social services, including adult day care, meals, and transportation." (McCarthy, 2015)
- "Interdisciplinary team meets regularly to design individualized care plans." (McCarthy, 2015)
- "Goal is to allow patients to live independently in the community." (McCarthy, 2015)
- "Patients receive all covered Medicare and Medicaid services through the local PACE organization in their home and community and at a local PACE center, thereby enhancing care coordination." (McCarthy, 2015)
- "Clinical staff are employed or contracted by the local PACE organization, which is paid on a per-capita basis and not based on volume of services provided." (McCarthy, 2015)

Outcomes

Well-being	Utilization	Cost
X	X	X

Notes

- "Fewer hospitalizations but more nursing home admissions." (McCarthy, 2015)
- "Better quality for certain aspects of care such as pain management, and lower mortality, than comparison groups." (McCarthy, 2015)
- "Cost-neutral to Medicare; may have increased costs for Medicaid—more research is needed." (McCarthy, 2015)

SOURCE: McCarthy, 2015

STANFORD COORDINATED CARE

Target population	Matched Segment
Top 20 percent of Stanford's employees and dependents with complex medical needs, who have two or more emergency room visits related to underlying medical conditions over the past year, and poor adherence to treatment recommendations. (Glaseroff, 2015)	Not used in matching exercise

Intervention Components

- "Upon joining the program, SCC patients are assigned to care teams and complete a comprehensive intake process that focuses on the question, 'Where do you want to be in a year?'" (CHCS, 2015)
- "Care teams include a physician, registered nurse or other provider, and a care coordinator/ medical assistant trained to act as a coach and navigator, as well as a social worker who specializes in trauma informed care, a physical therapist who specializes in chronic pain, and a clinical pharmacist." (CHCS, 2015)
- Care coordinators/medical assistants perform routine preventive services and chronic disease monitoring between clinic visits for a panel of 100 patients with the goal of encouraging patients to follow through on their action plans. (AHRQ, 2016)
- The care team focuses on improving each patient's self-management by supporting the patient's self-identified goals and assisting the patient to develop achievable action plans scaled according to the patient's PAM score. (CHCS, 2015)

Outcomes

Well-being	Utilization	Cost
X	X	X

Notes

- Surveys show staff and patient satisfaction ratings in the 99th percentile. Care coordinators working under protocol and informed by a care gap dashboard are effective at ensuring routine monitoring for prevention and chronic disease management. (AHRQ, 2016)
- PAM scores increased in 34 percent of participants, with a net improvement of 23 percent. Mental composite score increased in 50 percent of participants and physical composite score increased in 64 percent of participants. (Glaseroff, 2015)
- Care coordinators working under protocol and informed by a care gap dashboard are effective at ensuring routine monitoring for prevention and chronic disease management. (Glaseroff, 2015)

SOURCES: AHRQ, 2016; Center for Health Care Strategies, 2015; Glaseroff, 2015

REFERENCES

Agency for Healthcare Research and Quality. 2016. *Case Example #1: Stanford Coordinated Care.* http://www.ahrq.gov/professionals/systems/primary-care/workforce-financing/case-example1.html (accessed August 22, 2017).

Brown, R., D. Peikes, G. Peterson, J. Schore, and C. M. Razafindrakoto. 2012. Six features of medicare coordinated care demonstration programs that cut hospital admissions of high-risk patients. *Health Affairs 31(6):* 1156–1166.

CareFirst. 2014. *2013 PCMH Program Performance Report.* https://member.carefirst.com/carefirst-resources/pdf/pcmh-program-performance-report-2013.pdf (accessed September 8, 2017).

CareFirst. 2017. *CareFirst BlueCross BlueShield's Patient-Centered Medical Home Program: An Overview.* https://member.carefirst.com/carefirst-resources/pdf/pcmh-program-overview.pdf (accessed August 22, 2017).

Care Management Plus. 2017. *Oregon Health & Science University.* https://www.ohsu.edu/xd/education/schools/school-of-medicine/departments/clinical-departments/dmice/research/care-management-plus/ (accessed August 18, 2017).

CareOregon. 2014. *Health Resilience Program: Program Description.*

Center for Health Care Strategies, Inc. 2015. *Profiles in Innovation: Stanford Coordinated Care, Palo Alto, California.*

Centers for Medicare and Medicaid Services. 2016. *Independence at Home Demonstration Fact Sheet: July 2016.* https://innovation.cms.gov/Files/factsheet/iah-fs.pdf (accessed August 22, 2017).

Children's National. 2017. *Complex Care Program.* https://childrensnational.org/departments/complex-care-program (accessed August 17, 2017).

Cigna. 2014. Cigna Achieves Goal of 100 Collaborative Care Arrangements Reaching One Million Customers.

Cigna. 2017. *A Network That Fits Your Needs.* https://www.cigna.com/business-segments/medium-employers/network-that-fits-your-needs (accessed August 22, 2017).

Commonwealth Care Alliance. 2017. *Senior Care Options.* http://www.commonwealthcarealliance.org/become-a-member/senior-care-options (accessed August 17, 2017).

Counsell, S. R., C. M. Callahan, W. Tu, T. E. Stump, and G. W. Arling. 2009. Cost Analysis of the Geriatric Resources for Assessment and Care of Elders Care Management Intervention. *Journal of the American Geriatrics Society 57(8):* 1420–1426.

Coye, M. J. 2016. *Identifying the Design Elements of Successful Models.* Presentation at the January 19th NAM Models of Care for High-Need Patients meeting, Washington, DC.

Davda, R. 2015. Cigna Collaborative Care: Embedded Care Coordinator. Presentation at the July 7th NAM Models of Care for High-Need Patients meeting, Washington, DC.

Dorr, D., A. B. Wilcox, C. P. Brunker, R. E. Burdon, and S. M. Donnelly. 2008. The Effect of Technology-Supported, Multidisease Care Management on the Mortality and Hospitalization of Seniors. *Journal of the American Geriatrics Society* 56:2195–2202.

Furman, D. 2015. *Alignment Healthcare: Changing Healthcare One Patient at a Time.* Presentation at the July 7th NAM Models of Care for High-Need Patients meeting, Washington, DC.

Glaseroff, A. 2015. *Models of Care for High Risk, High Cost Patients.* Presentation at the July 7th NAM Models of Care for High-Need Patients meeting. Washington, DC.

Health Services for Children with Special Needs, Inc. 2016. *Health Services for Children with Special Needs Health Plan.* http://www.hschealth.org/health-plan (accessed August 17, 2017).

Hostetter, M. and S. Klein. 2016. Wiring New Models of Primary Care: The Role of Health Information Technology. The Commonwealth Fund.

Indiana University. 2017. *GRACE Team Care.* http://graceteamcare.indiana. edu/home.html (accessed August 17, 2017).

Johns Hopkins School of Medicine and Johns Hopkins Bloomberg School of Public Health. 2013. *Hospital at Home.* http://www.hospitalathome.org/ (accessed August 17, 2017).

Johns Hopkins University. 2014. *MIND at Home: About Us.* http://www.min-dathome.org/about-us.html (accessed August 22, 2017).

Kao, J. 2016. *2016 #OWHIC Summit Preview: Alignment Healthcare's John Kao on Population Health.* Interview with Oliver Wyman Health.

Klein, S. and M. Hostetter. 2016. In Focus: Redesigning Primary Care for Those Who Need It Most. The Commonwealth Fund.

LaPlante, B. 2015. *Minnesota's Health Care Home (HCH).* Presentation at the July 7th NAM Models of Care for High-Need Patients meeting, Washington, DC.

Maeng, D. D., J. Graham, T. R. Graf, J. N. Liberman, N. B. Dermes, J. Tomcavage, D. E. Davis, F. J. Bloom Jr, and G. D. Steele Jr. 2012. Reducing Long-Term Cost by Transforming Primary Care: Evidence From Geisinger's Medical Home Model. *American Journal of Managed Care* online.

Mangiante, L. 2015. *Intensive Outpatient Care Program.* Presentation at the July 7th NAM Models of Care for High-Need Patients meeting, Washington, DC.

McCarthy, D., J. Ryan, and S. Klein. 2015. Models of care for high-need, high-cost patients: An evidence synthesis. *Issue Brief (Commonwealth Fund)* 31:1–19.

Meltzer, D. O. and G. W. Ruhnke. 2014. Redesigning Care For Patients At Increased Hospitalization Risk: The Comprehensive Care Physician Model. *Health Affairs 33(5):* 770–777.

Minnesota Department of Health. 2017. *Health Care Homes.* http://www.health.state.mn.us/healthreform/homes/ (accessed August 17, 2017).

MissionPoint Health Partners. 2017a. *Our Health Partner Model.* http://missionpointhealth.org/members/our-health-partner-model/ (accessed October 23, 2017).

MissionPoint Health Partners. 2017b. *Our Story.* http://missionpointhealth.org/about-us/our-story/ (accessed August 22, 2017).

O'Brien, J. 2015. *CareFirst Patient Centered Medical Home Program.* Presentation at the July 7th NAM Models of Care for High-Need Patients meeting, Washington, DC.

Pacific Business Group on Health. 2015. *Intensive Outpatient Care Program.*

Partners HealthCare. 2016. *iCMP: Focusing on the Chronically Ill to Improve Care, Reduce Costs.* http://connectwithpartners.org/2016/06/29/icmp-focusing-on-the-chronically-ill-to-improve-care-reduce-costs.

Ramsay, R. 2015. *Health Resilience Program: Payer-Provider-Community Partnership to Improve Outcomes for High Risk/High Cost Medicaid Population in Oregon.* Presentation at the July 7th NAM Models of Care for High-Need Patients meeting, Washington, DC.

Samus, Q. M., D. Johnston, B. S. Black, E. Hess, C. Lyman, A. Vavilikolanu, J. Pollutra, J-M Leoutsakos, L. N. Gitlin, P. V. Rabins, and C. G. Lyketsos. 2014. A multidimensional home-based care coordination intervention for elders with memory disorders: the Maximizing Independence at Home (MIND) Pilot Randomized Trial. *American Journal of Geriatric Psychiatry* 22(4): 398–414.

Schilling, B. 2011. Boeing's Nurse Case Managers Cut Per Capita Costs by 20 Percent. *The Commonwealth Fund.*

Stremikis, K., E. Hoo, and D. Stewart. 2016. Using The Intensive Outpatient Care Program To Lower Costs And Improve Care For High-Cost Patients. *Health Affairs Blog.*

Tanio, C. and C. Chen. 2013. Innovations at Miami Practice Show Promise for Treating High-Risk Medicare Patients. *Health Affairs* 32(6): 1078–1082.

Taylor, E. F et al. 2015. Evaluation of the Comprehensive Primary Care Initiative: First Annual Report. Mathematica Policy Research.

The University of Chicago. 2017. *Comprehensive Care Program*. https://ccpstudy. uchicago.edu/ (accessed August 17, 2017).

US Department of Veterans Affairs. 2017. *Homeless Patient Aligned Care Teams*. https://www.va.gov/homeless/h_pact.asp (accessed August 17, 2017).

Wholey, D. R., M. Finch, N. D. Shippee, K. M. White, J. Christianson, R. Kreiger, B. Wagner, and L. Grude. 2015. Evaluation of the State of Minnesota's Health Care Homes Initiative: Evaluation Report for Years 2010–2014. Minnesota Department of Health: Saint Paul, MN.

xG Health Solutions. 2017. *ProvenHealth Navigator: Your Guide to an Effective Patient-Centered Medical Home*. https://xghealth.com/provenhealth-navigator-your-guide-to-an-effective-patient-centered-medical-home/ (accessed August 17, 2017).

APPENDIX B

WORKSHOP AGENDAS

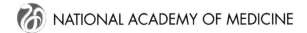 NATIONAL ACADEMY OF MEDICINE

MODELS OF CARE FOR HIGH-NEED PATIENTS

A National Academy of Medicine Workshop

. . . funded by the Peterson Center on Healthcare

July 7, 2015
Keck Center
Room 100
500 Fifth St, NW
Washington DC 20001

NAM LEADERSHIP CONSORTIUM FOR VALUE & SCIENCE-DRIVEN HEALTH CARE

Meeting objectives

1. What are the key characteristics of high-need patient populations, and which subgroups offer the greatest opportunity for impact?
2. What factors are most important in determining the match between a model of care and a patient population?
3. How can lessons learned from past experience with high-need patients be amplified and spread effectively?

AGENDA

8:00 AM   Coffee and light breakfast available

8:30 AM   Welcome and agenda overview

- *Michael McGinnis, MD, MPP*, National Academy of Medicine
- *Peter Long, PhD*, Blue Shield of California Foundation (*Chair*)

8:45 AM   Partner organizations: introduction and updates

- *Emily Zyborowicz, MPH*, Peterson Center on Healthcare
- *G. William Hoagland*, Bipartisan Policy Center
- *Katherine Hayes, JD*, Bipartisan Policy Center
- *Jose Figueroa, MD, MPH*, Harvard T.H. Chan School of Public Health

9:15 AM   Patient perspective

Brief opening presentation and discussion on the personal perspectives of a patient.

- *Jeromie Ballreich*, Johns Hopkins University

9:30 AM   High-need patients: introduction and overview

Presentations and discussion on the existing high-need patient literature, including definitions, categories, challenges, and other considerations. [Meeting Goal: What are the key characteristics of high-need patient populations?]

- *Melinda Abrams, MS*, The Commonwealth Fund
- *Alan Glaseroff, MD*, Stanford University

10:30 AM   Break (15 min)

10:45 AM   Identifying and defining high-need patients

Presentations and discussion exploring special considerations for key subgroups and mechanisms for identifying opportunities for improving quality and controlling costs. [Meeting Goal: Which subgroups offer the greatest opportunity for impact?]

- *David Meyers, MD*, Agency for Healthcare Research and Quality (moderator)
- *Bruce A. Chernof, MD, FACP*, The SCAN Foundation
- *Frank V. deGruy III, MD, MSFM*, University of Colorado, Denver
- *Lisa Iezzoni, MD, MSc*, Harvard Medical School
- *David Meltzer, MD, PhD*, University of Chicago

12:15 PM   Meeting goal 1: closing discussion

12:30 PM   Lunch

1:30 PM   Models that deliver: success stories

Case studies of successful interventions and care models that engage the priorities of high-need groups. [Meeting Goal: What factors are most important in determining the match between a model of care and a patient population?]

- *Arnold Milstein, MD, MPH*, Stanford University (moderator)
- *John O'Brien, PharmD, MPH*, CareFirst BlueCross BlueShield
- *Robert Master, MD*, Commonwealth Care Alliance
- *Bonnie LaPlante, RN, MHA*, Health Care Homes, Minnesota
- *Rebecca Ramsay, MPH*, CareOregon

3:00 PM   Break

3:15 PM   Comments from the NAM president

- *Victor J. Dzau, MD*, National Academy of Medicine

3:20 PM   Applying models of care to diverse circumstances

Presentations and discussion on the challenges that arise in the application and spread of models of care in diverse settings and for diverse patient groups. [Meeting Goal: How can lessons learned from past experience with high-need patients be amplified and spread effectively?]

- *Gerard Anderson, PhD*, Johns Hopkins Bloomberg School of Public Health (*moderator*)
- *Rajesh Davda, MD*, Cigna Healthcare
- *Don Furman, MD*, Alignment Healthcare

- *Lisa Mangiante, MPP, MPH*, Pacific Business Group on Health
- *Deborah Peikes, PhD, MPA*, Mathematica Policy Research

4:45 PM Summary and next steps

- *Peter Long, PhD*, Blue Shield of California Foundation (Chair)
- *Michael McGinnis, MD, MPP*, National Academy of Medicine

5:00 PM Adjourn

PLANNING COMMITTEE

Chair

Peter Long, PhD, Blue Shield of California Foundation

Members

Melinda Abrams, MS, The Commonwealth Fund

Gerard Anderson, PhD, Johns Hopkins Bloomberg School of Public Health

Tim Engelhardt, Centers for Medicare & Medicaid Services

Katherine Hayes, JD, Bipartisan Policy Center

Aparna Higgins, PhD, MA, America's Health Insurance Plans

Frederick Isasi, JD, MPH, National Governors Association

Ashish K. Jha, MD, MPH, Harvard School of Public Health

David Meyers, MD, Agency for Healthcare Research and Quality

Arnold S. Milstein, MD, MPH, Stanford University

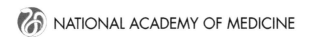

NATIONAL ACADEMY OF MEDICINE

MODELS OF CARE FOR HIGH-NEED PATIENTS

A National Academy of Medicine Workshop

. . . funded by the Peterson Center on Healthcare

January 19, 2016
National Academy of Sciences Building
Lecture Room
2101 Constitution Avenue, NW
Washington, DC 20418

NAM LEADERSHIP CONSORTIUM FOR VALUE & SCIENCE-DRIVEN HEALTH CARE

Meeting objectives

1. **Data and segmentation**. Review existing data sources on care delivery to high-need patients, and consider how the populations may be best characterized to design and target care more effectively.
2. **Design elements**. Explore successes and lessons learned from designing various models of care.
3. **Policy implications**. Consider policies particularly important to spreading the most successful models.

8:00 AM   Coffee and light breakfast available

8:30 AM   Welcome and agenda overview

• *Michael McGinnis, MD, MPP*, National Academy of Medicine
• *Jeff Selberg, MHA*, Peterson Center on Health Care
• *Peter Long, PhD*, Blue Shield of California Foundation (Chair)

8:45 AM   Patient perspective

• *Darcel Jackson*, Children's National Health System

9:00 AM   **Framing the conversation: utility of a segmentation strategy for high-need patients and implications for care and policy**

Perspectives on the issues and uses of different approaches to segmenting high-need patient populations, and the implications for care delivery and policy.

- *David Dorr, MD, MS*, Oregon Health & Science University
- *Craig Samitt, MD*, Anthem, Inc.
- *Simon Hambidge, MD, PhD*, Denver Health

9:30 AM   **The existing data on high-need patients**

Primary data sources and insights gleaned about the nature and care for high-need patients, including identification of the limits and opportunities of working with these data.

- *Gerard Anderson, PhD*, Johns Hopkins University
- *Ashish Jha, MD, MPH*, Harvard T.H. Chan School of Public Health
- *Paul Bleicher, MD, PhD*, Optum Labs

Q&A and Open Discussion

10:30 AM   Break

10:45 AM   Understanding the taxonomy of high-need patient populations

Synthesis of what we know about segmenting high-need patient populations, and the activities underway to build the taxonomy.

- *Melinda Abrams, MS*, The Commonwealth Fund

Q&A and Open Discussion

11:30 AM   Breakout sessions: interacting with the data and segmentation

Two small-groups discuss: 1) the use of a segmentation strategy for high-need patients; 2) challenges and opportunities in use of different approaches and data sources for segmenting patients; and 3) implications of groupings for design, organization, and financing of care delivery.

12:30 PM   Working lunch and report back from breakout sessions

1:30 PM   Identifying the design elements of successful models

Panelists explore attributes of successful models.

- *Molly Coye, MD, MPH*, Network for Excellence in Health Innovation
- *Randall Brown, PhD*, Mathematica Policy Research
- *Rahul Rajkumar, MD, JD*, Center for Medicare & Medicaid Innovation

Q&A and Open Discussion

2:30 PM   Replicating successful models through spread and scale

Panelists introduce policy strategies and opportunities to improve care for high-need patients.

- *Arnold Milstein, MD, MPH*, Stanford University
- *Katherine Hayes, JD*, Bipartisan Policy Center
- *Sandra Wilkniss, PhD*, National Governors Association

Q&A and Open Discussion

3:10 PM   Break

3:20 PM   Breakout sessions: policy implications

Two small-groups: 1) discuss key barriers to scaling new delivery models for high-need patients; and 2) identify essential elements for a policy framework that would mitigate these barriers.

4:20 PM   Report back

A facilitated large group discussion reviews outcomes and takeaways from the breakout.

4:45 PM   Summary and next steps

- *Peter Long, PhD*, Blue Shield of California Foundation (Chair)
- *Michael McGinnis, MD, MPP*, National Academy of Medicine

5:00 PM   Adjourn

PLANNING COMMITTEE

Chair

  Peter Long, PhD, Blue Shield of California Foundation

Members

  Melinda Abrams, MS, The Commonwealth Fund
  Gerard Anderson, PhD, Johns Hopkins Bloomberg School of Public Health
  Tim Engelhardt, Centers for Medicare & Medicaid Services
  Katherine Hayes, JD, Bipartisan Policy Center
  Aparna Higgins, PhD, MA, America's Health Insurance Plans
  Frederick Isasi, JD, MPH, National Governors Association
  Ashish K. Jha, MD, MPH, Harvard School of Public Health
  David Meyers, MD, Agency for Healthcare Research and Quality
  Arnold S. Milstein, MD, MPH, Stanford University

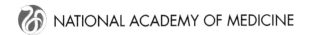 NATIONAL ACADEMY OF MEDICINE

MODELS OF CARE FOR HIGH-NEED PATIENTS

A National Academy of Medicine Workshop

. . . funded by the Peterson Center on Healthcare

October 21, 2016
Keck Center
Room 100
500 Fifth St, NW
Washington, DC 20001

NAM LEADERSHIP CONSORTIUM FOR VALUE & SCIENCE-DRIVEN HEALTH CARE

Meeting objectives

1. **Examine tools to improve care delivery for high-need patients**. Discuss a patient "taxonomy" matched to care models with the most potential to improve outcomes and lower costs, and the use of measures to enhance care delivery.
2. **Advance policy to support better care for high-need patients**. Consider a policy-level approach and other insights to support and accelerate the spread and scale of effective care models.
3. **Synthesize and identify future opportunities**. Provide a synthesis of the three-part workshop series and identify approaches and priorities for advancing progress.

8:00 AM   **Coffee and light breakfast available**

8:30 AM   **Welcome and agenda overview**

- *Michael McGinnis*, National Academy of Medicine
- *Jeff Selberg*, Peterson Center on Healthcare
- *Peter Long*, Blue Shield of California Foundation (*Chair*)

9:00 AM   **Patient perspective: A caregiver and clinical team example**

- *Eric De Jonge*, MedStar Total Elder Care
- *Veronica Humes Butler*, Long-time Caregiver
- *Gretchen Nordstrom*, MedStar Total Elder Care

9:30 AM   **A patient taxonomy and promising care models**

This session will examine a taxonomy of high-need patients matched to care models with the most potential to improve outcomes and lower the total cost of care for high-need patients.

- *Melinda Abrams*, The Commonwealth Fund, Planning Committee Member
- *Arnie Milstein*, Stanford University, Planning Committee Member

Q&A and Open Discussion

10:45 AM   **Break**

10:55 AM   **Policy opportunities for spread and scale of care models**

Introductory comments:
- *David Blumenthal*, The Commonwealth Fund

The planning committee offers insight on opportunities to advance policy.
- *Gerard Anderson*, Johns Hopkins School of Public Health, Planning Committee Member

Bipartisan Policy Center policy framework for implementation of effective care models for high-need patients, particularly Medicaid and Medicare eligible.
- *Katherine Hayes*, Bipartisan Policy Center, Planning Committee Member

Reactor panel:
- *Julian Harris*, Care Allies
- *Melanie Bella*, Formerly CMS and Independent Consultant
- *Carolyn Ingram*, Molina

Q&A and Open Discussion

12:30 PM   Lunch

1:00 PM   The use of measures in payment to enhance care

Experts discuss the use of measures in health care payment, and their role in enhancing and incentivizing high-value care for high-need patients.

- *Helen Burstin*, National Quality Forum
- *Shari Ling*, Centers for Medicare and Medicaid Services
- *Rick Kronick*, University of California San Diego

Q&A and Open Discussion

2:15 PM   Synthesis

A synthesis of suggestions and insight gleaned to date from the three-part workshop series.

- *Ashish Jha*, Harvard School of Public Health, Planning Committee Member
- *Peter Long*, Blue Shield of California Foundation, Planning Committee Chair

3:00 PM   Counsel on moving the field forward

A tightly moderated discussion of priorities for stakeholder action to improve care for high-need patients.

Moderator: *David Meyers, AHRQ*, Planning Committee Member

Reactor insight:
- Payer: *Aelaf Worku*, CareMore
- System representative: *Dave Chokshi*, NYC Health + Hospitals

- Patient: *MaryAnne Sterling*, Sterling Health IT Consulting and Connected Health Resources
- Physician researcher: *David Dorr*, Oregon Health and Science University

4:15 PM   Closing remarks

- *Michael McGinnis*, National Academy of Medicine
- *Peter Long*, Blue Shield of California Foundation (Chair)

4:30 PM   Adjourn

PLANNING COMMITTEE

Chair

   Peter Long, PhD, Blue Shield of California Foundation

Members

   Melinda Abrams, MS, The Commonwealth Fund

   Gerard Anderson, PhD, Johns Hopkins Bloomberg School of Public Health

   Tim Engelhardt, Centers for Medicare & Medicaid Services

   Jose Figueroa, MD, Harvard School of Public Health

   Katherine Hayes, JD, Bipartisan Policy Center

   Frederick Isasi, JD, MPH, National Governors Association

   Ashish K. Jha, MD, MPH, Harvard School of Public Health

   David Meyers, MD, Agency for Healthcare Research and Quality

   Arnold S. Milstein, MD, MPH, Stanford University

   Diane Stewart, MBA, Pacific Business Group on Health

   Sandra Wilkniss, PhD, National Governors Association

APPENDIX C

WORKSHOP PARTICIPANTS*

Christine Aguiar, MPH
Vice President, Medicare and Managed Long-Term Care
Association for Community Affiliated Plans

Chiledum Ahaghotu, MD
R. Frank Jones Endowed Professor and Chair of Urology
Howard University Health Sciences

Gretchen Alkema, PhD, LCSW
Vice President of Policy and Communications
The SCAN Foundation

Neeraj K. Arora
Senior Program Officer, Improving Healthcare Systems
Patient-Centered Outcomes Research Institute

David Atkins, MD, MPH
Acting Chief Research and Development Officer
US Department of Veterans Affairs

Jeromie Ballreich, MHS
PhD candidate for Health Economics
Johns Hopkins University

Jessica Bartell
Physician
Epic

*Position at the time of attendance.

Mary B. Barton, MD, MPP
Vice President for Performance Measurement
National Committee for Quality Assurance

Jayasree Basu, PhD, MBA
Senior Economist & Health Scientist
Agency for Healthcare Research and Quality

Melanie Bella, MBA
Former Director, Medicare-Medicaid Coordination Office
Centers for Medicare and Medicaid Services

Amy Berman, BSN, LHD
Senior Program Officer
John A. Hartford Foundation

Beth Berselli, MA, MBA
Program Officer
Gordon and Betty Moore Foundation

Arlene Bierman, MD, MS
Director, Center for Evidence and Practice Improvement
Agency for Healthcare Research and Quality

Leah Binder, MA, MGA
President and Chief Executive Officer
The Leapfrog Group

Laura Birchfield Kennedy
Director of Health Policy
National Partnership for Women & Families

Paul Bleicher, MD, PhD
Chief Executive Officer
Optum Labs

David Blumenthal, MD
President
The Commonwealth Fund

Peter Boling, MD
Professor and Chair of Geriatric Medicine
Virginia Commonwealth University Medical Center

Vence L. Bonham, Jr., JD
Senior Advisor to the Director on Genomics and Health Disparities, National
    Human Genome Research Institute
National Institutes of Health

Cynthia Boyd, MD, MPH
Associate Professor of Medicine, Division of Geriatric Medicine and Gerontology
Johns Hopkins University School of Medicine

Resa Bradeen, MD
Regional Medical Director for Children's Services
Providence Health & Services, Oregon Region

Randall Brown, PhD
Director of Health Research
Mathematica Policy Research, Inc.

Sheila Burke, RN, MPA, FAAN
Strategic Advisor
Baker, Donelson, Bearman, Caldwell & Berkowitz, PC

Helen Burstin, MD, MPH, FACP
Chief Scientific Officer
National Quality Forum

Rebecca Case, JD
Director, Medicaid Policy
America's Health Insurance Plans

Bruce Chernof, MD, FACP
President and Chief Executive Officer
The SCAN Foundation

Preeta Chidambaran, MD, MPH
Medical Officer for Quality
Health Resources and Services Administration

Gary Claxton
Vice President & Director of the Health Care Marketplace Project
Henry J. Kaiser Family Foundation

Chris Collins
Director, Office of Rural Health and Community Care
North Carolina Department of Health and Human Services

Molly Collins Offner, MHSA
Director for Policy Development
American Hospital Association

Amy Compton-Phillips, MD
Chief Quality Officer
Kaiser Permanente

Ceci Connolly
Managing Director, Health Research Institute
PricewaterhouseCoopers

Janet Corrigan, PhD, MBA
Chief Program Officer, Patient Care
Gordon and Betty Moore Foundation

Steven R. Counsell, MD
Mary Elizabeth Mitchell Professor & Chair, Geriatrics
Indiana University School of Medicine
Founding Director
IU Geriatrics

Molly Coye, MD, MPH
Social Entrepreneur in Residence
The Network for Excellence in Health Innovation

TjaMeika Davenport
Parent Navigator
Children's National Hospital

Rajesh Davda, MD
National Medical Director, Network Performance Evaluation
Cigna Healthcare

Frank V. deGruy III, MD, MSFM
Woodward Chisholm Professor & Chair
University of Colorado, Denver

K. Eric De Jonge, MD
Executive Director
MedStar Total Elder Care

Susan Dentzer
Senior Policy Advisor
Robert Wood Johnson Foundation

Don E. Detmer, MD, MA, FACMI, FACS
Professor Emeritus
University of Virginia School of Medicine

David Dorr, MD, MS
Associate Professor of Geriatrics and Vice Chair of Clinical Informatics
Oregon Health and Science University

Linda Dunbar
Vice President, Population Health/Care Management
Johns Hopkins HealthCare, LLC

Nancy E. Dunlap, MD, PhD, MBA
Scholar
University of Alabama at Birmingham

Victor J. Dzau, MD
President
National Academy of Medicine

Richard Elmore, MA
Senior Vice President, Corporate Development and Strategy
Allscripts

Jacqueline Erdo, MPH
Public Policy Manager
Cystic Fibrosis Foundation

Marcus Escobedo, MPA
Senior Program Officer
John A. Hartford Foundation

Suzanne Fields, MSW, LICSW
Senior Advisor for Health Care Policy and Financing
University of Maryland School of Social Work

Jose Figueroa, MD, MPH
Instructor of Medicine, Harvard Medical School
Hospitalist, Brigham and Women's Hospital

Lawrence J. Fine, MD
Branch Chief, Clinical Applications and Prevention Branch, National Heart,
 Lung and Blood Institute
National Institutes of Health

Elizabeth J. Fowler, PhD, JD
Vice President, Health
Johnson & Johnson

Susan Frampton, PhD
President
Planetree

Joseph Francis, Jr., MD, MPH
Director, Clinical Analytics and Reporting
US Department of Veterans Affairs

Richard S. Frank, MD, MHSA
Vice President, Health Care Management
Anthem, Inc.

Terry Fulmer, PhD, RN, FAAN
President
The John A. Hartford Foundation

Don Furman, MD
Chief Strategy Officer
Alignment Healthcare

Eric Gascho
Assistant Vice President, Government Affairs
National Health Council

Alan Glaseroff, MD
Clinical Professor, Medicine
Stanford University

B.K. Gogia
Managing Principal
Trigon Health

Donald Goldmann, MD
Chief Medical and Scientific Officer
Institute for Healthcare Improvement

Christine Grady, RN, PhD
Chief, Department of Bioethics
National Institutes of Health

Robert A. Greene, MD, MHCDS, FACP
Executive Vice President, Chief Population Health Management Officer
Dartmouth-Hitchcock Medical Center

Sheldon Greenfield, MD
Donald Bren Professor of Medicine and Executive Co-Director, Health Policy Research Institute
University of California, Irvine

Jim Hahn, PhD
Specialist in Health Care Financing and Health Economist
Congressional Research Service

Robert T. Hall, JD, MPAff
Director
American Academy of Pediatrics

Allison Hamblin, MSPH
Vice President, Strategic Planning
Center for Health Care Strategies

Simon Hambidge, MD, PhD
Chief Ambulatory Care Officer, Denver Health
Prof. of Pediatrics and Epidemiology, University of Colorado

Pastor Bruce Hanson, MDiv
Patient Advocate
PCORI, HSAG, PQA

Lauran J. Hardin MSN, RN-BC, CNL
Director Cross Continuum Transformation, National Center for Complex Health and Social Needs
Camden Coalition of Healthcare Providers

Julian Harris, MD, MBA
President
CareAllies

G. William Hoagland
Senior Vice President
Bipartisan Policy Center

Margaret Houy
Senior Consultant
Bailit Health Purchasing

Pamela S. Hinds, PhD, RN, FAAN
Director, Department of Nursing Research and Quality Outcomes and
  Associate Director, Center for Translational Science
Oncology Nursing Society

Richard Hodach, MD, MPH, PhD
Chief Medical Officer and Vice President of Clinical Product Strategy
IBM

Tom Hubbard, MPP
Vice President, Policy Research
The Network for Excellence in Health Innovation

Leighton Huey, MD
Associate Dean of Community and Continuing Education
University of Connecticut Health Center

Veronica Humes Butler
Caregiver

Lisa Iezzoni, MD, MSc
Professor of Medicine
Harvard Medical School

Carolyn Ingram, MBA
Vice President
Molina Healthcare

Darcel Jackson
Parent Navigator
Children's National Hospital

Paul Johnson, MD
Internal Medicine
Hennepin County Medical Center

Emily Jones, PhD, MPP
Office of Behavioral Health and Intellectual Disabilities
US Department of Health and Human Services

Lauren Jones
Engagement Coordinator
Aledade, Inc.

Rhys W. Jones, MPH
Vice President, Medicaid Advocacy
America's Health Insurance Plans

Sherrie Kaplan, PhD, MPH
Assistant Vice Chancellor of Healthcare Measurement and Evaluation and
    Executive Co-Director, Health Policy Research Institute
University of California, Irvine

Joy Keeler Tobin, MBA
National Patient Safety Partnership
The MITRE Corporation

Leslie Kelly Hall
Senior Vice President, Policy
Healthwise

Meredith L. Kilgore, RN, PhD
Professor & Chair
Department of Health Care Organization and Policy
University of Alabama School of Public Health

Ira M. Klein, MD, MBA, FACP
National Medical Director, Clinical Thought Leadership
Aetna

Kellen A. Knowles
Medical Student
Johns Hopkins University

Richard G. Kronick, PhD
Professor, Department of Family Medicine & Public Health
University of California at San Diego

Joel Kupersmith, MD
Former Chief Research and Development Officer
US Department of Veterans Affairs

Ronald Lampert, MSW, ACSW
Vice President of Health Care Strategies
Thresholds Inc.

Bonnie LaPlante, RN, MHA
Certification and Capacity Building Supervisor
Health Care Homes, Minnesota

Kevin Larsen, MD, FACP
Medical Director, Meaningful Use
Office of the National Coordinator for Health IT

Eva K. Lee, PhD
Director, NSF-Whitaker Center for Operations Research in Medicine and
    HealthCare, and Professor, Industrial and Systems Engineering
Georgia Institute of Technology

Russell B. Leftwich, MD
Chief Medical Informatics Officer
State of Tennessee

Rebecca Leibowitz
Director, Accountable Care & Value-Based Strategy
American Gastroenterological Association

Charlotte M. Lewis
Quality Lead, Exchanges
US Office of Personnel Management

Shari M. Ling, MD
Deputy Chief Medical Officer
Centers for Medicare and Medicaid Services

Teresa Litton, MPH
Senior Policy Advisor
National Association of ACOs

Kathy Lockhart
Office of Quality, Safety and Value
US Department of Veterans Affairs

Joanne Lynn, MD, MA, MS
Director, Center for Elder Care and Advanced Illness
Altarum Institute

Ellen Makar, MSN, RN-BC, CCM, CPHIMS, CENP
Senior Policy Advisor
Office of the National Coordinator for Health IT

Lisa Mangiante, MPP, MPH
Director, Intensive Outpatient Care Program
Pacific Business Group on Health

Robert Master, MD
Chief Executive Officer
Commonwealth Care Alliance

Ercelle Mayner
Federal Employees Health Benefits Program
US Office of Personnel Management

Kaitlin McHenry
Student
Johns Hopkins University

David Meltzer, MD, PhD
Chief, Section of Hospital Medicine
University of Chicago

Susan Mende, BSN, MPH
Senior Program Officer
Robert Wood Johnson Foundation

Mark Miller, PhD
Executive Director
Medicare Payment Advisory Commission

Nancy Miller, PhD
Senior Advisor, Healthcare Delivery Research Program
National Cancer Institute
National Institutes of Health

Parsa Mirhaji, MD, PhD
Research Associate Professor
Yeshiva University Albert Einstein College of Medicine

Russ Montgomery
Director, Office of Population Health Improvement
Maryland Department of Health and Mental Hygiene

Ben Moulton, JD, MPH
Senior Vice President, Advocacy and Policy
Healthwise

Lauren Murray
Director, Consumer Engagement and Community Outreach
National Partnership for Women & Families

Amol Navathe, MD, PhD
Assistant Professor of Medicine and Health Policy
Perelman School of Medicine

Debra Ness, MS
President
National Partnership for Women & Families

Chelsea Newhall
Director, Corporate Strategic Medical Initiatives
The AmeriHealth Caritas Family of Companies

Marci Nielsen
Chief Executive Officer
Patient-Centered Primary Care Collaborative

Gretchen Nordstrom, MSW
Chief Social Worker
MedStar Total Elder Care

John J. O'Brien
Director, Health Care and Insurance
US Office of Personnel Management

John M. O'Brien, PharmD, MPH
Vice President, Public Policy
Carefirst

Sally Okun, RN, MMHS
Vice President of Advocacy
PatientsLikeMe

Ann S. O'Malley, MD, MPH
Senior Fellow
Mathematica Policy Research

Alexander Ommaya, DSc
Senior Director, Clinical Effectiveness and Implementation Research
Association of American Medical Colleges

Egondu Rosemary Onyejekwe, PhD
Contributing Faculty
Walden University

Alexandra E. Page, MD
Orthopaedic Surgeon, Health Services Consultant
American Academy of Orthopaedic Surgeons

Herbert Pardes, MD
Executive Vice Chairman of the Board of Trustees
New York-Presbyterian Hospital

Deborah Peikes, PhD, MPA
Senior Fellow
Mathematica Policy Research

Mai Pham, MD, MPH
Chief Innovation Officer & Acting Director, Policy and Programs Group
Center for Medicare and Medicaid Innovation
Centers for Medicare and Medicaid Services

Steve Phillips, MPA
Senior Director, Health Policy & Reimbursement
Johnson & Johnson

Philip Posner, PhD
Ambassador and Member of Patient Engagement
Advisory Panel
Patient-Centered Outcomes Research Institute

Terri Postma, MD
Medical Officer, Center for Medicare
Centers for Medicare and Medicaid Services

Andreas Preising
Director, Government Affairs
Johnson & Johnson

Matthew Press, MD, MSc
Senior Advisor and Medical Officer
Center for Medicare and Medicaid Innovation

Ronald Przygodzki, MD
Director, Biomedical Laboratory Research and Development Service
US Department of Veterans Affairs

Amir Qaseem, MD, PhD, MHA
Director, Clinical Policy
American College of Physicians

Lynn Quincy, MA
Director, Healthcare Value Hub
Consumers Union

Ted D. Quinn
Chief Executive Officer and Cofounder
ACT.md

Melanie Raffoul, MD
Family Physician
American Academy of Family Physicians

Rahul Rajkumar, MD, JD, FACP
Deputy Director
Center for Medicare and Medicaid Innovation

Rebecca S. Ramsay, BSN, MPH
Director, Community Care
CareOregon

Carol Raphael, MPA
Senior Advisor
Manatt Health Solutions

Amita Rastogi, MD, MHA
Medical Director, Cost of Care Programs
Health Care Incentives Improvement Institute

Carol Regan, MPH
Senior Advisor, Center for Consumer Engagement in Health Innovation
Community Catalyst

Alison Rein, MS
Senior Director for Evidence Generation and Translation
AcademyHealth

Tiffany N. Roberson, MBA, MSHA
Health Planner
Anne Arundel County Department of Health

Maiaras Rodrigues dos Santos
Doctoral Candidate and Volunteer at Children's National Medical Center
University of Sao Paulo

Eric Rollins, MPP
Policy Analyst
MedPAC

Larry Roshfeld, MEd
Chief Executive Officer
Trigon Health

Josh Rubin, JD, MBA, MPH, MPP
Executive Program Officer
University of Michigan Medical School, Department of Learning Health Sciences

Victoria Sale
Clinical Director, Cross Site Learning and Workforce Development
Camden Coalition of Healthcare Providers

Craig Samitt, MD
Executive Vice President and Chief Clinical Officer
Anthem

Vinod K. Sahney, PhD
Distinguished University Professor
Northeastern University

Claudia Salzberg
PhD Candidate
Johns Hopkins Bloomberg School of Public Health

Lucy Savitz, PhD, MBA
Assistant Vice President for Delivery System Science, Institute for Healthcare Delivery Research
Intermountain Healthcare

Jeffrey D. Selberg, MHA
Executive Director
Peterson Center on Healthcare

Katherine Scher, RN, CCM
Director of Population Health Management
Henry Ford Health System

Mary Jean Schumann, DNP, MSN, RN, MBA, CPNP, FAAN
Senior Associate Dean for Academic Affairs
The George Washington University School of Nursing

Anne Schwartz, PhD
Executive Director
Medicaid & CHIP Payment & Access Commission

David C. Seaberg, MD, CPE, FACEP
Dean & Professor
University of Tennessee College of Medicine

Nicoleta Serban
Associate Professor
Georgia Institute of Technology-Industrial Systems and Engineering

Tanya Shah, MBA, MPH
Senior Program Officer, Delivery System Reform Program
The Commonwealth Fund

Melissa Shannon, JD
Director of Government Relations and Public Affairs
Commonwealth Care Alliance

Ruth Shea, MSW
Social Worker
MedStar Total Elder Care

Bruce Sigsbee, MD, FAAN
President
American Academy of Neurology

Joel Slackman, MS
Executive Director, Legislative and Regulatory Policy
Blue Cross Blue Shield Association

Kirsten Sloan
Senior Director, Policy Analysis and Legislative Support
American Cancer Society Cancer Action Network

Scott R. Smith, PhD
Director, Division of Health Care Quality and Outcomes
US Department of Health and Human Services

William D. Smucker, MD
Primary Care Physician
Summa Health System

Richard Snow, DO, MPH
System Vice President, Clinical Transformation
OhioHealth

Donald M. Steinwachs, PhD
Professor
Johns Hopkins University Bloomberg School of Public Health

Mary Anne Sterling, CEA
Cofounder
Connected Health Resources

Diane Stewart, MBA
Senior Director
Pacific Business Group on Health

Christina Strubbe
Director of Sales & Marketing
ACT.md

Regina Szylit Bousso, PhD, RN
Associate Professor and Volunteer at Children's National Medical Center
University of Sao Paulo

Susan Tanaka
Senior Policy Advisor
Peter G. Peterson Foundation

Marit Tanke, MD, PhD
Harkness Fellow
Harvard T.H. Chan School of Public Health

Kenneth E. Thorpe, MA, PhD
Professor of Health Policy
Emory University

Emilia Thurber
Medical Student
Johns Hopkins University

Trissa Torres, MD, MSPH, FACPM
Senior Vice President
Institute for Healthcare Improvement

Cori E. Uccello
Senior Health Fellow
American Academy of Actuaries

Bret Voith
Associate/Summer Intern to Dr. Don Furman
Alignment Healthcare

Kristal Vardaman, MSPH
Principal Analyst
MACPAC

Timothy Westmoreland, JD
Professor
Georgetown University

Wes Walker, MD
Chief Medical Officer, East Region
Cerner Corporation

Timothy J. Ward
Interim Chief, Performance Improvement Office
US Navy, Office of the Surgeon General

Anne Watson, MSc, PhD, BSN, RN
Research Nurse Coordinator
Children's National Medical Center

C. Edwin Webb, PharmD, MPH
Associate Executive Director
American College of Clinical Pharmacy

Barbara Wells, PhD
National Heart, Lung, and Blood Institute
National Institutes of Health

Ashlie Wilbon, RN, MS, MPH
Managing Director, Quality Measurement
National Quality Forum

Sandra Wilkniss, PhD
Program Director, Health Division
National Governors Association

Aelaf Worku, MD
Regional Medical Officer for Clark County, Nevada
CareMore Health System

Katie Wright
American Cancer Society Cancer Action Network

Samuel Wu, PharmD
Public Health Advisor
US Department of Health and Human Services

Baligh Yehia, MD, MPP
Senior Advisor to the Secretary for Health
US Department of Veterans Affairs

Sharon Zalewski
Executive Director
Regional Primary Care Coalition

Emily Zyborowicz, MPH
Manager, Research and Identification
Peterson Center on Healthcare

APPENDIX D

BIOGRAPHICAL SKETCHES

Planning Committee Biographies

Peter V. Long, PhD (*Chair*), is president and CEO of Blue Shield of California Foundation, a health foundation established in 2002 to ensure access to quality, affordable care for all Californians, and to end domestic violence. Dr. Long has an extensive background in health policy, working on issues affecting underserved communities at the state, national, and global levels. Previously, Dr. Long served in leadership roles at the Henry J. Kaiser Family Foundation and The California Endowment. He received a BA from Harvard University; an MS in health policy from The Johns Hopkins University School of Hygiene and Public Health; and a PhD in health services from the University of California, Los Angeles.

Melinda K. Abrams, MS, is a vice president for The Commonwealth Fund's Health Care Delivery System Reform program. Since coming to the fund in 1997, Ms. Abrams has worked on the fund's Task Force on Academic Health Centers, the Child Development and Preventive Care program, and, most recently, she led the Patient-Centered Primary Care Program. Ms. Abrams has served on many national committees and boards for private organizations and federal agencies and is a peer-reviewer for several journals. Ms. Abrams holds a BA in history from Cornell University and an MS in health policy and management from the Harvard School of Public Health.

Gerard F. Anderson, PhD, is a professor of health policy and management and director of the Johns Hopkins Bloomberg School of Public Health's Center for Hospital Finance and Management. Prior to coming to Johns Hopkins in 1983, Dr. Anderson worked in the Office of the Secretary of the US Department of Health and Human Services from 1978 to 1983. Dr. Anderson is currently conducting research on chronic conditions, comparative insurance systems, medical education, health care payment reform, and technology diffusion. He has directed reviews of health care systems for the World Bank, World Health Organization, and USAID in multiple countries and has directed more than 100 research projects. He has authored two books on health care payment policy, published more than 250 peer-reviewed articles, testified in Congress 50 times, and serves on multiple editorial committees.

Tim Engelhardt, MHS, is the director of the CMS Medicare-Medicaid's Federal Coordinated Health Care Office. The office was created in the Affordable Care Act to improve services for individuals dually eligible for Medicaid and Medicare. Prior to joining CMS in 2010, Mr. Engelhardt was a consultant with The Lewin Group, where he supported a variety of health and long-term care initiatives for federal, state, and local government agencies. He previously served as the deputy director for long-term care financing at the Maryland Department of Health and Mental Hygiene (the state Medicaid agency). Mr. Engelhardt received a BA in sociology from the University of Notre Dame and an MHS from the Johns Hopkins Bloomberg School of Public Health.

Jose Figueroa, MD, MPH, is an instructor of medicine at Harvard Medical School and an associate physician at Brigham and Women's Hospital (BWH). He is also currently a research fellow at the Harvard Initiative for Global Health Quality (HIGH-Q) and the Harvard Global Health Institute (HGHI). He graduated from Harvard Medical School and the Harvard School of Public Health in 2011 with a concentration in health policy. He completed his residency in internal medicine at Brigham and Women's Hospital in July 2014, where he now serves as faculty director of the BWH Residency Management & Leadership Track. He has previously worked for the Disparities Solutions Center at the Massachusetts General Hospital (MGH), Best Doctors Inc., and the GAVI Alliance in Geneva, Switzerland. Currently, his main research interests include (1) understanding the needs of high-cost, high need patients; (2) improving quality of care for vulnerable populations, including racial/ethnic minorities; and (3) understanding the impact of federal and state regulation on health care quality and costs.

Katherine Hayes, JD, is the director of health policy at the Bipartisan Policy Center (BPC). Prior to joining the BPC, Ms. Hayes worked as an associate research professor in the Department of Health Policy at the George Washington University School of Public Health and Health Services and served as codirector of Health Reform GPS: Navigating Health Reform Implementation, a website jointly sponsored by the Robert Wood Johnson Foundation and GW's Hirsh Health Law and Policy Program. She also taught graduate courses in federal advocacy and policy making and the federal budget process. Prior to joining GW, Hayes served as vice president of health policy for Jennings Policy Strategies, Inc. Other private-sector experience includes legal practice as a member of the health and legislative practice groups at Hogan & Hartson, LLP (now Hogan Lovells); policy director for two large Catholic health systems; and policy director for Cardinal Glennon Children's Hospital. Her government experience includes serving as legislative counsel to Senator Evan Bayh (D-IN); legislative assistant to Senator John H. Chafee (R-RI) and Congressman Mickey Leland (D-TX); and as a program consultant for the State of Missouri Medicaid agency. Ms. Hayes also worked as a health and education policy adviser for the State of Texas, Office of State-Federal Relations. She received a BA in international studies from the University of North Carolina at Chapel Hill and a JD from The American University Washington College of Law.

Frederick Isasi, JD, MPH, is the current executive director of Families USA. He previously served as the health division director with the National Governors Association Center for Best Practices (NGA Center). In that role, he oversaw the entire Health Division portfolio, including work related to: health care service delivery and payment reform; Medicaid reform and cost containment; state employee and retiree health benefits; maternal and child health; public health; prescription drug abuse prevention; health information exchange and analytics; behavioral health and the social determinants of health; and health insurance coverage issues such as insurance market reforms and health insurance exchange planning and operations. Previously, he served as the vice president of health policy at The Advisory Board Company, where he founded the health policy division focused on surfacing insights related to transforming the quality and efficiency of health care with a particular focus on risk-based payments, accountable care, population health, patient engagement, and payment bundling. Mr. Isasi also served for 5 years as the senior legislative counsel for health care to Senator Jeff Bingaman, working on both the Finance Committee and the Health Education Labor and Pension (HELP) Committee. During his time in the Senate, Mr. Isasi authored numerous health care laws related to Medicare, Medicaid, the State Children's Health Insurance Program (SCHIP), payment transformation and accountable care, quality, health information technology, health care workforce, oral health care, public health, and the Food and Drug Administration. He also worked extensively on the Affordable Care Act, including the development of new health insurance exchanges and insurance market reforms. Mr. Isasi graduated with a JD from Duke University Law School and received an MPH from the University of North Carolina at Chapel Hill with honors. He also has published research on the adherence of HIV-positive patients to antiretroviral treatments and has extensive biomedical research experience.

Ashish K. Jha, MD, MPH, is director of the Harvard Global Health Institute, and K.T. Li Professor of International Health & Health Policy, at the Harvard T.H. Chan School of Public Health, professor of medicine at Harvard Medical School, and a practicing internal medicine physician at the VA Boston Healthcare System. Dr. Jha received his MD from Harvard Medical School and trained in internal medicine at the University of California, San Francisco, where he also served as chief medical resident. He completed his general medicine fellowship from Brigham and Women's Hospital and Harvard Medical School and received his MPH from Harvard T.H. Chan School of Public Health. Dr. Jha's major research interests lie in improving the quality and costs of health care with a specific focus on the impact of policy efforts. His work has focused on a broad set of issues, including transparency and public reporting of provider performance, financial incentives, health information technology, and leadership, and the roles they play in fixing health care delivery systems.

David Meyers, MD, FAAFP, a board-certified family physician, serves as chief medical officer for the Agency for Healthcare Research and Quality (AHRQ). Prior to his appointment to this new position, he directed AHRQ's Center for Evidence and Practice Improvement, where he led AHRQ's Improving Primary Care initiative, oversaw the center's work supporting the US Preventive Services Task Force, the Agency's Evidence-based Practice Center initiative, Health IT portfolio, Decision Sciences group, and Practice Improvement Division. From 2011–2012 he also served as the Acting Scientific Director for the US Preventive Services Task Force. His recent publications have focused on primary care transformation, the evidence base for the patient-centered medical home, the primary care physician workforce, and foundational thinking about building capacity for ongoing and systematic quality improvement in primary care. Before joining AHRQ in 2004, Dr. Meyers practiced family medicine, including maternity care, in a community health center in southeast Washington, DC, and directed the Georgetown University Department of Family Medicine's practice-based research network, CAPRICORN. He is a graduate of the University of Pennsylvania School of Medicine and completed his family medicine residency at Providence Hospital/Georgetown University. After residency, he completed fellowship training in primary care health policy and research in the Department of Family Medicine at Georgetown University.

Arnold S. Milstein, MD, MPH, is professor of medicine and the director of the Clinical Excellence Research Center (CERC), which is housed in the Center for Advanced Study in the Behavioral Sciences at Stanford University. CERC designs and demonstrates, in multistate locations, scalable health care delivery innovations that provide better care with less health care spending. His research spans positive value outlier assessment, human-centered health care design, and, in partnership with Stanford's AI Lab, the development of technology-based cognitive aids to boost the yield from health care spending. Before joining Stanford's faculty, Dr. Milstein founded a national health care performance–improvement firm that he expanded globally after its acquisition by Mercer. He subsequently cofounded three nationally influential public benefit initiatives, including the Leapfrog Group and the Pacific Business Group on Health. As a congressional MedPAC commissioner, he originated two legislative changes to align health care provider revenue with value to patients. Dr. Milstein was elected to the National Academy of Medicine and cochaired its analysis of opportunities to safely slow national health spending growth.

Diane Stewart, MBA, joined the Pacific Business Group on Health in January 2001. She serves as the senior director for the Redesigning Care portfolio for PBGH. Ms. Stewart created PBGH's health care improvement initiative, California Quality Collaborative, a statewide collaborative program to reengineer care in the outpatient setting in partnership with commercial health plans, medical groups, and employers. She serves as the lead for PBGH's CMMI Innovation Award for changing care for high-risk patients, the Intensive Outpatient Care Program, and a CMS-funded Practice Transformation Network program. She also leads the Better Maternity Care program, which applies a combination of payment reform and QI to reduce C-Section rates. Ms. Stewart was a founding member, and now a board member, for the Network for Regional Health Improvement, a national organization of multistakeholder regional health initiatives to promote transparency and system improvement across local health care systems. Previously, she led the technical development team for the Integrated Healthcare Association's (IHA) Pay for Performance program, which collects and reports measures of clinical performance, patient experience, and IT functionality for 215 medical groups caring for 6 million patients. Prior to joining PBGH, Ms. Stewart was director of quality and planning at the Palo Alto Medical Foundation, where she initiated the quality program driving improved outcomes in patient satisfaction, clinical performance, financial performance, and staff satisfaction. She has also held management positions at Harvard Community Health Plan as well as other IPAs and medical groups on the East Coast. Ms. Stewart received a BS in biology from Dartmouth College and an MBA from the Yale School of Management.

Sandra Wilkniss, PhD, serves as program director for the National Governors Association (NGA) Center for Best Practices' Health Division. Dr. Wilkniss focuses on issues related to behavioral health and social determinants of health and the innovative integration of these into health system transformation efforts. She leads the NGA Center's technical assistance work with states advancing programs for high-need, high-cost populations. Prior to joining NGA, Dr. Wilkniss worked for 3 years in the US Senate as senior legislative assistant for health care to Senators Jeff Bingaman and Martin Heinrich. She joined Senator Bingaman's staff after serving 1 year as an American Association for the Advancement of Science/American Psychological Association Congressional Fellow in his office. Before her career transition to the health policy field, Dr. Wilkniss worked for 15 years as a scientist-practitioner in adult psychopathology, specializing in serious mental illness. She served as the director of Thresholds Institute at Thresholds Psychiatric Rehabilitation Centers, the research and training arm of the Chicagoland's largest psychiatric rehabilitation provider. She also served as adjunct assistant professor at Dartmouth Medical School, assistant clinical professor at the University of Illinois at Chicago, and the chief psychologist on the inpatient unit at the University of Illinois at Chicago hospital. Dr. Wilkniss completed her fellowship training at the Weill Medical College of Cornell University & New York Presbyterian Hospital/Payne Whitney Psychosis Clinic and her clinical internship at the San Francisco Veterans Affairs Medical Center. She holds a PhD in clinical psychology from the University of Virginia and a BA in psychology from Princeton University. Dr. Wilkniss also holds a certificate in nonprofit management from the Kellogg School of Management at Northwestern University. She is licensed to practice psychology in the State of Illinois. She received a Chicago Community Trust Emerging Nonprofit Leader Fellowship Award and the Carol T. Mowbray Early Career Research Award from the US Psychiatric Rehabilitation Association.

Taxonomy Workgroup Biographies

Melinda J. Beeuwkes Buntin, PhD, is the chair of the Department of Health Policy at Vanderbilt University's School of Medicine. She previously served as deputy assistant director for health at the Congressional Budget Office (CBO), where she was responsible for managing and directing studies of health care and health care financing issues in the Health, Retirement, and Long-term Analysis Division. Prior to joining CBO, Dr. Buntin worked at the Office of the National

Coordinator for Health IT, where she established and directed the economic analysis, evaluation, and modeling group while on leave from RAND. At RAND, Dr. Buntin served as deputy director of RAND Health's Economics, Financing, and Organization Program, director of Public Sector Initiatives for RAND Health, and codirector of the Bing Center for Health Economics. Her research at RAND focused on insurance benefit design, health insurance markets, provider payment, and the care use and needs of the elderly. She has an AB from the Woodrow Wilson School at Princeton and a PhD in health policy with a concentration in economics from Harvard University.

Dave A. Chokshi, MD, MSc, is an assistant vice president at the New York City Health and Hospitals Corporation—the largest public health care system in the United States—where he leads the Office of Ambulatory Care Transformation. He practices primary care (internal medicine) at Bellevue Hospital and is an assistant professor of population health and medicine at NYU Langone Medical Center. Previously, Dr. Chokshi was director of population health improvement at NYU Langone. In 2012–2013, he served as a White House fellow at the US Department of Veterans Affairs, where he was the principal health adviser in the Office of the Secretary. His prior work experience spans the public, private, and nonprofit sectors, including positions with the New York City and State Departments of Health, the Louisiana Department of Health, a start-up clinical software company, and the nonprofit Universities Allied for Essential Medicines (UAEM), where he was a founding member of the board of directors. Dr. Chokshi has written on medicine and public health in *The New England Journal of Medicine, JAMA, The Lancet, Health Affairs,* and *Science.* He has also contributed to *The Atlantic* and *Scientific American.* He serves on the board of Advisors for the Parkland Health & Hospital System. In 2015, Dr. Chokshi was elected a fellow of the New York Academy of Medicine, and in 2016, he was elected a fellow of the American College of Physicians. He trained in internal medicine at Brigham and Women's Hospital, where he practiced primary care at the Southern Jamaica Plain Health Center, and he was a clinical fellow at Harvard Medical School. During his training, he did clinical work in Guatemala, Peru, Botswana, Ghana, and India. He received his MD with Alpha Omega Alpha distinction from Penn, an MSc in global public health as a Rhodes Scholar at Oxford, and graduated summa cum laude from Duke.

Henry Claypool, policy director, Community Living Policy Center, University of California, San Francisco, having sustained a spinal cord injury in a snow skiing accident in college, has spent his career advocating for the rights and needs of people living with disabilities. Most recently, he served as the executive vice president of The American Association of People with Disabilities. He was also the senior advisor to the Secretary of Health and Human Services where he was a principal architect of the administration's efforts to expand access to community living services, which culminated in the creation of the Administration for Community Living. He served as a commissioner on the 2013 Commission on Long-Term Care.

David A. Dorr, MD, MS, serves as professor and vice chair of medical informatics for the Department of Medical Informatics & Clinical Epidemiology as well as a professor of general internal medicine/geriatrics at Oregon Health & Science University. Broadly, Dr. Dorr's interests lie in care management, coordination of care, collaborative care, chronic disease management, quality, and the requirements of clinical information systems to improve and support these areas. His current primary concentrations are Transforming Outcomes for Patients through Medical home Evaluation & re-Design, or TOPMED (funded by The Gordon & Betty Moore Foundation), Risk Stratification in Primary Care (funded by The Commonwealth Fund and AHRQ), and further dissemination and evaluation of the Care Management Plus project (initially funded by The John A. Hartford Foundation). Dr. Dorr is interested in policy and payment reforms to help provide better-coordinated patient-centered care and support efficiency in the health care system. He was chosen as the New Investigator of the Year by the American Medical Informatics Association in 2007. Dorr earned his BA in economics and his MD from Washington University in St. Louis. He then completed internal medicine residency at Oregon Health & Science University, and earned an MA in medical informatics and health services administration from the University of Utah.

David Labby, MD, PhD, was the founding chief medical officer of Health Share of Oregon, a Coordinated Care Organization (CCO) that is financially and clinically accountable for the physical, behavioral, and dental care of 260,000 Medicaid enrollees in the tri-county region around Portland, Oregon. He was at Health Share from 2012, when CCOs were launched as the key element in the state's health care transformation efforts, until retiring in July 2015. He continues to work with Health Share as their health strategy adviser as well as consulting with other CCOs. Before coming to Health Share, Dr. Labby was medical director for CareOregon, the state's largest Medicaid Managed Care Plan. While at CareOregon, he was responsible for developing and overseeing the health plan's care management program for members with complex conditions.

Starting in 2006, he initiated and led the plan's Primary Care Renewal initiative to support key network providers in moving to a "medical home" model of care that includes integrated behavioral health. Dr Labby directed Health Share's "Health Commons" program, a 3-year federally funded Innovations Grant initiative focused on creating a regional system of care for high- needs/high- cost individuals. Dr. Labby is a general internist who practiced in primary care and was medical director in both primary care and multi-specialty settings before coming to CareOregon in 2000. He received his PhD in cultural anthropology.

Prabhjot Singh, MD, PhD, is director of the Arnhold Institute for Global Health at the Mount Sinai Health System. His work combines systems engineering and social mobilization principles, with an emphasis on how the US health care system can learn from other industries and low-resource settings to improve health and health care. He cofounded the One Million Community Health Workers Campaign, an initiative of the African Union and the UN Sustainable Development Solutions Network. This inspired the launch of City Health Works, a Harlem-based social enterprise that develops scalable health coaching services for high- need patients, of which he is the founding technical adviser. In 2016, his Arnhold Institute team, in partnership with the UN Secretary General Special Envoy's Office, planned to launch the Health Equity Atlas of Africa, an open framework to drive collaboration among data scientists, health system experts, and frontline health workers.

CPSIA information can be obtained
at www.ICGtesting.com
Printed in the USA
BVHW06s1123280918
528714BV00003B/3/P

9 781947 103061

WILLIAM HUTCHINSON ROWE

The MARITIME
HISTORY
of MAINE

THREE CENTURIES OF
SHIPBUILDING & SEAFARING

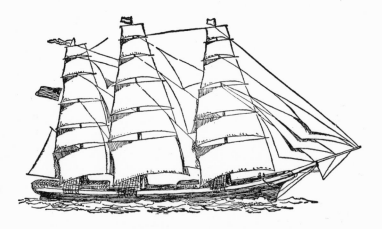

THE BOND WHEELWRIGHT COMPANY • *Maine*

PRINTED IN THE UNITED STATES OF AMERICA
By Halliday Lithograph Corporation, Hanover, Mass. 02339

TO
A. D. R.

The MARITIME HISTORY *of* MAINE

THREE CENTURIES OF
SHIPBUILDING AND SEAFARING

CONTENTS

[7]

ILLUSTRATIONS

[9]

Illustrations

FOREWORD

ALONG THE MAINE COAST people are born with salt in their blood. From Kittery on the Piscataqua to Calais on the St. Croix, twenty-five hundred miles of shore line and tidewater have been the scene of shipbuilding and seafaring for more than three centuries. Today a great change has taken place. While there are small craft—coasters, fishermen, and their like—in abundance, the tall wooden ships have gone. And with them has departed a way of life. Gone, as Lincoln Colcord has so beautifully written:

> ". . . like a high squall sinking beyond the horizon, wind and sea, motion and color, romance and aspiration, a whole range of human endeavor, all vanishing to leeward with the tall ship in their midst, done with life and bound for the seas of story."

This recounting of the rise and the decline of the wooden ship has been a large but fascinating task. Like the Maine seacoast boy in the days of the wooden ship, I have been progressively ambitious. Sailing first in my local waters with *Shipbuilding Days in Old North Yarmouth*, then on a coastwise voyage in *Shipbuilding Days in Casco Bay*, I now make this bolder venture into blue water. In this undertaking I wish to acknowledge my debt to the late Lincoln Colcord for his invaluable counsel. To Howard I. Chapelle I am grateful for his criticism of the technical aspect of shipbuilding. Robert Farlow

Foreword

has contributed from his experience in the creation of other maritime books. To Dudley Cammett Lunt I am indebted for his assistance in the preparation of the manuscript itself.

To those many other friends who have contributed valuable and generous assistance I am deeply grateful, and my appreciation is no less deep because I but list their names: Mr. Myron H. Avery, Mr. Walter B. Allen, Miss Reina M. Blanchard, Dr. Nathaniel B. T. Barker, Mrs. Fannie S. Chase, Mrs. Frances Brooks Colcord, Miss Joanna Carver Colcord, Mr. Walter G. Davis, Miss E. Marie Estes, Mrs. Fannie Hardy Eckstorm, Miss Mary Gilman, Captain William H. Gooding, Mr. Chester E. Hathaway, Dr. Allison Hunt, Mr. Samuel M. Holway, Mr. William C. S. Ingraham, Mrs. Evelyn C. Johnson, Mr. William W. Loring, Mrs. Mary D. Marshall, Miss Ida B. Mitchell, Mr. Horace Mitchell, Mr. Charles J. Nichols, Captain Charles C. Oakes, Mrs. Abbie Buxton Oakes, Mr. William D. Patterson, Miss Elizabeth Freeman Reed, Mr. George Wharton Rice, Miss Elizabeth Ring, Mrs. Anna Dubois Rowe, Miss Marion B. Rowe, Mrs. Arlene G. Storer, Mr. Joseph T. Sylvester, Miss Margaret J. Thompson, Miss Florence Kingston Vose, Miss Louise Woodbury Vose, Mr. George S. Wasson, Captain Francis E. Young, Mr. A. J. Huston, and Mr. Charles S. Morgan.

WILLIAM HUTCHINSON ROWE

Yarmouth
Maine

CHAPTER ONE

The MAINE COAST

From gray sea-fog, from icy drift
From peril and from pain
The home-bound fisher greets thy lights
O hundred-harbored Maine!

John Greenleaf Whittier,
The Dead Ship of Harpswell

THE QUAKER POET violated no principle of the Friends when he gave to Maine the sobriquet "hundred-harbored." He indulged in no poetic license, let alone hyperbole, in ascribing to her so modest a number. A thousand would have hit nearer the ·truth. The rock-bound coast, the legions of ledges stretching their treacherous lengths far out into the sea, the high, knobby little islands called "Pound of Tea," "Pumkin Knob," or "Junk of Pork" on account of their shape and size, the tides racing through thoroughfares and gurnets with a rise of from ten to thirty feet—all these, together with fifteen to thirty hours of pea-soup fog every week, would make this coast an impossible one for mariners but for the refuge to be found in these little harbors.

Then there are the islands. They range along the coast almost like a breakwater or a barrier reef. Thus long stretches, such as from Portland to Mount Desert, have an inner passage where the waters are relatively quiet and there are harbors with depth and holding ground adequate for any craft. So handily are they placed that it would be a sudden storm that could surprise a down-east skipper on a lee shore. The mainland, too, is a very nursery for ships, with deep coves for their cradles and clustering islands and high promontories to shelter them and break the force of the winds.

It was the glaciers of the Ice Age that first molded Maine into a habitation fit for men who would build, sail, and love wooden ships. These glaciers rising to the height of Katahdin's lofty saddle traveled southerly and southwesterly, ploughing out broad and deep channels far out into the sea. On either side they left the rugged islands which today mark out their paths. Of these the islands in Casco Bay are typical. They lie in three parallel rows known as the Outer, Middle, and Inner ranges. Thus it is interesting to reflect that Cushing's Island may once have formed a part of Mere Point, just as the Outer Green and Jewell's Island did of Harpswell Neck, or again Half Way Rock of Bailey's or Sebascodegan.

The Labrador Current swirled close in around Cape Sable to eddy in the Gulf of Maine. For ages its arctic waters, laden with icebergs, were destined to beat against the shore until the coast became as ragged as a fringe. Thus ground by glaciers and swept by strong tides, a coast line that measures in a straight line from Kittery to Calais some two hundred and twenty miles today has a tidal length of more than twenty-five hundred. This is near to half of the Atlantic Coast. Then there is height also. You can travel all the way down the Atlantic seaboard to Rio and not sight a seamark such as Mount Desert, where Cadillac rises almost sheer out of the ocean to a height of 1,532 feet. Here has been fashioned a shore unlike any other in the world. The vast rise and fall of the tides in the narrow bays and the prevalent northwest winds keep all of the harbors free of ice the greater part of the year. And some of them, from Portland to Penobscot Bay and as far as Winterport, Eastport, Lubec,

The Maine Coast

Cutler, and Machiasport are clear throughout the whole twelve months.

He who would paint a picture of maritime Maine must have a wide canvas and a palette holding many colors. The multiplicity of its harbors, the ragged contour of the coast with its wide estuaries and penetrating rivers, endow it with a commercial history which has many facets. It is unlike that of Massachusetts, whose maritime history coils in shipshape fashion around a few ports such as Boston, Salem, and New Bedford, each of which makes its own contribution of unique interest. In Maine there are no focal points conveniently at hand for the telling of its maritime development. The Maine coast is so dissected by salt water that the route by land between communities is oftentimes seven and even ten times the distance that separates them as the crow flies. While this tended to isolate the towns and to hinder their development, it also threw each upon its own resources and thus engendered development along unique and individual lines.

At Bath the stocks producing the great ships that carried cargoes to the ends of the earth crowded one upon the next along the shore. A bit to the eastward is the town of Boothbay. Her harbor was filled with fleets of seiners and bankers, as befits a port whose wealth is founded upon fisheries. Then there is Searsport, again to the eastward. Here after the building, in the days of small schooners, brigs, and barks, of two hundred vessels, it was discovered that her beaches were too shoal for the launching of the larger ships of later generations. The energies of her menfolk turned to seamanship and ship operation, and there came into being that glorious company of great captains who have made Maine ships known in every deepwater port in the world. Then just up the Penobscot is Bangor. Here was the strategic point for the shipment of timber. For many a year Bangor was the greatest lumber port of the world. And downstream, still on our way eastward, are communities which have fattened on the humble porgy and the small and multitudinous sardine. And all along the coast are the harbors whose coasters long sustained the burden of common carriage by sea and gave us the phrase "the coastwise trade."

Nature has divided the Maine coast into four distinct parts. There is the Western, which extends from the Isles of Shoals to Cape Elizabeth near Portland. Then there is Casco Bay with its great cluster of islands. The Middle Coast is next, running from Cape Small Point to the eastern bank of the Penobscot. Finally there is the Eastern, reaching thence on through the Passamaquoddy to Calais. Each of these coast lines has unique and distinct features. The earliest settlements were made all along the shore. Of these the traces are meager, save in the form of problems for the historian. The later development of the coast took its direction precisely contrary to the course of empire. It has ranged from west to east.

The Piscataqua River forms the western bound of Maine and marks the beginning of the Western Coast. Here began the lumber industry in America. For two centuries rafts of the King's masts or great gundalows brought down the ship timber from the hills of Maine and New Hampshire to the royal dockyards, and later to the navy yards at Kittery. On this part of the coast Whittier was wrong, for there is not a first-class harbor in all its sixty-mile length. But there is Agamenticus, whose green dome is one of the oldest and best-known seamarks of the coast. The flat shore that reaches eastward in long stretches of white sand and river marshes, with here and there a jutting promontory of granite, was never attractive to the shipbuilder. Nonetheless in early times every town found a creek wide enough to carry a vessel to the ocean on a flood tide. The Kennebunks, by thus working their small rivers to the uttermost, achieved an enviable place in the history of the American merchant marine. The wide beaches of fine white sand coupled with the warm water have turned the whole region into an aquatic playground and summer resort. Here is located Old Orchard Beach. The name derives from the ancient fruit orchard which once lined the hillside in back of the beach. In its early days it was a fashionable resort.

Contained within the outstretched arms of Cape Elizabeth and Small Point lies Casco Bay. It is in a class by itself. The shining white sand has disappeared. In its stead are small shingle beaches. The shore is high, but it is not rocky. A triple line of islands protects the inner reaches of the Bay from the violence of the open sea. There are four small but deep rivers which run inland to mingle with the fresh water from the lakes and ponds up country. Here were located the best sites for the building yards. During the era of the wooden ship these yards formed a line around the grassy shores which was almost unbroken. The ringing blows of the adz and the mallet were silenced only when the bells of the white churches in the villages announced a day of rest. While few vessels were built at Portland, this city was the center for the many trades which attended the outfitting of a ship.

It is the Middle Coast that is the heart of maritime Maine. This is the land of the great forested rivers. "A great river is equivalent," it is said, "to a great key unlocking the resources of a country." The middle coast has a ringful of these keys to the treasure chest that is central Maine. There is the Kennebec, navigable forty-five miles up from the sea and tapping a back country rich with timber. At her mouth she conjoins with the Androscoggin at Merrymeeting Bay. Then there are the deep, wide tidal rivers with harbors at every turn. These are the Sheepscot, the Damariscotta, the Medomac, and the St. George's. But the greatest of these is the Penobscot. Here for many a year the lumber schooners sailed in unbroken line to take to the markets of the world the timber that had been driven down through the gorges of the West Branch and the white water of Sourdnahunk to Bangor.

This also is the workaday part of the coast, this land of the pointed firs. The beaches are few. The shore is ragged and rocky and the water is cold, bitter cold. But nature is generous. In addition to the lumber there was lime and granite and ice and brick clay. All these had to be got to markets which lay by way of the sea. Hence we find here some of the oldest and the largest of the building yards. Bath is without peer, but close in the running came Bowdoinham, Richmond, Thomaston, Waldoboro, Camden, and Rockland. All along this shore the Camden hills looked down upon hundreds of frames rising from almost every shingle beach of this stretch.

Thus we come at last to the coast of the towering headlands. From the Penobscot through Passamaquoddy is the really bold coast of the Atlantic states with towering cliffs and deep still bays. "In hundreds of places, the conditions of sea permitting," it is said, "an ocean liner could run up to the very rocks, make fast to a hardy spruce and land passengers and cargo without scratching the paint of her underbody." Here the recurrent thunder of the surf is never silent, and the tides, responding to the pull of the near-by Bay of Fundy, rise to tremendous heights with sea fall and whirlpool in their paths. Who can blame those ancient voyagers who, when they saw the rocky ramparts that guarded the coast from Mount Desert to Quoddy Head, felt that it was entrenched against civilization?

The pioneer Yankee was not daunted by this forbidding aspect. Men from the western towns found that the Union and Narraguagas rivers and Machias and Cobscook bays opened up the vast riches of virgin timber. They came there and settled, in quiet river towns. Here they built the ship and found the cargo. Calais on the St. Croix became one of the foremost lumber ports of the world. Little Robbinston sent out some of the fastest clippers of her day. In later days the rushing tide rips of the innumerable bays bore the Quoddy boats laden with silver herring to factories where, by some subtle alchemy of mustard and cottonseed oil, they are transformed into French sardines. Perhaps the greatest change is in the character of Mount Desert. In the days of the brig and the topsail schooner it was almost a wilderness. Then within a few short years it became the summer home of the wealthy and the resort of the fashionable.

This place of itself from God and nature affordeth as much diversitie of good commodities as any reasonable man can wish. . . . Here are more good harbours for ships of all burthens than England can afford and far more secure from all winds and weathers than any in England, Scotland, France or Spain. . . . on both sides every half mile very gallant Coves, some able to contain almost a hundred sail, where the ground is excellent soft ooze with a tough clay under for anker hold, and where ships may lie without either Cable or Anker only moored to the shore with a Hauser. Here are made by nature most excellent places, as Docks to grave or Careen ships of all burthens; secured from all winds. . . .

Besides, the bordering land is a most rich neighbour trending all along on both sides. . . . The wood she beareth is not shrubbish fit only for fewell, but goodly tall Firre, Spruce, Birch, Beech, Oke . . . like stands left in our pastures in England, good and great, fit timber for any use. . . . Upon the hills grow notable high timber trees, masts for ships of 400 ton; and at the bottom of every hill, a little run of fresh water. . . . We saw great store of fish, some great, leaping above water, which we judged to be Salmons. . . . The farther we went, the more pleasing it was to every man, alluring us still with expectation of better. . . .

So runs James Rosier's *True Relation* of the discovery of the St. George's River in Maine by Captain George Waymouth in the month of June and in the year of our Lord 1605.

CHAPTER TWO

The WINTER FISHERIES

In March, Aprill, May and halfe June, heere is Cod in abundance; in May, June, July and August, Mullet and Sturgion whose Roes do make Caviare and Puttargo. Herring, if any desire them: I have taken many out of the bellies of Cods, some in nets; but the Salvages compare their store in the sea, to the haires of their heads, and surely there are an incredible abundance on the Coast. In the end of August, September, October and November, you have Cod againe to make Corfish or Poore John: Hake you may have when the Cod failes in summer, if you will fish in the night, which is better than Cod. Now each hundred good you take here is as good as two or three hundred in Newfoundland.—Captain John Smith, *The Description of New England*, 1616.

The Coast aboundeth with such multitudes of Codd that the inhabitants of New England doe dung their ground with Codd; and it is a commodity better than the golden mines of the Spanish Indies; for without dried Codd, the Spaniard, Portugal and Italian would not be able to vittel a ship for the Sea.—Thomas Morton, *New English Canaan*, 1632.

THE FIRST PIONEERS of Maine were fishermen. The settlers and planters came afterward. These early fishermen came ashore, not that they might sow and reap, but that they might exercise their "privilege of salting and drying of their fish and drying of their nets." Not only the maritime but the whole history of Maine stems from the discovery of the winter fisheries.

It was some unknown and unsung voyager who discovered

that in the winter months in search of their spawning ground the cod shift from the cold depths of the offshore banks to the warmer waters of the shore of Maine. Unnumbered European fishermen had dropped their hooks in this "strangest fish pond" and pulled in a bountiful reward many a year before the seventeenth century. It is from this later period that the written record has survived, and prominent in it are the writings of the energetic and enthusiastic Captain John Smith.

The practical captain, coming to Monhegan in April 1614, "to make tryalls of a Mine of Gold and Copper," soon turned from these "costly conclusions" and set his men to "making fish." He recurs to the subject of the fisheries again and again. He appeals to his readers' thrift, hoping to entice them to settle by promising them the advantage over their European competitors of a double season and an earlier market. With this he couples that great advantage to the home-loving Englishman that he might have "fishing before your doors and may every night sleep quietly ashore with good cheer and what fires you will, or when you please with your wives and families." Smith's example was as good as his precept. On his flakes at Monhegan he made 40,000 dry fish as well as corning another 7,000, and by sending one shipload to England and the other to Spain he cleared £1,500 from his six-month voyage.

Stirred by Smith's success and his writings, English fishermen and merchants soon evidenced a new interest in the coast of Maine. But not in the founding of colonies, as the disappointed admiral of New England had hoped. Their desire was for "voyages of profit." "One might as well try to hew rocks with oyster shells," said the Captain, "as to induce merchants and others to furnish funds for colonization." From March to June the little harbor at Monhegan now presented a busy scene, with boats going in and out for abundant catches to be dried along its shores. Captain Michael Cooper came with a part of Smith's old crew, accompanied by four vessels, one a ship of 300 tons. In 1616 came Richard Hawkins, then president of the Plymouth Company, with two vessels, while at the same time ten more fished in the waters round. Sir Ferdinando Gorges invested in a vessel and sent her to the coast for fish. On board was Gorges' close friend Richard Vines, who landed at Winter Harbor at the mouth of the Saco River, and spent the winter in the wigwams of the Indians. Of all this activity Monhegan was the center.

In 1620 James I, by the Great Patent of New England, at the instigation of Sir Ferdinando Gorges conferred upon him and his associates in the Plymouth Company a monopoly of the fishing in the seas adjoining their domain. This was a severe blow. It affected not only the merchants of Bristol and other western ports of England, whose fishermen made annual voyages to the teeming waters around Monhegan and Damariscove, but also the colonists of Virginia, who stored their boats at Monhegan during the winter. Now their voices were raised in common protest that "fishing is free."

The monopoly meant that each fishing vessel must pay a license fee of some 83 cents a ton. Considering the average size of the craft, this would equal fully $100 each today. Few fishermen could afford to have this costly paper nailed to their foremasts. For four years a battle royal was waged in Parliament for free fishing. In vain did Sir Ferdinando strive to sell these licenses on the Maine coast, finding the fishermen to be "stubern Fellows." In 1624 the voice of these people was heard through the House of Commons. The upshot was that all were allowed to continue their fishing, dry their nets, split and salt their catches, and cut the timber necessary for building their stages, boats, and habitations on any unoccupied shore.

When the Pilgrims settled in Plymouth, nothing but fishing stations existed to the eastward. But these swarmed with vessels, thirty making their headquarters in the little wedge-shaped harbor of Damariscove in 1622. The winter of this year was one of distress for the settlers at Plymouth, who had not then learned either to harvest the fields or to fish in the seas. Although the people had long been living on short rations, their food supply was so nearly spent that in May they decided that they must seek help from the fleet to the eastward. Of this they had been told by the men of the shallop which had visited them from Weston's ship *Swallow.* Edward Winslow set out for Damariscove. He received a kind welcome in the fleet and so abundant and free a supply of food for the famishing colony that he returned much pleased. He has left a grateful tribute to these early fishermen with the words, "What they could they did freely, wishing their store had been such as they might have in greater measure expressed their love, and supplied their necessities; for which they sorrowed provoking one another to the utmost of their abilities."

When John Pory, Secretary for Virginia, touched at Damariscove, he noted that Gorges kept thirteen fishermen and two shallops there to provide fish for commerce the year round. For protection against the French and Indians they had built a strong palisade of spruce trees, and in addition to their small arms they kept ten good dogs. Pory did not mention any settlement, but about this time Abraham Jennings, a prominent merchant of Old Plymouth, obtained possession of the island of Monhegan and established a trading station and fishing business. Some idea of the business done may be gained from the affidavit of one Thomas Piddock, that during June and July there were shipped to Bordeaux in the *Jacob* 173,700 dry fish weighing 3,042 quintals. A quintal being 112 pounds, this amounted to upwards of 300,000 pounds of fish of a value estimated at $10,000.

When Captain Christopher Leavitt ranged up the coast in 1624, he found no settlements from the Piscataqua to Newagen. The fishermen had set up their stages on the outer islands of

Casco Bay, and several vessels from Weymouth, England, were fishing there. Two had stationed themselves at the Sagadahoc and nine more around Southport and Boothbay Harbor. Noting that four sturgeon had been taken during the season by the herring boats, the captain foresaw what later became a profitable trade. But what most impressed him was the need of organization and protection for the fishermen.

Some two years before this they had been attacked by the Indians. More than twenty schooners had been seized and some of the crews killed. Most of the vessels were soon afterward recaptured and the crews redeemed, but this condition was too terrible to be endured. Not only was there this danger from the savages, but boats left stored on shore and the stages and flakes to which their builders hoped to return the next season were torn down, destroyed, or pre-empted by others whose only claim was the right of possession.

When Captain Leavitt returned to England he had perfected a well-thought-out plan for the protection of the fisheries from July to December, when the fleets were not on the coast. One harbor to which all the boats along the coast could be brought for storage and protection must be fortified. For this he had in mind what is now Portland Harbor. Then there must be a police patrol. For this four vessels were needed, which he guaranteed would pay their own way by the fish and oil they would take. Leavitt's plans reached the ear of King Charles, who ordered all churches in the realm to take up a contribution to aid this enterprise on the Maine coast. What sum was raised or how it was used in carrying out his plans is not recorded. All that we know is that Leavitt died at sea in 1630.

The rugged coast and the uncompromising features of soil and climate, coupled with the fact that Maine was destined to serve as a buffer in the half century of conflict between the French and Indians and the English colonies at the south, made these dreams of Captain John Smith and Christopher Leavitt slow of fulfillment. However, a new phase in the fisheries developed. Hitherto vessels from the ports of western England had come, set up temporary flakes on the outer islands, and stayed only long enough to catch and cure their fish. They then rushed off with their cargo to market with no definite thought of returning the next year. Merchants to whom the waste of such methods was abhorrent now began to establish stations which they maintained from year to year. In this manner fishing as well as fur trading might be carried on in a more systematic manner. All up and down the coast at the Isles of Shoals, Kittery Point, Winter Harbor, Stratton's Island, Richmond's Island, Sagadahoc, Damariscove, Pemaquid, New Harbor, Monhegan, Saint George and Matinicus, such stations gradually began to take form.

The largest of these stations was located at Richmond's Island off Cape Elizabeth. It is described in great detail in the letters of John Winter, the agent resident there, to his employer Robert Trelawney, a merchant in Plymouth, England. From them there may be reconstructed the daily life of the enterprise that was springing up all along the coast from Piscataqua to Matinicus at the foot of Penobscot Bay. We see the various buildings go up, the boats' crews arrive from England and go out with their lines and bait, returning with their fare, sometimes good, sometimes light. We hear of the making of cor-fish (whole cod pickled in brine) and the splitting and salting of the dry cod and trying out the fish oil or "traine." We read Winter's orders to his patron for clothing, strong waters, and fishing gear, or the iron work of a vessel he is building. We know the names of his workmen and his accounts with them, which show the amount of aqua vitae or "cyder" demanded by each. He even tells how much of each man's wages are paid to his wife in England. Mrs. Winter comes to be with her husband

and to feed the men. The quarrels about food and slothful servants enter the correspondence. Tragedy stalks when a favorite maidservant is caught by the tide and drowns on the bar.

On the mainland bears carry away the pigs and the cattle are disturbed by the Indians. Rival fishermen from Barnstable break down the flakes, and unfaithful servants plan to steal away the newly built vessel and sail off with it. There are rumors of the pirate, Dixie Bull, and his depredations at Pemaquid. Winter fears that Richmond's Island will be the next to suffer. The Reverend Richard Gibson comes to minister to the spiritual needs of the station. He disregards the charms of Winter's daughter Sarah, who finds consolation upon Gibson's departure, when Robert Jordan comes to take his place. The long enumeration of the varied products of Winter's kitchen garden even reminds one of the modern seed catalogue.

At this time more fish could be taken within two leagues of this little island off Cape Elizabeth than at any other place on the coast. Winter found it very profitable to keep boats at sea the year round. Richmond's Island being a port of call for vessels coming on the coast, dried fish were constantly being shipped in them to European ports. In Winter's accounts there is mention of *Angel Gabriel, James, Fellowship, Hercules, Hunter, Lion, Margery,* and other vessels and their masters. Later two vessels were built on the island and the fish was carried to Europe direct or to "the Bay" for shipment. Also a considerable coasting trade was carried on from the Kennebec to Virginia.

The average fishing boat of this time was of about 200 tons burden. It carried some fifty men. Each member of the crew put in 20 shillings toward provisions, and, as has always been the custom of fishermen, they "went on shares." The vessel had one third. The second was allowed for "victuals," salt, nets, lines, hooks, and other implements for the taking and making of fish. This cost about £800. The remaining third was divided among

the crew. As a rule, full fares amounted to around 4,000 quintals. At that time in Mediterranean ports fish brought from
36 to 45 Spanish reals a quintal. On an average of 40 reals or
£1 sterling, this provided a "share" of some £26 to each man.

In the latter half of the seventeenth century, when the shore
fisheries had become well established, smaller boats, or shallops,
were used. These carried four men. There was the master, who
steered, a midshipman, a foremastman, and a shoreman, who
acted as cook and also attended the fish on shore, washing, salting, and turning them on the flakes. The larger proportion of
the fish were salted and dried. Some, called "cor-fish" or corned
fish, were packed whole in brine. Mackerel and herring were
salted in hogsheads to be used as bait or sold as food for slaves.
The oil was carefully tried out and as "traine" made a valuable
export.

Each year three voyages were averaged, and at the end of
each voyage the catch was sorted according to quality. First
in value were the merchantable fish, full-grown, well shaped,
and with flesh as clear as "lanthorn horn." These sold in the
Catholic countries of Europe for 30 to 45 reals a quintal. In a
second class were the so-called "refuse fish," wholesome and
sweet, but not so full-fleshed and finely formed. These might
here and there be salt-burned and spotted. They were a staple
in the West India trade as a food for the Negroes and brought
the fishermen 9 or 10 shillings a quintal. A third variety, known
as "dun" or dark fish, became known in the early eighteenth
century. So popular did it become that in 1745 a quintal would
sell in Spain and the Mediterranean even on a low market for a
guinea. Only pollock were used. The fish were caught in the
summer season and cured on the rocks by drying them carefully without much salt. Their flavor was improved by piling
them together in a dark place or covering them with marsh hay.
This was an art peculiar at first to the Isles of Shoals.

It would be interesting to know something of the personalities of these fishermen. Generous-hearted we have found them to be, with a readiness to help that impressed even the cold Winslow. They were merry at times, and after a hard voyage ready to cut loose with their revels. The records reveal a glimpse of a Maypole dance which antedates the famous one at Merrymount. It was set up by the men of the fishing fleet on Damariscove Island. Their earnings were good, but the bumboatman was the curse of the coast. Josselyn tells of it in his racy style: "it does some of them but little good, for the merchant to increase his gains comes in with a walking tavern, a bark laden with the legitimate blood of the rich grape which they bring from Phial, Maderia, Canaries with Brandy, Rhum, the Barbadoes strong water, and tobacco. Coming ashore he gives them a taste or two which so charms them that for no persuasion that their employers can use will they go out to sea, although fair and seasonable weather, for two or three days, nay sometimes a whole week, till they are wearied with drinking. When the day of payment comes they may justly complain of their costly sin of drunkeness for their shares will do no more than pay their reckoning."

Up to the second quarter of the eighteenth century fish formed the principal staple of export from Maine as from Massachusetts. Trade was based on the "New England Silvermine," as the fisheries were called. The trade with the French West Indies became so great between 1713 and 1730 as to alarm the merchants and planters in the English islands. A multitude of little brigs and topsail schooners carried out the products of every community along the coast, "refuse fish," lumber, horses, butter, and country produce. Then it brought back all kinds of West India goods, such as sugar and molasses, and some specie.

The outlying islands, near the fishing banks, had been first occupied by colonists. These were well protected from the

Permanent,

License of a VESSEL above 20 Tons, to carry on the Cod-Fishery, for one year:

N. *Seventeen.* DISTRICT of the PORT of *Portland & Falmouth*

Nath Fosdick

IN PURSUANCE of an Act of the Congress of the United States of America, entitled " An Act for enrolling and licensing Ships or Vessels to be employed in the coasting trade and fisheries, and for regulating the same," *Elias Thomas Merchant of Portland, William Dingley Mariner of Durham and Isaac McLellan Merchant of Portland, in the County of Cumberland & State of Massachusetts*

having given bond that the Schooner called the *Molly* whereof the said *William Dingley* is Master; burthen *Twenty one — 39/95* Tons, as appears by her enrollment dated at *Portland & Falmouth May second 1798 No. sixteen*

shall not be employed in any trade while this license shall continue in force, whereby the revenue of the United States shall be defrauded; and having also Sworn — that this license shall not be used for any other Vessel, or for any other employment than is herein specified, LICENSE IS HEREBY GRANTED for the said Schooner — called the *Molly of Portland* to be employed in carrying on the COD-FISHERY for one year from the date hereof, and no longer.

Port of Portland & Falmouth GIVEN under my hand and seal of office, at the this *fifth* — day of *May* — in the year One thousand Seven hundred and ninety seven,

License to fish for cod issued in 1797 to the schooner *Molly* of Portland.

Indians by the stretches of open water. Later arrivals, finding these occupied, settled on the protected headlands jutting from the coast itself. Finally they penetrated the rivers far from their mouths and founded fortified trading stations on their banks. These were called "houses on the rivers." Here, although fur trading was the first consideration, the fisheries had an important place. As early as 1632, Thomas Purchase carried on a considerable business at Brunswick Falls in the taking and curing of salmon for the London market, where they were highly esteemed. Dr. Noyes, one of the Plymouth proprietors, engaged in the sturgeon fishery at Ancient Augusta near Small Point Harbor and employed, it is said, no less than twenty ships in taking and transporting these fish to market. Alewives and shad fairly crowded the brooks. At Wolomontogus Stream in Pittston even swine and bears came to the banks and ate their fill.

Within a generation's time permanent fisheries came to be established here and there along the coast. The Pepperell family is a case in point. The first of this name, William, came to the Maine Coast as an apprentice boy on an English fishing schooner. Upon the completion of his term of service he set up for himself on Star Island in the Isles of Shoals. Here he caught and dried his own fish, making a specialty of the "dun fish" which was much in demand among the epicures of Europe and brought three times the profit of dried cod. Frequent trips to Kittery Point brought him into contact with John Bray, an English shipwright and boatbuilder who had established a yard there in the 1660's.

In 1682 he moved to the mainland, at Kittery Point. Here, having married Bray's daughter Margery, he laid the foundation of one of the earliest fortunes in America. Here today stands what remains of the beautiful Pepperell mansion. His is said to have been the largest commercial establishment in New England prior to the Revolution. There were stores, warehouses, building yard, gardens, a deer park, and the inevitable block house for defense against marauding Frenchmen and Indians.

The fisheries were the most extensive and the most lucrative part of "The William Pepperells" business. The firm kept a hundred or more boats on the banks. Their cargoes rarely failed to return a profit, whether they went to the South to be exchanged for corn, tobacco, and naval stores, to the West Indies for molasses and tropical products, or to England, Spain, and Portugal for dry goods, salt, iron, cordage, wines, and fruit. William Pepperell's six daughters shared their father's trading ability and often sent adventures to England and the West Indies in the form of fish and furs for exchange for the dresses and finery which are dear to the heart of a woman. Bills of sale have survived which show their ownership of shares in the Pepperell fleet.

Those engaged in the fisheries along the coast in these early days lived in fear of attacks by the Indians. One of their prominent chiefs was a savage known by the unpleasant name of Mugg. At Ticonic Falls he is reputed to have told his braves: "I know that we can even burn Boston and carry all the country before us, but to do this we must go to the fishing islands and take all the white men's vessels." The Indians were neither sailors nor good oarsmen. None the less they stealthily entered the harbors after nightfall, and coming upon the fishers unaware, they succeeded in capturing in the month of July 1677 some twenty fishing vessels on the coast from Wells to Casco Bay. The bulk of these hailed from Salem. A large vessel was equipped as a man-of-war and sent out from there to retake the prizes. This was easily accomplished, for the ketches had already been stripped and abandoned. The savages had found them too heavy to be managed with paddles, and they did not understand the use of sails.

A more serious outrage occurred in 1724. Again the Indians

appeared suddenly on the seacoast and seized all the vessels they could find. In a few weeks' time they took twenty-two vessels —two shallops on the Isles of Shoals, eight fishing vessels taken in Fox Island Thoroughfare, one large schooner armed with two swivels, and twelve other craft surprised in various places. In these piratical attacks they killed twenty or more men and took many more prisoners. These latter were the masters and the more skillful seamen. The savages compelled them to navigate this ill-assorted squadron. Then with the help of the Micmacs of Cape Sable they terrorized all who sailed along the eastern coast. Several underarmed expeditions were sent against them. It was not until three vessels manned by sailors and commanded by officers of the man-of-war *Seahorse*, then on the Boston Station, were sent out that the Indians tired of naval warfare and disappeared.

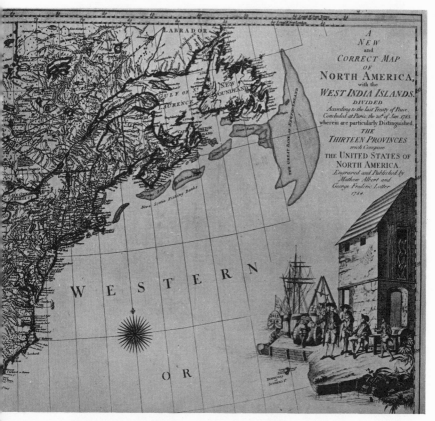

The North Atlantic Coast, the fishing grounds, and a vignette of the early West India trade—1784. *Courtesy Dudley C. Lunt.*

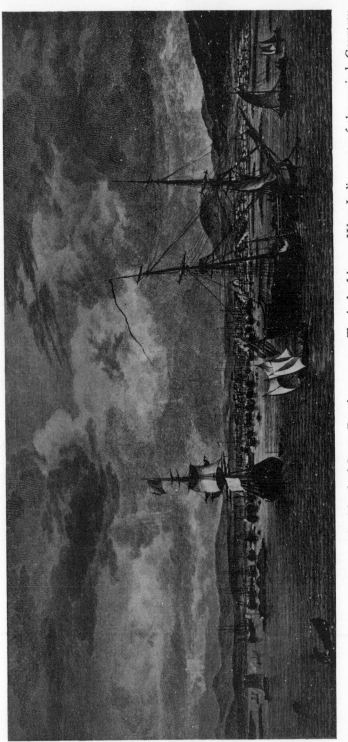

The anchorage at Port au Prince in the island of Santo Domingo—1780. Typical of larger West India ports of the period. *Courtesy Dudley C. Lunt.*

CHAPTER THREE

The KING'S BROAD
ARROW

There is also the very good newes comes of four New England ships come home safe to Falmouth with masts for the
King; which is a blessing mighty unexpected, and with out
which, if for nothing else, we must have failed the next year.
But God be praised for thus much good fortune, and send
up the continuance of his favor in other things! So to bed.—
The Diary of Samuel Pepys, December 3, 1666.

THE COAST OF MAINE was the easterly border of the vast tract
of forest land which for nearly a century and a half was to furnish the Royal Navy with great masts. It formed a part of the
unbroken forest which skirted the Atlantic coast from the
Straits of Belle Isle to the Rio de la Plata. The portion which
came to be known as the white pine belt bordered the sea from
Nova Scotia to New Hampshire and reached back into the
country west of the Connecticut and Hudson rivers.

The earliest record of taking a mast on this coast was on
Henry Hudson's first voyage in 1609, when he cut and stepped
a foremast in the *Half Moon* in the southern part of Penobscot
Bay. Other voyagers than Captain Smith were impressed more
by its growth of timber than by its "mynes of gold and cop-
per." Almost every early account stresses its value to the Royal
Navy as a source of oak and pine. Thus, as Rosier relates,
Waymouth found at the mouth of the St. George's River in

[33]

1605 "spruce trees of excellent timber and height able to mast ships of great burden." Oak he also mentions, but not pine, for this is a fir country. On the Camden and Union hills he observed "notable high timber trees, masts for ships of four hundred tons." It was from this region that England received her first cargo of masts. These were cut in the summer of 1634 and shipped in the *Hercules* of Dover. Attracted by this rich and gigantic forest growth, it was customary for many English vessels returning from Massachusetts to head east in order to cut and ship their return cargo on the shores of Maine.

With the approaching depletion of England's native growths her shipbuilders turned first to the Baltic region for naval timber and masts. Then the Dutch wars of the seventeenth century all but cut off this supply. Great masts had been brought from New England to the English dockyards, but there was no system co-ordinating supply and demand. The quotation at the head of this chapter is evidence of the anxiety of the Lords of the Admiralty as reflected in this entry of their clerk in his famous diary. In desperate straits, England turned to the colonies, and in 1652 there began a regular supply of these great sticks that were to furnish the largest masts of the Royal Navy for a century and a quarter.

This business of furnishing masts is reflected in curious connections. In 1665 the General Court of Massachusetts softened its refusal at the behest of the Commissioners of the Crown to furnish troops for a proposed attack on the French by a resolution to present to the King the best commodity the colony afforded for the accommodation of the Royal Navy. This turned out to be masts. Of the cargo sent two years later a part was from the Maine woods. Two of the committee were Captains Clark and Lake. Since 1650 they had been carrying on an extensive business at Arrowsic in fur, lumber, and shipbuilding. The two great masts which they delivered to Sir William Warren were indeed royal. They measured 101¼ and 100 feet in length, and crosswise at the butt 36½ and 38 inches.

The first step taken by the Crown to control the forests in the interest of British sea power was the appointment in 1685 of a Surveyor of Pine and Timber. Edward Randolph's commission called for a survey of the Maine woods within ten miles of any navigable river. He began at the Penobscot and reported large fir trees—20 to 34 inches in diameter—on Mount Desert Island and the Sheepscot. There was an almost untouched tract on the Kennebec where forty or fifty vessels might load with pine or fir and masts, boards, and plank. Good trees were to be had along the rivers from the Kennebec westward to the Piscataqua, but here "the saw mills had made great havoc in the tymber." From Pemaquid south he found "vast, very vast quantities of oak tymber, both straight and compass," and near-by convenient places where sixty sail of from 200 to 500 tons might be built yearly.

This was soon followed by a restriction placed in the new charter of Massachusetts in 1691. There was a reservation to the Crown of all white pine with a diameter of twenty-four inches at a foot above the ground, standing on any land not previously granted to a private individual. A penalty of £100 was imposed for the felling of such trees without a royal license. A surveyor was appointed for the province, and the forests near the coast were carefully surveyed. Then it was that all trees suitable for masts or bowsprits were blazed with the King's broad arrow. With his marking hatchet the surveyor made three cuts through the bark, resembling the barbed head of an arrow or the track of a crow, the ancient sign of naval property.

Up to the outbreak of the Indian wars, which laid waste the eastern towns of the province, many cargoes of masts and other ship timber were cut along the Maine rivers for the dockyards in England and those at Jamaica and Antigua as well. For a long time, because of the influence of the Wentworths, Benning and his nephew John, who successively held the office of surveyor, the trade centered at Portsmouth. Thus in the seventeenth century the "Piscataway" furnished most of the great masts for the Royal Navy. As early as 1700, however, it was necessary to go twenty miles back into the country to find a good mast. This distance increased year by year until the mountain ranges of New Hampshire presented an insurmountable barrier. Then the choppers extended their operations toward the east, and in 1727 Falmouth on Casco Bay, the site of present-day Portland, became a regular shipping port for the King's masts. Dunstans Landing at the head of the Scarborough Marshes was also a mast depot.

This lucrative business meant much to Falmouth and was of great benefit in building up the commercial enterprises of the town. A Boston paper, the *New England Weekly Journal*, of May 8, 1727, observed, "Captain Farles in one of the mast ships now lays at Casco Bay, who, we hear, is not a little pleased with the commodiousness of that fine harbor to carry on said business. And as this must tend very much to encourage settlements in those parts of the country, especially the flourishing bay that will be the center of it; so there is no reason to fear but that our government will in their wisdom, look upon it very much to their interest to protect and encourage it."

The Admiralty did not buy its masts and timber direct, but through contractors, who in turn had mast agents in New England. There were four of these who were well known in Maine—Samuel Waldo, Thomas Westbrook, George Tate, and Edward Parry. A typical establishment was that of Thomas Westbrook at Stroudwater on Fore River in back of Portland. Here the site of his mast landing is today clearly revealed by the three main streets of the village. The roads from a wide surrounding region converge toward this landing. Over them the enormous white pines of Cumberland County were "baulked"—that is, dragged from the woods to the waterside. From here they were floated down to the mast houses nearer the harbor where they were hewed "sixteen sides" and loaded on the waiting mast ships.

The business steadily extended eastward. Not even the danger from hostile Indians was allowed to interfere with it. Bands of soldiers guarded the cutters and teamsters along the banks of the Presumpscot and on the shores of Sebago Lake. One of the finest stands of white pine lay between the waters of the Little Androscoggin and the upper sources of Royall's River. From this region the masts were floated down to the landings in Yarmouth, or baulked to Mast Landing on Harraseket River in Freeport. The peculiar shape of Freeport's town square today bears witness to the room needed to turn these great sticks. At the landing a block house was built of rejected masts to shelter the soldiers stationed there. This structure was still standing a few years ago. At these smaller stations either the mast ships called to take on their cargo, or the masts, carefully lashed together, were towed along the shore to the larger harbor at Falmouth.

In the month of September 1687, Samuel Sewall, on a visit to Salmon Falls, made the following record in his journal: "Ride into a swamp to see a mast drawn of about twenty-six inches or twenty-eight; about two and thirty oxen before, and about four yoke by the side of the mast between the fore and hinder wheels. 'Twas a notable sight."

When we remember that the trees were often three feet in diameter at the butt and sometimes a hundred and twenty feet in height, the skill required to fell these great columns can be appreciated. Frequently each was worth five hundred dollars, and a slight error of judgment by the axmen might ruin the tree for use as a mast. Then the loss would be borne by the contractor. The time usually chosen for cutting was when the snow was deep, filling the hollows and covering the knolls. A bed was prepared by leveling all the inequalities in the ground and bedding down the place with other trees, whose springy branches would soften and break the violence of the thundering fall.

The hauling or "baulking" of these huge sticks to the nearest waterway called for great skill and heavy labor on the part of the mastmen. For a description we turn to the now forgotten pages of Elijah Kellogg. A sailor in his youth, he was for many years pastor of the Mariners' Church and Sailors' Home in Boston and of the Harpswell Church, the members of which to a man followed the sea. His name was a byword in American homes two generations ago. His stories for boys contain an authentic record of life along the Maine coast and in the fisheries and the West India trade. Thus does he tell of the "baulking" of masts in the Township of Gorham in *Good Old Times:*

> The party had in the first place to break the road with heavy sleds, it being all the oxen could do to get through the deep snow; then they took light loads of the small spars which they continued to haul for some days, in the meantime carefully examining the road, cutting off all roots that projected into it, putting poles in soft places and treading down the snow into them that they might freeze and make a hard road and making all necessary bridges in the gulleys till all the way was hard and smooth as glass. They now put a bowsprit on to try, which from its different shape was much less difficult to haul than a mast. As the road bore this without slumping they now loaded one of the large masts. Men were stationed by the middle cattle to keep them from getting down or getting the chain over their backs in crossing gullies or knolls; for they were sometimes hung up by the neck for a moment and a chain straightened over a creatures back would break it instantly. Men were also stationed by the sled with ropes to keep it from turning bottom up.

The King's Broad Arrow

The government paid a bounty of £1 a ton, that is, for fifty cubic feet of rough or forty of hewn timber. So profitable was the work that many of the new settlers spent their time "masting" to the neglect of their farms and brought famine on themselves. In 1770 the price paid for the largest masts, 36 inches at the butt and 36 yards long, was £110. Bowsprits 38 inches by 25 yards long brought £48, and yards 25 inches by 35 yards, £25. It will be noticed that masts were so hewed that they measured as many yards long as they were inches at the butt. The size of these masts from New England made a deep impression on the shipwrights of the great English dockyards of Deptford, Woolwich, Chatham, Sheerness, Plymouth, and Portsmouth. So large were they that one of them served to make a lower mast for a first-rate ship of the line. This was far better than the largest sticks of Baltic fir, which had to be pieced together and formed into a made mast.

Their great size required especially constructed mast ships for their conveyance, and these were often built in the colonies. It is known that one was built in Falmouth in 1734, and others followed. They were usually from 400 to 600 tons burden, but at least one is reported to have measured 1,000 tons. They were built with large ports for taking in their bulky cargo and could carry from fifty to a hundred of the largest sticks, as well as many other pieces—bowsprits, yards, spars, oar rafters, etc.

The arrival and departure of a mast ship was an event to be recorded in the diaries of the day, for they served almost as the regular liners of the period, bringing passengers, troops, freight, and mail. So important were they and their cargoes that they were often convoyed by a frigate to protect them from French privateers or Dutch capers. In 1772, Maine had taken the lead in the trade over Portsmouth. In that year 382 masts, 69 bowsprits, and 451 spars were shipped. As a side line to this a great lumber business was built up that continued to flourish long after the separation. Shipbuilding was also encouraged.

The protection of the trees bearing the King's mark was particularly difficult in Maine. In the first place, there was a long dispute as to whether the words "private property" in the exception exempting trees which stood on tracts of land granted before October 7, 1690, did or did not apply to all the forests in Maine. The contention was that they were included in the private grants which Massachusetts had purchased from the Gorges heirs. Furthermore, the proceeds from the lumber from the smaller trees were greater than the fees paid for the great masts, and those whose living depended on lumbering and milling could not wait for the mast pines to be cut. Then, too, other settlers who wished to clear the land found that the great trees occupied ground needed for agriculture.

Thus reports went repeatedly to the Navy Board similar to this one in 1747, that "to the eastward at York, Wells, Kenibunk, Saco, Scarborough, Casco Bay, Keinbeck and Pemquid they cut and saw at pleasure and send them where they choose." Or this from Scammel, writing from Falmouth as late as 1772: "Shingle and clapboard makers are the greatest destroyers of white pines, for extremely delicate in their choices, they chop into great trees to see if they split well continuing this illegal process until they find such as are suitable. The trees thus wounded soon perish, to the great detriment of His Majestie's navy."

Many and devious were the means used by the settlers to defy the King's officers and destroy the marked trees. Mysteriously kindled fires burned them and made them unfit for masts. All the smaller growth would be cleared from around them. Then, being exposed to the full force of the wind, they were soon uprooted and ruined. When sawed into lumber they were carefully cut down so that the width of the boards would not furnish evidence of illegal cutting. This fact one may verify for himself by searching houses built prior to the Revolution for floor or roof boards more than twenty-three inches in width.

Deputy surveyors attempted to surprise the choppers at work in the woods, and they searched in the mill ponds and shipping ports for logs scaling the damning twenty-four inches. But they had little success in enforcing the law. John Wentworth, who succeeded his uncle Benning as Surveyor General, was a conscientious administrator. By his good sense, pleasing personality, and tact, he came the nearest to succeeding. An American born and bred, he knew how to deal with frontiersmen, and he gained their respect and obedience.

In the country that surrounded and lay back of Casco Bay great fires in 1761 and again in 1762 destroyed vast quantities of the finest timber on the pine stands that were furnishing masts. The fire of 1761 burst out early in July in the New Hampshire woods. Driven by the wind toward the east, it traversed many of the back towns and entered Scarboro, Gorham, and at last New Casco—the present Falmouth—where it was extinguished by a flood of rain after it had raged uncontrolled for nearly two months. The following year six houses, two sawmills, and several barns were destroyed in Scarboro and six families burned out in ancient North Yarmouth. There extensive fenced fields were destroyed by the flames, which were so violent that the cattle in the pastures could not escape. This was the beginning of the end of the masting business in this vicinity. Then the regions farther east were developed for this trade.

In song and story British "walls of oak" are synonymous with the strength of her navy. With the red oak of the English hedgerows "unwedgeable and gnarled," American white oak could never compete. The early builders were unaccountably neglectful of that finest of ship timber, southern live oak. But when this was built into "Old Ironsides" the English were soon convinced of its quality. The white oak from Casco Bay that Surveyor General Bridger sent early in the eighteenth century to the English dockyards as a sample received an unfavorable official report. It did not have the required firmness and weight; it did not have enough compass (i.e., curved) pieces, for it grew in thickets and was therefore too straight; it rotted in transportation, et cetera, et cetera. When English oak was scarce about 1740, the Naval Board used a few cargoes. This, with the supply sent from Casco Bay during the Seven Years' War, comprised about all that was used by the Royal Navy. The *Faulkland* and the *Bedford Galley*, built at Kittery in the 1690's, were also disparaged. However, the former was in active service until 1768 and the latter did not disappear from the records until around 1723.

The very existence of the North American forests played a vital part in the struggles for Continental supremacy in the eighteenth century. Louis XIV protested that the cession of Maine would ruin the commerce and navy of France. The relative position of Britain, bottomed as always upon sea power and maritime commerce, depended in large measure upon the forests of Maine. This dependence in the day of the wooden ship was an element of weakness during the American Revolution and constituted an important factor in the outcome of the seven years' struggle for American independence. This was clearly apparent to the members of the First Continental Congress in 1774.

The enforcement after Concord and Lexington of their predetermined policy of nonintercourse with Great Britain immediately deprived the Royal Navy of its supply of yards and masts, upon which it had depended since Cromwell's time. In Boston all the spars and naval stores collected on Noddle Island were burned. At Portsmouth three hundred patriots towed the masts up the Piscataqua out of the reach of H.M.S. *Scarborough,* which was in port to receive them. The men of Georgetown, now Bath, surprised the ax men at work at the King's dock and commanded them "in the name of the people of America, not to strike another blow." Then they drove them to the transports waiting below.

It was Falmouth, now Portland, that suffered under British retaliation for such measures. In June 1775, two ships came into the harbor with orders from Admiral Graves to secure all the masts possible. They, of course, had been towed out of reach. On seeking to load in the Presumpscot River, the British encountered an aroused citizenry who seized their boats, guns, and men. Thus the mast ships were forced to sail without a cargo. Admiral Graves warned a prisoner, Captain Philip Crandall of Harpswell, that if the masts were not given up he would "beat the town down about their ears." In October this threat was made good. Captain Mowatt and his fleet bombarded the town of Falmouth and reduced it to ashes.

The news of Bunker Hill and the last cargo of colonial masts reached England at about the same time. Strong arguments were heard in Parliament for retaining the source of supply. The necessity of holding as much of Maine as possible for this purpose was the chief factor in the British occupation of Castine throughout the Revolution. The interest of Britain in the Penobscot country was to be evidenced a generation later by her occupation of Castine again in 1814. Disappointed in both instances, however, she was forced to turn to the pine forests east of the St. John.

Many a famous man-of-war crossed Maine spars alow and aloft. The *Victory,* Nelson's flagship at Trafalgar, had Maine-grown masts. Then there is the frigate *Constitution,* popularly known as *Old Ironsides.* With a keel of white oak from New Jersey, timbers of live oak and red cedar from Georgia, she was equipped with white pine masts from Maine. These sticks were cut in the town of Windsor on the north side of the Augusta road, between Cooper's Mills and Bryant's Corner and within half a mile of the corner. Thomas Cooper of Newcastle and one Gray, who afterward settled in Windsor or Whitefield, cut the trees. Then they swamped a road to Puddle Dock in Alna in the winter of 1796–97, and hauled them into the Sheepscot. In the lumberman's vernacular, to swamp a trail or road is to clear it. In the spring they were floated down to Wiscasset, where government agents yoked them at both ends with pieces of white oak, slipped through mortices in the three trees. They were towed to Boston, where, on the twentieth of September, 1797, the frigate was launched.

The American Revolution rendered King George's broad arrow meaningless. France then became a good market for American masts. The Minister of Finance, Calonne, abolished all duties on ship timber, and the old masting ports took a new lease on life. Masts were brought to these ports from all the forest-lined rivers of Maine. In the latter days of wooden men-of-war all the navies of the world flew their pennants at the peak of a Maine mast. The great white pine became more and more difficult to find, and as early as 1820 those cruising the woods for masts were forced to travel deep into the forests to find proper timber.

CHAPTER FOUR

SHIPBUILDING *in* COLONIAL MAINE

SIR: With much trouble I have gotten men and sent them for the sloop, and desire you to dispatch them with all speed, for, if all things be ready they may be fitted to leave in two days as well as seven years. If you and the carpenter think it convenient and the ground has not too much descent, I think it may be safer to bend the sails before you launch her, so that you may be able to leave immediately. But I shall leave it to your management and desire you to hasten them day and night; for, Sir, it will be dangerous tarrying there on account of hostile savages in the vicinity and it will be very expensive to keep the men on pay. I send you a barrel of rum and there is a cask of wine to launch with. So with my services to yourself and lady hoping they are all in good health, as I am at present, who am your humble servant at command.—*William Pepperell to Captain John Hill at Saco, Nov. 12, 1696.*

WITH A SURE MARKET in the ports of Europe and the West Indies for their fish and for the furs brought downriver by Indians eager to "truck," the settlers along the shore of Maine soon turned to shipbuilding on a considerable scale. Indeed, shrewd merchants found that there should be at their stations at least one man skilled in the building and rigging of ships.

Any account of shipbuilding in colonial Maine must of necessity be fragmentary. Very few records remain to tell of the number of craft built along the shore, for local use and foreign sale. How numerous they were may be judged from the fact that even in the bloody years of Indian warfare from 1693 to 1714, when the entire coast east of Wells was laid waste, forty-seven vessels of 30 tons and more were launched in Kittery and York alone. A plentiful supply of timber handy to the waterside, low wages, and a work day lasting from sunup to sundown gave an advantage to our builders that much disturbed the master carpenters of England. On more than one occasion they petitioned Parliament not to encourage shipbuilding in the colonies.

The record of the first ship has survived. At the mouth of the Kennebec in the summer of 1607 the Plymouth Company had established a settlement. In the company of adventurers was one Digby, a London shipwright. On the twenty-first of August, one day after the work on the settlement was commenced, he gathered about him those men who were familiar with shipbuilding and began to cut timber for the construction of a small craft. This was the first vessel to be built by Englishmen in the New World. She is believed to have been launched early in September, for on a plan of the settlement drawn by one of the colonists on the eighth there is to be seen under the guns of the fort a representation of a vessel thought to be the "pretty pinnace *Virginia*."

Although of but 30 tons burden, the *Virginia* of Sagadahoc justified the foresight of the Plymouth proprietors. She was used for voyages up- and downriver and on coastwise trips to collect furs for the *Mary and John* to take back to England. After the departure of the larger vessel, she made longer voyages, one as far south as the Jamestown settlement, with that New England staple, salted cod. In the spring of 1608, when the colony was finally given up, she set sail in company with the *Gift of God* for Plymouth, with a cargo of furs and sassafras root. Then for some twenty years she plied between England and Virginia until, returning with a cargo of tobacco, she was wrecked on the Irish coast.

In the early fragmentary allusions to the Maine coast there is a hint that about 1620 George Richmond built a vessel on the Island, off Cape Elizabeth, which bears his name and where he headed up an enterprise employing shipbuilders and fishermen. Much more is known of the building there of the bark *Richmond* seventeen years later by John Winter, who was agent for the proprietors, Trelawny and Goodyear. This little vessel, of 25 or 30 tons burden, was built and launched early in 1637. She sailed at once to Massachusetts Bay with a cargo of wine, oil, and earthenware. Under Captain Narius Hawkins she had an adventurous life in the coasting trade sailing "for the Bay, or the Dutch plantation or Keynetticot," and as far south as Chesapeake Bay. In the summer of 1639 he was sent across from Casco Bay to England with a cargo of pipe staves. These staves were made of oak for the great puncheons or casks used for the storage of wines and long known as pipes. We catch some glimpses of her for a few years in the Public Record Office of London, until she was confiscated for the use of Parliament along with the other property of the cavalier, Robert Trelawny.

Shipbuilding was apparently intended to be one of the regular industries of Richmond's Island, for in 1640 Stephen Sargent, Winter's master builder, was drawing the plans of a ship to be called the *Richmond* to take the place of the bark. The work on the vessel went slowly, on account of the lack of skilled labor, and it was two years before she was launched. However, when she slid into the water in July, 1641, her builder was pleased. He wrote home to England, "She swimbed as upright as might be when she was launched and was very stiff on her side." Her dimensions are given as 50-foot keel and 18½ foot to the beam. She had two decks, a forecastle and quarterdeck, a 9-foot hold and 4½ feet between decks. The first cargo was put in as soon as the deck was caulked and while the carpenters were finishing the vessel. It consisted of salt fish, traine, i.e., fish oil, and "fish peas." Under the command of her builder, Stephen Sargent, she sailed for Bilbao, Spain.

The trading posts or "truck houses" established along the coast and on the rivers in the seventeenth century trafficked in fish, furs, and lumber. One of the largest and most active was that of Thomas Clark and Thomas Lake of Boston, set up around "Arowsick Town" on the Sheepscot River in the 1650's. It was a large undertaking. Saw and grist mills were in operation, and a large stockaded fort was built with bakehouses, smithies, and cooper shops. Workmen came there for permanent settlement with their families and cattle. The cost of the establishment has been estimated to be £20,000. Here at Spring Point on the Sassanoa River several boats and vessels were fitted out, victualed, and loaded for Boston and other ports. It was in this yard that Maine's distinguished shipbuilder, William Phipps, made his start as an apprentice.

Born on what is still known as Phipps' Point in the present town of Woolwich, young Phipps, after spending a few years in the Clark and Lake yard, went to Boston and spent four years with the builders in the yards there. His character and ability were such that he won the confidence of a group of Boston merchants, who contracted with him to build a vessel. He returned to Maine, where he knew he would find every kind of timber needed near at hand. The vessel had been launched and was nearly finished when the Indian outbreak of 1676 fell upon the Maine settlements. One of the first attacks was upon Arrowsic Fort, not more than two miles from young Phipps' yard. The completion of the vessel was rushed, the workmen and the Phipps family hurried aboard, sails were bent, and the vessel carried its builders out of Hocamock Bay and

The Log of the *Dash*—September 7-8, 1813. *Original in Maine Historical Society.*

[Remarks on Tuesday, Sept. 7th: "Commences with pleasant weather. At 1 PM sent up the royal yard & set the sail. At 3 PM saw a sail to the S. & W. At 4 she had got nearly in our wake. At 5 PM she bore down before the wind and gave chase with a press of sail. She proved to be a schooner. Still kept on our course all hands to quarters. At 8 PM lost sight of her. At 9 PM jibed ship & shifted studding sails. At 2 AM heard a gun fired on the larb. quarter & directly after a false fire & blue lights were shown astern. At 5 AM discovered 3 men of war in chase of us, one on the larb. quarter & 2 on the starb. quarter about 3 miles distant. Made all sail before the wind. At 9 had seen one of them out of sight. At 11 the 2nd gave up the chase being about 8 miles dist.; the other still in chase about 6 miles distant. Weather very squally & variable accompanied with rain. At ½ past 11 AM hove over the spare topmast, gaff & jibboom & made & shortened sail occasionally." **Remarks on Wednesday, Sept. 8th:** "Begins with strong breezes from the N. & W. Found we left the chase very fast. At 4 observed her to take in her light sails, reef her topsails & haul on a wind. At 5 PM lost sight of her. Took in some of our light sails. At 6 PM 3 reefed the mainsail. Mid part squally with rain. Made & shortened sail occasionally. At 5 AM saw a sail on the starb. beam standing on a wind to the W——. Ends pleasant"]

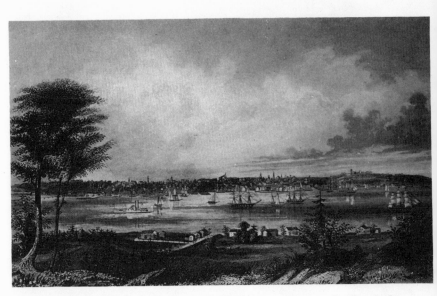

Portland from Purpooduck (South Portland)—1850. *Courtesy Dudley C. Lunt.*

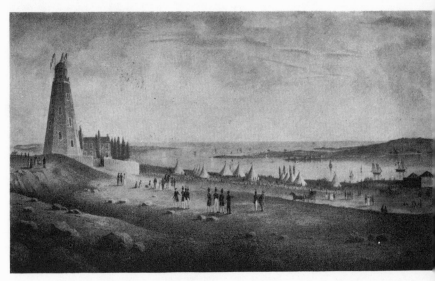

The main ship channel from the Observatory on Munjoy Hill, Portland—1830. *From a painting by Charles Codman.*

down the Sheepscot to safety. Phipps went on to fame and fortune, which included retrieving a treasure lost on a Spanish galleon off the Bahamas, becoming Governor of Massachusetts, and being knighted by King James.

★　★　★

At the western end of the Maine settlements a similar development took place at the mouth of the Piscataqua river. Here a straight channel free of shoals, six fathoms and more deep, and a quarter mile wide, leads into a long tidewater basin, the shores of which are nearly one hundred miles long. Near the head of it the name Pipe Stave Landing attests its antiquity. Its broad, deep mouth is today flanked by Portsmouth to the westward and the Navy yard at Kittery Point to the eastward. This body of water saw the native development of a type of river craft both indigenous and unique. This was the gundalow.

It developed out of the use in the early days of a flat-bottomed square-ended scow propelled by poles. Then a rudder, generally with a tiller, was added, platforms were built at each end, and there appeared a square sail hung on a removable mast. The final model and definite type was a spoon-bowed, round-sterned vessel, completely decked over and capable of some 35 tons of cargo, though she drew but 12 to 16 inches when light and up to 4½ feet when laden. Her top hamper was a high peaked lateen sail. This was just the thing to catch the uncertain breezes which came in gusts from the hills down through the high irregular banks.

This sail was bent to a long yard hung on a rotating stump mast about ten feet high and so arranged with tackle and counterweights that it could easily be lowered to pass under a bridge. With one or more large lee boards a gundalow could make good time even to windward or against the current; down one tide and back with the next was her rule of thumb. For generations and up into the present century this picturesque gundalow was the common carrier here and on all tidal rivers that sweep, now shallow, now deep, in and out of the marshes and flats on this eastern coast. In the time of Sarah Orne Jewett some twenty-odd gundalows were owned at Pipe Stave Landing in South Berwick.

It was here at the mouth of the Piscataqua that the firm which came to be known at its height as "The William Pepperells" early combined shipbuilding with fishing. The founder of the family, William, had started as an apprenticed fisherman. His son became a baronet. They built ships on both the Piscataqua and the Saco, as the letter at the head of this chapter bears witness. At the headwaters of the Piscataqua were great forests from which seemingly inexhaustible stores of lumber were floated down to the Point. The ease with which ironwork, cordage, and canvas could be brought here made Kittery an ideal location for shipbuilding. Its population increased faster than that of any other town in the province, and by 1746 it was paying nearly one-half the tax assessed for the whole province of Maine.

The William Pepperells built up a princely fortune by an ingenious cycle of operations, each bearing a profit. The lumber and carpenter work in their building yards was paid for out of their own stores of merchandise, provisions or English goods acquired by sale or exchange in their voyages. Often the proceeds of a voyage would be deposited with bankers in Plymouth or London. Then bills of exchange would be drawn on them in favor of Boston merchants who were glad to buy them at a considerable advance, the Pepperells taking their pay either in goods to replenish their stores or in provincial money. This money in turn was used to purchase at a low price real estate that was rapidly increasing in value. So extensively did they buy that it is said that their landed estate was larger than any other in America, with the exception of those of the royal patentees, such as the Penns or the Fairfaxes. It has been said that William Pepperell could travel from the Piscataqua to the Saco without stepping off his own soil.

Any account of the Pepperells is incomplete without a reference to the famous expedition against Louisburg, on the southeast side of Cape Breton Island. Here the French had spent a vast sum in fortifying this naturally commanding position. One of the strongest fortresses in the world, hardly surpassed by Quebec or Gibraltar, it effectually blocked the entrance to the St. Lawrence to any English vessel, afforded a base for French squadrons which might threaten the ports of the Atlantic coast, and sheltered privateers that gave the greatest possible annoyance to the eastern colonists and especially to the fishing fleets. "Louisburg must be destroyed" was a slogan which deepened into a war cry along the Maine coast in the winter of 1744–45.

When the call to arms came, Maine responded with two regiments numbering nearly three thousand men, which were quickly raised along shore from Kittery to the Sheepscot. Colonel William Pepperell was put in command, a choice demanded by his character, energy, good judgment, and personality. He contributed £5,000 toward the expedition. The fleet, consisting of thirteen vessels carrying 204 guns, was under the command of Captain Edward Tyng, a merchant of Falmouth, as Commodore. To the rendezvous in Nantasket Roads in Boston Harbor there came from all the little towns along the coast sloops filled with men. Some eighty transports in all carried the troops on to Louisburg. What was at first regarded as a "mad scheme" became a brilliant victory that "struck the civilized world dumb with amazement."

The Louisburg expedition is an integral part of the maritime history of Maine. The scheme was conceived and fostered by William Vaughan, whose lumbering and fishing operations on the Damariscotta River identify him with the Maine Coast. Its commander, Colonel Pepperell, the District's first citizen, received a commission as Colonel in the British Army and in consequence of the destruction of Louisburg was created a baronet. In addition to Commodore Tyng, the third in command was General Samuel Waldo, who also was a prominent figure on the Maine Coast.

In those early days there were others besides the Pepperells building ships on the Piscataqua. The first William's father-in-law, John Bray, was well established there as early as 1660. Upriver at Crooked Lane, Robert Cutts—who lived like a lord, it is said, and employed slaves in his yard—built for the fisheries and the West India trade. After his death his yard was continued by his son Richard. In the next century the names of John Diamond, William Tytherly, Peter Dixon, and Samuel Winkley figure in this calling.

Men-of-war have been built there for over two hundred and fifty years. To sustain the heavy losses in their successive struggles with the French, the British Admiralty initiated the policy of constructing naval vessels where ship timber was near at hand. The frigate *Falkland*, of 637 tons, the first ship of war to be built on this side of the Atlantic, was launched in 1690 here from Badger's Island yard. In 1690 she was followed by the galley *Bedford*, of 372 tons, mounting 32 guns. These were the first of the long line of naval construction which has lasted into our own time. It is claimed that up to the time of the Civil War more government vessels were built on the Maine shore of the Piscataqua than at any other place on the continent.

Many a provincial shipbuilder laid his keel and built his vessel on the shore surrounded with growing timber, from which he cut, so to speak, both ship and cargo. He and his men often did their day's work in constant fear of an Indian attack. Near Wells in June 1692, the crews of two vessels numbering fourteen men armed with muskets staved off an attack of French and Indians of several times their number. From 1676, despite successive treaties, the settlements in western Maine from the Piscataqua to the Kennebec were time and again overrun and destroyed by the savages. None the less, throughout this period vessels were successfully built and launched, often under the protection of armed guards.

In 1713 the peace of Utrecht marked the close of forty years of this intermittent barbarous warfare. In the comparative peace that followed, the settlements of western Maine began anew. Indeed, in some instances villages were rebuilt for the third time. With this came a resurgence in the fisheries, the traffic in furs, and dealing in lumber—then the three staples of early Maine commerce.

By 1736 the fishermen numbered some six hundred men. With the Indians in retreat into Canada, the "truck houses" pushed year after year farther up the rivers. In lumber, in addition to the masting trade with England, there was a ready market in Caribbean and European ports for pipe staves, boards, shingles, and ship timber. Hence the demand for ships. All along the shore was to be heard the ring of the broadax, the tapping of the caulker's mallet, and the rush of the launching vessel.

There were building at one time on the Maine Coast in the year 1742 forty "topsail vessels." By this phrase is meant the square-rigged, in contradistinction to the schooner-rigged, vessel, or fore-and-after, as it was generally called in the early days. A complete picture of this industry is an impossibility. Although contract building was not unknown, the construction of a ship was usually a man's own affair. It should be borne in mind that railroads and highways were nonexistent and that the few roads were little more than trails. The great bulk of transportation was water-borne in the sloops, shallops, schooners, and brigs of the day. The building of a vessel on the shores of a farm, the produce of which it would later take to market, was no more to be noticed than is the acquisition of a truck today.

This early maritime activity in the District in colonial times was the forerunner of the shipbuilding which in the nineteenth century became the outstanding aspect of the State of Maine's share in the American merchant marine. Any organized or consistently kept records that there may have been in these early days are now simply non-existent. Such records do not begin until after the establishment of the federal government and the erection of customs districts. The picture must be assessed and pieced together from sporadic entries in diaries and manuscripts. For example, with respect to Falmouth—the site of the modern city of Portland—in the eighteenth century, a valuable source of information is the Journal of the Reverend Thomas Smith, covering the years from 1720 to 1787. In March 1727 Parson Smith recorded: "About this time Mr. Reddin came down with a considerable quantity of goods to build a sloop." Five months later he reports that the "sloop built before my door was launched to-day." Since he lived at the foot of King, now India, Street, where Clay Cove made up to the foot of the street, the location is established.

This site is now lost, a circumstance which illustrates the difficulty in reconstructing the maritime past of a water front. Clay Cove has long since been filled in. This is true of the entire water front in the modern city of Portland. In 1850, in order to give railroad connection between the eastern and western parts of the city, a granite retaining wall was constructed and the space within it was filled in. The right of way created was given the name of Commercial Street.

Thus at one stroke all the little coves and breastworks where so many vessels had been built were wiped out. Here had been "the black wharves and the slips" of Longfellow's "Lost Youth." Today the water's edge is practically straight. To trace the original water front one must pass along the winding turns of Fore Street, many rods inland, which originally followed the shore line.

The Clay Cove yard was the property of Lemuel and Ezekiel Dyer. Lemuel lived in a large house at the head of the shipyard and actually built and launched his vessels in his own back yard. The master carpenter was James Gooding, whose name was known in the trade for over half a century. Among those whom he trained were James Milk and Samuel Cobb, who were famous shipbuilders in the mid-eighteenth century.

The town was situated on a promontory which in those days was all but surrounded by water, and which was known as the Neck. There were yards at Stroudwater on the shores of Fore River, at Ferry Village, which is now South Portland, and on around along the shores of Casco Bay. A contemporary affidavit on file in a lawsuit refers unmistakably to a shipyard on Royall's River in Yarmouth as early as 1740. At about the same time John Lemont was building small vessels on his farm at New Meadows. At Middle Bay one Robert Dunning is known to have been building before the Revolution. One of the first entries on the Register in Bath is of the schooner *Betsey*. She was built at Harpswell in 1781.

The tonnage owned in Falmouth amounted to 1,367 tons in 1752. This comprised seven schooners and fifteen sloops, the largest being 80 tons. In the following year it dropped to 1,344 tons, including a 100-ton brig. Twenty years later the total was 2,020 tons, and the year following it rose to 2,555. The prominent shipowners of the period comprised such names as Jedediah Peeble, Enoch Ilsley, Jeremiah Pote, Benjamin Titcomb, Robert Pagan, Simon Mayo, and Thomas Sanford.

Down around Bath on the Kennebec was the country that was destined to become, and indeed to be at the present day, the great center of shipbuilding in Maine. That portion of the river known as the Long Reach, which was a stretch of three miles unequaled in the world for easily sloping shores on which to lay a keel and a channel that was wide and deep to receive a launching ship, put Bath out in front. It is claimed with respect to the yards at the north end of the city that "more ships have been built on that strip of Bath shore front than on any other of equal area in the world."

Jonathan Philbrick was the pioneer builder in Bath. With the help of his two sons he launched a schooner in 1743 near the site of the present Custom House. The man remembered as the first to establish shipbuilding as a business was Captain William Swanton. In 1762 he built on contract the first full-rigged ship launched in Bath. She was constructed in a yard situated at the foot of Summer Street and was named the *Earl of Bute*. The next year Captain Swanton built another ship for an English merchant named Jenness, and the following season still another, the *Rising Sun*, for a Mr. Ayles. This was followed by the *Moon*. He continued to launch about one ship a year until the Revolutionary War. In 1776 he put over the first ship built in Bath for war. This was the privateer *Black Prince*.

In 1762 Joshua Raynes, another shipbuilder, had built the sloop *Union* here, and six years later John Patten, John Fulton, and Adam Hunter launched the 90-ton sloop *Merry Meeting*. This was the first of many Kennebec vessels built above the Chops. In 1772 they constructed the *Industry*. With a cargo of boards, shingles, and four masts, she is said to have been the first vessel to sail out of the Kennebec for the West Indies. Topsham and Bowdoinham may both claim these vessels, for Sampson's Point, in the vicinity of which they were built, has belonged at different times to both towns. Farther up the Kennebec Reuben Colburn and Thomas Agry, the latter a Cape Cod shipbuilder from Barnstable, were building as early as 1763 near Agry's Point, in the present town of Pittston. The names of their vessels are lost, but their yards will always be remembered, for in them were built the batteaux hauled up the Kennebec and through the Dead River country by Arnold's men on the famous expedition to Quebec.

The early days of Bath were akin to those of other towns all along the shore. It was after the Revolution and in the next century that its name became known all over the seafaring world for the wooden ships of Maine.

The next river beyond the Kennebec is the Sheepscot. Here Wiscasset Point early became the center of an extensive lumber trade. No harbor was better suited for it. Here, thirteen miles from the ocean, with a bold, deep approach averaging a third of a mile in width, the Sheepscot spreads out in a broad bay where a hundred ships could anchor in twelve to twenty fathoms. Vessels were early built on its shores—the first of which we have a record being in 1737. As early as 1750 a Spanish man-of-war had loaded a cargo of masts here, and a considerable export trade in lumber to England, Scotland, and the West Indies gradually developed. In 1794 the village was surpassed in tonnage by the port of Portland alone, and that by only 1,400 tons. When Dr. Paul Coffin visited the Point in 1796 it was a place of much trade and navigation and had grown two-thirds in six years. Had he returned four years later, he would have found some thirty square-rigged vessels owned here, aggregating 10,000 tons. So important were the financial transactions between the village and England that the house of Anderson, Child and Child of Liverpool kept two of its members resident here for several years.

General Abiel Wood was Wiscasset's outstanding shipbuilder and owner in the early days. He came to the Point from Middleboro, Massachusetts, as early as 1766 and at once set up a yard, probably on Bradbury Cove. The names of his early vessels are lost, but between 1795 and 1806, with his son Abiel,

Jr., he launched at least twenty-six. The Woods were largely busy with the spar and salt trade to Liverpool. The outward cargo was "ton timber," that is, large trees hewed square, for in protection of its own sawyers England would not import finished lumber. This was cut on the Kennebec and floated down on the ebb of the tide in rafts, the hard wood atop of the pine. All salt for the fisheries had then to be imported, and the return cargo was mainly of that article. In a letter to Captain Spencer Tinkham of the ship *Astrea*, General Abiel directed him to bring salt "common and blown" and "fill in with a mixed cargo" of nails, paint, nautical instruments, such as compasses, wood and brass, spy glasses, boat hooks, quadrants, ship scrapers, screws, shovels, locks and thumb latches, warming pans, bellows, blankets, broadcloth, silk handkerchiefs, men's black hats, carpeting, pocket knives, Bibles, and some forty-odd other articles.

At this period six long wharves extended from the shore to the channel of the river. One of these was built by General Wood, and another was owned by his son, Joseph Tinkham Wood. The latter was a large shipowner in his own right of the famous "continent" ships—the *Europe*, *Asia*, *America*, and *Africa*. The third wharf was owned by Moses Carlton, who had come from Head Tide in Alna and who held a prominent place among the shipowners of the town. His ships were built on the upper river. Near the foot of Maine Street was the yard of Major Seth Tinkham, and in a salt cove that then flowed in back of the Congregational vestry was that of Colonel John Kingsbury.

Wiscasset is a classic example of the Maine coastal town which has enjoyed its generation of remarkable creative growth. Inevitably the tide goes out; conditions change, and the days of its greatness are in the past. Here the embargo in the early years of the next century marked the beginning of the end.

Shipbuilding in Colonial Maine

While the Sheepscot is a small river and could not compete with the Kennebec to the west and the Penobscot to the eastward, both of which reach far up into the vitals of the north of Maine, in the next century it was the scene of some notable shipbuilding. Wiscasset's stately and beautiful mansions facing on Maine and High Streets are worthy memorials of the days of its roaring trade in lumber.

Within a very few miles to the eastward is the Damariscotta. Here at Newcastle, when the town meeting was offering "thirty shillings for every gray wolf that shall be catched and killed," full-rigged ships of 300 tons were being launched. Before the Revolution, George Barstow, a ship's carpenter from Hanover, Massachusetts, was building here. Later his son, Colonel George, established a yard and did a considerable business building on contract for Salem merchants. At about this time Nathaniel Bryant came from the South Shore in Massachusetts and laid down his ways. These yards were the forerunners of several at Newcastle and Damariscotta whose builders—William Hitchcock, Abner Stetson, Algernon S. Austin, Ebenezer Haggett, Metcalfe and Norris, and others—were to make some notable contributions to the fleets of clippers and down-easters in the next century.

On the St. George there are evidences in the early eighteenth century of the lime burning which would later develop into a thriving industry and keep the yards in the region busy supplying schooners for many a year. The first vessel built was a coaster, probably a sloop, in the town of Cushing. She was named the *Industry* and was lost on her first voyage in a November snow squall off Cape Ann. In 1775 the Lermonds launched at their mills on Oyster River in Warren, the *Dolphin*. She fared in better luck. It was four years before she was cast away.

In the Penobscot Bay country the 60-ton sloop *Hannah* was

the first vessel built. She was launched by Colonel Jonathan Buck, who had come from Haverhill on the Merrimac to Bucksport in 1762. The *Hannah* was burned in 1779 by the British ship *Nautilus*. This significant fact marks a terminal point to the colonial period of Maine shipbuilding. It also ushered in a hiatus in the development of eastern Maine.

British forces soon seized all of eastern Maine, and thereafter they controlled the Penobscot region throughout the war. From this vantage the ill-fated Penobscot expedition, organized from Boston, failed to dislodge them. The conditions of war brought great changes on the Maine coast. While the majority of those engaged in seafaring activities—and this, in these days, meant almost the entire population—supported the war, there were not a few names well known at the time who adhered to the Crown.

It was not long after the outbreak of hostilities that British men-of-war standing on and off the coast brought seafaring and shipbuilding to a standstill. The first naval engagement of the war was fought off Machias. The infamous Mowatt fired the little town of Falmouth after a squabble over masts. At Kittery on the northwest end of Langdon's Island, naval vessels were built and launched.

The *Raleigh* was the first. In May 1777 there was launched the *Ranger*. Under command of John Paul Jones she carried the news of Burgoyne's surrender to Europe and received there in Quiberon Bay the first salute ever given to the American flag. Five years later there came off the ways the *America*, a gift to the French government, and the first line-of-battle ship to be built in this country.

All along the coast merchants and fishermen took to privateering. This was a speculative venture in which, if you lost, you stood to lose your life or spend the next few years of it in a prison hulk. But when Lady Luck favored, the fortunes established from the sale of prizes were enormous. With the close of the war, the merchant fleet was reduced to next to nothing. A great depression impended, and the years ahead were those of scarcity, hard struggle, and reconstruction.

CHAPTER FIVE

The WAR YEARS

The Commodore's patience seemed now exhausted and, taking the trumpet, he hailed and said, "I am now going to hail you for the last time. If a proper answer is not returned, I will fire a shot into you." A prompt answer came back, "If you fire a shot, I will return a broadside." Preble then hailed, "What ship is that?" The reply was, "This is His Britannic Majesty's ship *Donegal*, eighty-four guns, Sir Richard Strahan, an English Commodore. Send your boat on board." Under the excitement of the moment, Preble leaped on the hammocks and returned for answer,

"This is the United States Ship *Constitution*, forty-four guns, Edward Preble, an American Commodore, who will be damned before he sends his boat on board of any vessel." And turning to the crew, he said, "Blow your matches, boys!"

The conversation here ceased, and soon after a boat was heard coming from the stranger, and arrived with a lieutenant from the frigate *Maidstone.*—*The Autobiography of Charles Morris.*

Too lightly built and too heavily sparred, the privateer was never a comfortable or a safe vessel. Beautiful beyond anything then known in naval construction, such vessels roused boundless admiration, but defied imitators. . . . Americans were proud of their privateers, as they well might be; for this was the first time when in competition with the world, on an element open to all, they proved their capacity to excel, and produced a creation as beautiful as it was practical.—Henry Adams, *History of the United States.*[1]

[1] Vol. VII. Charles Scribner's Sons.

The War Years

THE GENERATION from the Revolution through the war of 1812 lived at the high tide of the romance and adventure of the sea. This was the time for a Tom Cringle's Log, had Michael Scott been born a Yankee. Those were the days of the Algerine Corsairs, the undeclared war against France with its concomitant spoliation claims, the British press gang, free trade, and sailors' rights; running the embargo and smuggling; the dash, the excitement, and the prizes to be had in privateering. The period comes alive in the pages of Elijah Kellogg's forgotten tales for boys, in James Fenimore Cooper's *Ned Myers*, *The Pilot*, and *The Red Rover*, and in the historical romances of Kenneth Roberts. Indeed, in *Ned Myers, or Life before the Mast*, Cooper told of his experiences in the *Sterling* out of Wiscasset on a voyage that touched the ports of Carthagena, London, and Philadelphia, in the course of which the ship was visited by press gangs, stopped by a pirate felucca, and chased by a privateer.

Take the case of Edward Preble for the "chance and change of a sailor's life." Born in 1761 in the Town of Falmouth and District of Maine, he ran away from his father's farm to sea on a privateer out of Newburyport at the age of sixteen. His father, General Jedediah Preble, who had seen service at Louisburg, got the boy a commission as a midshipman in the Massachusetts State Marine. He served in the Revolution and survived the horrors of a prisoner of war's life aboard the prison ship *Jersey*. Then followed fourteen years in the merchant marine. In 1798 he was appointed a lieutenant in the United States Navy and served in the war against France. The incident described at the head of this chapter took place off Gibraltar in 1803, just prior to his campaign before Tripoli. He was later to be known as the father of the United States Navy, as so many officers later to make their name in the War of 1812 had served and trained with and under him.

The Revolutionary War was concluded by the Peace of

Paris in 1783. Shortly thereafter came New England's first and greatest depression. Maine felt the "embarrassment" severely. There was little hard money in circulation, and the effect of that little was seriously diminished by the great influx of foreign goods. The merchant marine had been swept from the seas by the war. The vessels that remained were small and worn-out privateers which had been built on too sharp lines to be good cargo carriers. Even if England had not slammed shut the doors of her ports in our faces, there was insufficient money in the country to build suitable full-bodied craft or even to fit out fishermen with boats and gear for their work. Even as late as 1787 there was not a single vessel owned in Portland.

The states on the seaboard were fighting a commercial war among themselves. It is a sad story of monopoly and sectional jealousy. Connecticut threw her ports wide open to the British, but laid heavy duties on Massachusetts. New York obliged every Yankee sloop that came through Hell Gate to pay entrance fees. The adoption of the federal Constitution put an end to these abuses. It is interesting to note that of the forty-six delegates from Maine to the Massachusetts convention, the only one to speak in favor of adoption was a Captain Snow, a shipmaster and shipbuilder of Harpswell. On the final question of ratification, however, twenty-five voted in the affirmative. The majority would have been larger had the delegates been able to foresee its effect on the District of Maine. The first measure adopted by Congress under the Federal government encouraged American shipping by affording protection in the form of differential duties levied on imports in American and foreign vessels. Moreover, in tonnage duties an advantage of almost 50 per cent was granted.

Under this stimulus the shipping business began to thrive. All along the Maine coast tools were taken up in the yards to meet the demand for vessels. Lumber from the foothills of the

White Mountains began to move swiftly down the Piscataqua, the Kennebunk, and the Saco. The great demand was for bottoms to carry it to market. The busy mills in the neighborhood of Casco Bay were piling the wharves at Portland, North Yarmouth, and Freeport with deals, i.e., heavy sawn timbers, as well as masts, spars, and staves. The falls of the Androscoggin at Brunswick could hardly take care of the logs that came down the river, where twenty-five saws awaited them. Wiscasset was entering upon the golden age of her prosperity. Although the great forests of the Penobscot had not as yet been opened, the shores near tidewater had numbers of little mills.

Migration to the eastward reached its height. Between 1783 and 1826 there were 226 new towns incorporated in Maine. This was five and a half times as many as there had been up to the time of the Revolution. The streams of new settlers moved in two directions, up the great rivers into the interior and along the coast from the Penobscot to the St. Croix. In this region, the present-day counties of Hancock and Washington, some fifty-five mills were operating as early as 1800. New towns were laid out in the midst of the forests on rivers, both little and big. They were the only routes over which the lumber could be carried to market. Ships just had to be built.

In order to regulate the collection of duties on imports and tonnage, the new government classified the coasts and seaports of the District in nine commercial districts. In 1799 they were arranged anew into ten. This arrangement, with added ports of delivery, stood unchanged well into the next century. They were:

1. York, with Kittery and Berwick as its annexed ports
2. Biddeford and Pepperelborough (Saco), with Wells, Kennebunk, Cape Porpoise, and Scarborough
3. Portland and Falmouth, with North Yarmouth, Freeport, and Harpswell

4. Bath, with Pittston, Topsham, Georgetown, and Brunswick
5. Wiscasset, with Boothbay
6. Waldoborough, with Bristol, Nobleboro, Warren,
   Thomaston, Cushing, Camden, and Ducktrap (Lincolnville)
7. Penobscot, with Frankfort, Blue Hill, Hampden, and
   Deer Isle
8. Frenchman's Bay, with Union River (Ellsworth)
9. Machias
10. Passamaquoddy

Some notion of the growth of maritime interest in the state
may be gathered by a comparison of the figures of 1794 with
those of 1812, at the commencement of the war with England.
In 1794 there were owned in the District of Maine 49,769 tons
of shipping. By 1812 this figure had risen, despite discourage-
ments and opposition, both foreign and domestic, to 148,876
tons. This was a gain of 300 per cent.

The gain was particularly noticeable in the Penobscot region.
By 1800 shipbuilding had become as firmly established here as
elsewhere in the District. While in 1794 only 3,683 tons were
owned there, this had increased more than fivefold in 1812, to
20,480 tons. The shores of this beautiful bay and river were
settled rapidly after the Revolution, and shipyards multiplied
apace. By the opening of the second war with England in 1812,
16 schooners and 3 large sloops had been built at Isleboro; 2
ships, 15 schooners, and a sloop at Hampden; and 3 ships, 4
brigs, 7 schooners, and 2 sloops at Bucksport. Here as early as
1800 Captain James Ginn had founded a yard, and a family of
shipbuilders continuously engaged in the business in it until
1883. In 1799 Castine owned 3 ships, 1 brig, 10 schooners, and
2 sloops, all built in the town. The next decade there were

added to them 2 ships, 6 brigs, 6 schooners, and 2 sloops. Bangor's yards had been opened by Deacon William Boyd in 1789 or 1790. In the next twenty years he, with Robert Treat and Captain Samuel Lowder, had launched 1 ship, 12 schooners, and 2 sloops.

An example of how shipbuilding was stimulated at this time is to be had in the opening up of what is known as the "old China trade." The arrival in New York in May 1785 of the *Empress of China* with a rich cargo from Canton and the voyage two years later of Elias Hasket Derby's privateer of the Revolution, the *Grand Turk*, gave notice to all and sundry of the fabulous cargoes and profits to be had in the Far Eastern ports. No longer were Americans to be dependent for their teas and silks on the Dutch and English East India Companies. Maine's share in this trade was for the greater part confined to shipbuilding, and Maine-built vessels formed a large part of the Boston and Salem fleets. Twenty-seven of William Gray's large fleet were built in Maine yards, while Theodore Lyman, J. and T. H. Perkins, Joseph Peabody, and Preble and Company owned goodly numbers of vessels launched from the ways in the District.

Two Portland shipowners, Ebenezer Preble, who was the brother of the commodore, and Joseph Jewett, a merchant of the town, decided to build a ship for this trade. They persuaded William Gray, Jr., of Salem to join them. Gray had relatives in town and was bringing his cargoes of Russian hemp into Portland to be spun at his large ropewalk. At a cost of more than $60,000, the *Portland* was launched in the spring of 1796. She sailed from Boston early in the summer for Bombay with Captain Seth Storer of Saco as master. Preble was ship's husband.

No invoice of this outward voyage has come to light. It was probably similar to that of her second voyage in late December, 1797, when it consisted of 75 barrels of prime beef, 480 quintals of salt cod, 225 barrels of pickled salmon (at this time Maine salmon was a rival of salt cod on fish days in the Mediterranean countries), 17,000 white oak staves, 5,700 barrel staves, and 131 hogsheads of "shugar." This cargo was to be sold in the wine islands or the Mediterranean ports and wine or specie secured for trade at Bombay or Calcutta. On this voyage the owners changed. Seth Storer, her former captain, bought out Jewett's third from his widow, and "Billy" Gray sold his share to Nathaniel Silsbee of Salem, who went as master. In the papers recording these transfers we have a list of the *Portland's* cargo on her first voyage home from Bombay. Bandanna handkerchiefs, Beerboom Gurrahs, fine and coarse Policates, Allabad blue and Chittabudy Baftas, together with a confusing list of East India cotton piece goods, make up this curious invoice.

During Captain Nathaniel Silsbee's first voyage as master and part owner of the *Portland* in 1798, he was captured by a French privateer and taken into Malaga. Only his resolute determination and a forty-eight hour vigil in the office of the French consul got his ship released. A few days later the *Portland* was again seized in the harbor of Genoa. She was then forced to join the fleet that was to take Bonaparte's army to Egypt, and because of her superior accommodations she was chosen to transport the "Staff of the army." Despite the boast of the French officer who boarded her that "if God had one ship here and the Republic wanted it, he must give it," Captain Silsbee by a little Yankee trading with some barrels of beef and pork, which were badly needed by the French, regained possession of his ship.

Two years later Captain Silsbee in the Portland-built *Herald*, when returning from Calcutta in company with four other American vessels and the British East Indiaman *Cornwallis*, escaped from the French privateer *La Gloire*. The *Friendship*, also Portland-built, was attacked and captured by Malays when in the Sumatra pepper trade off Quallah Battoo. To avenge this, Captain John Downes in the frigate *Potomac* stormed the place in 1832, destroying its forts and killing the Sultan Po Mahomet with 150 of his followers. This is said to have been the first American naval battle in the Pacific.

Theodore Lyman, one of Boston's foremost merchants in the northwest fur and China trade, was born in York and came to Kennebunk to work in the store of Waldo Emerson. Here he laid the foundation of his fortune in the West India trade in 1790; he then moved to Boston and was among the first to send ships to the Pacific coast. His home in Kennebunk was a mansion in those days. Many of his vessels were built at Kennebunk in the Bourne shipyard. Here in 1800 was launched the *Atahualpa*, named for the Peruvian hero and martyr. Her career is one of the classics of the old China trade.

Captain William Sturgis took her to the northwest coast, where he traded with the Indians for sea otter skins. These he turned over in Canton for a rich return cargo. On his second voyage he sailed direct for China, having on board some 300,000 Mexican dollars. In Macao Roads he was forced to anchor in a calm. Here were sixteen pirate junks waiting for just such an opportunity. They swarmed about the ship flinging firebrands aboard, this being the favorite method of attack of their famous leader Appotesi. With the few cannon he had, Captain Sturgis held them off until with the help of a light breeze he gained the protection of the Portuguese fort at Macao. During this encounter Sturgis stood by with a lighted brand near a powder keg, resolved to blow his ship to eternity rather than surrender.

On the return voyage three Boston ships, the *William*, the *Mandarin*, and the *Atahualpa*, left Canton within three days of each other. On the thirteenth of April, 1810, all three came into Boston Harbor almost within sight of each other. This was the forerunner of many a famous deep-sea derby. An interest-

ing sidelight on the harsh relationship between masters and
owners at that time is the fact that in settling the voyage Lyman
forced Sturgis to pay freight on the cannon with which he had
beaten off the pirates and saved Lyman's ship, because he had
taken them along without orders.

BARBARY PIRATES—FRENCH SPOLIATIONS—PRESS GANGS

The merchant marine of the infant republic was subject to
attacks at this time from several quarters. For many years the
Barbary states Tunis, Algiers, Tripoli, and Morocco had levied
tribute on vessels trading in the Mediterranean. Even the English and French paid from one to three hundred thousand dollars a year on the theory that it was easier to buy them off than
to fight them. While the states on the seaboard were British
colonies, American ships had been furnished with passports and
had not been molested. The Barbary pirates looked upon the
United States with contempt and on the American merchant
marine as an easy mark for their corsairs.

Between 1785 and 1793, there were taken and confiscated
fifteen American vessels. One hundred and eighty officers and
seamen were held captive and worked in chain gangs in the
shipyards and mines or bending an oar on the benches of the
galleys. The ransom prices for these unfortunates were $2,000
for a captain, $1,500 for a mate, and $725 for a seaman. In its
earlier years the government was too poor either to pay for
their redemption or to secure their safety by tribute. The
captain of one of Colonel Jonathan Hamilton's Berwick brigs
which had been captured within five leagues of Lisbon tells of
the poor food, hard labor, and great suffering to which he and
his crew were subjected. He predicted that "in case something
is not done soon the whole Western Ocean will be infested
with 'Algerian cruizers.'"

Here is the story of another vessel hailing from the District of Maine. In 1783 the sloop *Squirrel* of Saco, having sailed from Casco Bay, was some weeks out when she was overhauled by a corsair from the Algerian Mole. She was captured and Captain Alexander Paine and his crew were taken into Algiers. Brought before the Dey, they had their choice of becoming Mohammedans or slaves. On their refusal to change their religion, he ordered that the captain and first mate be sent to the mines, and that the second mate and crew of eighteen be chained to the benches of a cruising galley armed with twenty-six eight-pounders. With no covering for their heads and but little for their bodies and on short allowances of bran bread and goat's meat, they endured the sun and rain of the Mediterranean for nearly five years.

In Christmas week of 1787, a French frigate of forty-eight guns commanded by John LeCotte engaged their vessel. Several broadsides were exchanged. At last the frigate was able to grapple the corsair. The Algerians, seeing that they were about to be taken, fell upon their prisoners with bayonets and cutlasses. They butchered them until they were overpowered by the French. Only seven remained alive. They were taken into Bordeaux, and when their wounds were healed, they were sent on to New York. Here they arrived in February 1790. Immediately they set out on foot for Saco, begging their food on the way. They arrived home seven years after they had sailed. Captain Paine and the first mate remained in the mines.

The District of Maine played a part in bringing the Barbary states to their bearings. The frigate *Crescent*, which the Deÿ demanded as a part of the tribute of 1797, had been built on Badger's Island at Kittery. When Commodore Preble forced Tripoli to sign the treaty of 1805, he had in his fleet the *Enterprise*, which was later to worst the *Boxer* in the famous sea fight off the mouth of the Kennebec. Then rigged as a schooner she captured a ketch which was later named the *In-*

trepid. This vessel was used in blowing up the *Philadelphia* in Tripoli harbor, one of the most spectacular events in American naval history, and on board the *Intrepid* a Maine boy lost his life. This was Lieutenant Henry Wadsworth. He was the uncle of the poet who bore his name.

★ ★ ★

In 1793 France declared war on Great Britain. Almost immediately the United States proclaimed its neutrality. This aggravated the raids of French men-of-war and privateers on American commerce which gave rise to the well-known "spoliation claims." The envoys—John Marshall, Elbridge Gerry, and Charles Cotesworth Pinckney—who were sent to France to negotiate a settlement of these claims were confronted with Talleyrand's official attempt to extort a bribe from their government. This called forth Pinckney's blunt retort, "Millions for defense, but not one cent for tribute." This was indignantly echoed throughout the nation, and it was with difficulty that the Adams administration prevented war. Nonetheless undeclared hostilities began on the sea, and for three years and more French privateers and cruisers continued their despoliation of our commerce, especially in the West India trade.

A voyage to the West Indies in those days could bring as much adventure and mishap as one around the world. Witness the record of the snow *Neptune* of Portland, skippered by John Codman. On the fourteenth of March, 1798, she was taken by the French and ordered into Guadeloupe. On the fifteenth she was retaken and carried into Antigua. After being detained here for sixteen days she was released upon the payment of salvage equal to one-eighth the value of the ship and cargo. Sailing from there, she was taken yet again on the second day out and carried to St. Martins. Here she was held another month. Then after a trial before the tribunal of Guadeloupe and Basse-Terre she was finally released. Leaving behind her mate and two seamen, she finally made Portland on the twenty-second day of May.

Many stories are told of Maine captains and mates who turned the tables upon their captors and retook their vessels. This was accomplished aboard the schooner *Apollo* of Wiscasset. When about five days out on the home voyage from Nevis in the Leeward Islands, she was boarded by a French privateer. Captain William Clifford was held prisoner. The mate and the entire crew were taken out, with the exception of one seaman, Solomon Trask. He pretended to be so sick that he was not removed. Then a prize master and five seamen were put on board. They held possession for only twenty-four hours.

Coming alongside another prize, a schooner from the Kennebec, which had been taken at the same time as the *Apollo*, the French prize master leaned over the quarter for a chat with the master of the schooner. He left his cutlass and pistols lying on the binnacle. Suddenly he turned and saw Captain Clifford with his cutlass. Springing to the binnacle for his pistols, he was confronted by Trask, who had them in his hands. He shouted to the master of the schooner to fire on the *Apollo*. Captain Clifford ordered him to countermand the order or Trask would blow him through. Then Trask drove four of the seamen down into the forecastle. The fifth put up a fight but was soon piped down. The prize master was kept on deck. Five days later they fell in with a Philadelphia schooner bound for Jamaica. Two of the sailors were put aboard her, but the other four Frenchmen were brought back to Wiscasset as prisoners and turned over to the authorities.

In 1800 Captain Samuel Whitney of Castine had his ship *Hiram* taken four times by the French. After the third capture he retook her almost single-handed from the prize master and nine seamen. He was making good his escape to the United States when he was again taken, on this occasion by a French frigate. He was left aboard his ship with a guard of eighteen men and a lieutenant. He managed to put all the nautical instruments on board out of order except his own sextant. In the confusion thus caused he almost succeeded in sailing the *Hiram* into Savannah harbor. But the crew became suspicious, and his little plan failed. Turning to sea once more, they were under way, as the French supposed, toward Guadeloupe. But under the navigation of Captain Whitney they arrived instead in Martinique. This port was then held by the British. After some time and expense the captain recovered his ship, this time for keeps.

The French spoliations were heavy blows to the ports of western Maine. Portland and Casco Bay lost some thirty vessels, of an estimated value of $354,967. Colonel Thomas Cutts of Saco counted his losses at $90,000. Kennebunk lost twenty-three vessels, Wiscasset nine, and Kittery and the Piscataqua region still more. When the treaty covering the Louisiana Purchase was concluded, one of the considerations was that the United States should assume the claims of its citizens against the French for these losses. They amounted to some $3,750,000. Until 1885, when the matter was finally referred to a court of claims, every Congress had before it a bill calling for payment. The court finally adjudicated several thousand of these cases, and awarded $4,800,000. But many claims still remain unsettled.

★   ★   ★

While France was stealing our ships and their cargoes, England was stealing our men. Jefferson put it this way: England had become "a den of pirates and France a den of thieves." England was fighting for her life. Her great defense was her navy, for which she must have men. The British were unwilling to surrender to a young and weak nation like the United States their long-claimed "right" to search the ships of other nations for those who were claimed to be subjects of the Crown. Thus the press gang boarded such merchant ships as were encountered at sea and with gag and pistol lay in wait ashore for the crews of ships enjoying the pleasures of the waterfront.

Modern historians disagree as to the number of these outrages or how serious they were. The numbers of the impressments gleaned from contemporary sources are notoriously unreliable, mixed as they are with political motives. There is no doubt that the insolent methods of British officers, and their contemptuous disregard of human rights, were more than irritating and were a just cause of war. Certain it is that they caused the hatred and bitterness toward the British which lingered for generations on the coast of Maine.

The District suffered severely. The columns of the Portland Gazette and of the Argus are filled with news items and letters describing these seizures. Captain Stone of Kennebunk lost his entire crew to the press gang of a British frigate as he lay in harbor in Kingston, Jamaica. Captain Smith of the Portland schooner *Friendship* was unable to move his ship from harbor because the captain of the brig *Port Mahan* had seized all of his crew except the mate. American sailors carried certificates of their birth and a description of their physical characteristics; but these "protections," as they were called, received but scant attention from the boarding officer.

Many a Maine man served in the British fleet during the French wars. Sylvanus Snow of Orrington served under Nelson at Trafalgar and on other ships until he made his escape at Minorca and got home in the Nobleboro-built ship *Monk*. John Allen of Topsham lost a leg in his impressment. He was turned out of the hospital when it was healed, a human derelict. Robert Randall and James Cotterill of Wiscasset were in the service eleven years before they were discharged as invalids. John Andrews of Wiscasset and Stephen Thompson of Boothbay were taken by a frigate off Cape Ann in July of 1796. Soon after, a

PASSPORT AND ROLL OF EQUIPAGE.

AGREEABLY to the Fourth Article of Convention between FRANCE and the UNITED STATES OF AMERICA. Made the third day of September, in the year of our LORD, one thousand eight hundred, for the Relief and Protection of American Seamen; with a list and description of the Officers and Crew of the American _____, _____ — of _____ _____ tons; and bound for _____ _____ Master, of the burthen of _____ _____ Portland, in the year of our LORD, one thousand eight hundred and _____

Time of Entry.	Names.	Rank.	Place of Birth.	Place of Residence.	Age.	Height.	Complexion.	To what Nation.
1807 Aug. 9	Zebediah Cheston	Mate	Newburyport	Portland	42	5 8	Dark	United States
Aug. 9	Benj. Phinney	Seaman	Scarborough	Scarborough	21	5 6	White	United States
Aug. 9	Nathaniel Seaman	Seaman	Newburn	Portland	25	5 5	Light	United States
Aug. 9	William Lane	Seaman	Newburn	Portland	36	5 6	Dark	United States
Aug. 9	Robt. Phinney	Seaman	Scarborough	Portland	20	5 32	Light	United States
Aug. 9	John Costa	Seaman	Portuguese	Portland	10	5 0½	Brown	United States
Aug. 9								

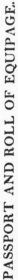

COMMONWEALTH OF MASSACHUSETTS

CUMBERLAND—

BE IT KNOWN AND MADE MANIFEST, That on this _____ day of _____ in the year of our LORD, one thousand eight hundred and _____ , before me, JOSEPH COFFIN BOYD, Esq. a Notary Public, by legal authority admitted and sworn, and dwelling in PORTLAND, personally came _____ of _____ and made oath that the above is a true ROLL or EQUIPAGE, of the _____ _____ , of which he is at present master.

IN TESTIMONY WHEREOF, I hereunto set my Hand, and affix my Seal Notarial, at Portland aforesaid, the day and year last above written.

Passport for the "Relief and Protection of American Seamen" aboard the brig
Cumberland of Portland, issued in 1807.

French frigate appeared, and in the ensuing action near George's Bank Andrews was killed.

A particularly vicious instance of the practice occurred on board H.M.S. *Macedonian*, 38, a new strong frigate commanded by Captain Samuel Carden "known in his own service as a heavy flogger and a great hand at impressing Yankees." There were seven Americans in the crew, of whom two hailed from Maine—John Card of Woolwich, who had been taken off the Wiscasset ship *Mount Vernon*, and John Wallis of Phippsburg. On October 25, 1812, when some six hundred miles broad off the Canaries, the *Macedonian* encountered the *United States*, commanded by Stephen Decatur. When the order to clear for action was given, Card, speaking for himself and Wallis, went aft to Captain Carden with the request that they might not be forced to fight against their flag. It is fair to state that this permission was often granted by British commanders. Captain Carden ungenerously ordered him to his quarters and threatened to shoot him if he made the request again. He then stationed midshipmen at all of the gangways with orders to shoot any man who left his station. In less than two hours the *Macedonian* struck her flag. John Card and John Wallis lay with the dead on her deck.

The early records reflect an occasional touch of humor. Upon entering the harbor of St. Thomas, Captain Theodore Wells' vessel was boarded by an officer of the British *Galletee*. This officer was, in the language of the captain, "a hard customer." He examined the ship's papers and the seamen's protections. Challenging them as Englishmen in disguise he made them strip that he might see if their bodies showed scars where they had been flogged aboard a man-of-war. He inquired from one of the seamen where he hailed from. Upon receiving the answer: "from Wells," he exclaimed, "There, I knew you were a Welshman." Notable instances of these outrages are recorded in the log book of the Wiscasset ship *Sterling*, in which during 1806–07 James Fenimore Cooper made his first voyage. Even her captain, John Johnston, "Captain Jack," was seized in London by the King's officers because, though born in America, he still talked a pretty broad brand of Scotch.

The peak of British naval arrogance was reached in the unprovoked, unwarranted, and unlawful attack of H.M.S. *Leopard* on the *Chesapeake*. Late in June, 1807, the *Chesapeake* was proceeding to sea off Cape Henry under command of Commodore Barron. The *Leopard* approached her down wind and, rounding to, hailed the American frigate stating that she had dispatches for the Commodore.

The upshot of this was that a boat came alongside and Barron was shown an order of Admiral Berkeley at Halifax requiring the searching of the *Chesapeake* for deserters. Barron replied in writing he knew of no such men as were described. He added: "I am also instructed never to permit the crew of any ship that I command to be mustered by any other but her own officers."

This was delivered on board the *Leopard*. Then after an exchange of hails and within less than a quarter hour, the *Leopard* opened fire with her full broadside on the helpless *Chesapeake*. Twice again this was repeated. The belated effort of the *Chesapeake* to clear for action resulted in the firing of one gun before she struck. British officers came on board, mustered the crew and seized three Americans, whom they imprisoned, and one Englishman, whom they later hanged at Halifax. The business left the American waterfront in a raging flame of indignation.

EMBARGO AND NONINTERCOURSE

In the titanic struggles between the British and the French which were to culminate at Waterloo, the young American republic was in the middle. For seafaring Americans the first decade of the new century was destined to be divided between prosperity and ruin. While the profits to be had in the neutral carrying trade were little short of fantastic, each belligerent endeavored by devious modes to control that trade for its own purposes and to suppress it in so far as it benefited the enemy. And this is where the ruin part of it came in.

Fully to understand the intricacies of the various moves of the contestants on a board which comprised the wide Atlantic and more, requires the combined capacities of a sea and a Philadelphia lawyer. For example, in June 1805 Sir William Scott, the celebrated admiralty judge, handed down his decision in the case of the *Essex*. It worked this way: An American vessel takes on a neutral cargo in Martinique and clears for Wiscasset. There the goods are landed and the duties are paid. Thereafter these goods are transported to London. Under the existing decisions of his own court, there had been a *bona fide* importation into the United States and the goods were not liable to seizure. Now at one stroke of the judicial pen all was changed. In the Essex decision he set aside his former ruling. Immediately vast numbers of cargoes in American bottoms became liable to seizure and were seized by the British as good prize. The *Essex'* maneuver was a part of a general scheme to gather all the West Indian trade into British hands.

A year later there was announced the so-called Fox blockade. Thereby the coast of Europe from the Elbe to Brest was declared to be blockaded. To this Bonaparte responded in kind in November 1806 with his famous Berlin decree. Thereby in turn the British Isles were declared to be in a state of blockade. Order in council succeeded order in council, that of Nov. 11, 1807, being the most important. It purported to exclude American commerce from any port closed to the British. The Napoleonic counter to this was the Milan decree—that all vessels

The Maritime History of Maine

which had been searched by or had paid duty to or had come to or from a British port were good prize.

There were no more neutrals. To all this the administration of Jefferson gave a characteristic answer. The "long" embargo went into effect on Dec. 22, 1807. For the next fourteen months no vessel could clear for a foreign port, and the coastwise trade was required to give bond that its cargoes would be landed in United States ports. At first the sentiment among some prominent Maine merchants and masters was in favor of the measure. William King of Bath and Abiel Wood of Wiscasset hoped that its purpose might be attained. But as the spring passed and the summer came, with no signs that either England or France would yield, the embargo became more and more unpopular.

Every effort was made to evade the law. Despite Jefferson's vigorous attempts at enforcement, with troops on the Canadian border and gunboats patrolling the coast, trade went right on with England through the Canadian provinces and with France by way of Florida. Then again many a coaster blown off the coast was forced to put into a European port on the other side of the Atlantic "in distress." This may have been the experience of Samuel Hadlock of Little Cranberry Island. When fishing off the Newfoundland Banks, instead of bringing his cod home he split and cured them on the rocks of Labrador. Then he sailed direct for Portugal. Evading the cruisers and privateers of France and England, he sold his cargo in Oporto for a good round sum and returned home with an equally valuable cargo of salt and lemons. Out of the proceeds he had Israel Higgins build a new schooner for him at Bar Harbor. Characteristically, he called her the *Hazard*.

Maine was the greatest offender. Ever since the close of the Revolutionary War, to avoid burdensome restrictions, many a cargo had been transferred from an American to an English bottom in Passamaquoddy Bay, or on the shores of Campobello or some other neutral island. Yankee skippers now surmised that if a desirable cargo was brought to this frontier a purchaser was certain to be found and also a way to get it across the border. British statesmen were quick to see the opportunity. In May effective aid was given by opening up the ports of New Brunswick to all such cargoes. Overnight Eastport became one of the busiest ports in the Union.

Even before the first of June large cargoes of flour began to arrive from the south. Fourteen vessels were at anchor in the harbor at one time. In one week 30,000 barrels were received, and by the lowest computation the quantity for the year was 160,000 barrels. No adequate warehouses or wharves existed, so caches were made along the shore or on the uplands from which led the shortest, the easiest, and the safest route to the international line. All along the shores from West Quoddy to Machias River such places of deposit ranged, convenient for purchasers from Grand Manan.

Despite the sentinels who were posted within twenty or thirty rods of each other all along the coast, the flour disappeared. There was no such thing as keeping it at Eastport at $4.00 a barrel, when a sea voyage of two miles increased its value 300 per cent. Boats of every size and description, from Indian canoes to English wherries, thronged the beaches. As the risk of transportation increased, the price for ferrying rose until $3.00 a barrel was charged. A good day's or night's work netted one some $40.00 or $50.00.

But finally prohibition did prohibit. A company of troops arrived, and a little later came the famous frigate *Chesapeake*, with Captain Stephen Decatur in command. Four of the little Jeffersonian gunboats were stationed in the rivers. On the English side of the line were anchored the British sloop of war *Squirrel* and the cutters *Pogge* and *Hunter* to aid the boats transporting the flour once they arrived in English waters. But despite dereliction of duty in many of the guards and the willingness of some of the officials higher up to take a nap to oblige a generous friend, the firm hand of the national government at last reduced the inducements of contraband trade. In August 1809 the ports of St. John and Halifax were again closed to American produce. But it was a great racket while it lasted.

Despite the hazard, adventurous spirits were willing to take the risk of getting a vessel to sea. Men of high standing in their communities thought it altogether right to break so unpopular a law. Some of these had cause to regret it in after years, when they found the memories of their political opponents a mite too accurate. With flour selling at Jamaica for $25.00 a barrel, potatoes at $7.50, and lumber which could be bought at the mills on the Maine runs for $8.00 bringing $60.00 a thousand in the West Indies, Yankee enterprise could not be restrained.

Some found "stress of weather" a good excuse for landing their cargo in a foreign port. A case in point was the *Ploughboy* of Bangor. She cleared at Newport, in October 1808, with provisions for Castine. But she was "blown off," touched at Antigua, and arrived in Castine late in February minus her cargo. Others, without clearance papers of any kind, sailed out boldly and sold both the ship and her lading. Or like Captain Benjamin Thomas of Camden, they returned with an empty hold but with no evidence of profit from the voyage. The proceeds had been hidden from the eyes of the law in holes bored in the stanchions of the vessel.

The ship *Sally* went out of the Kennebec one winter night in February 1809. She passed the fort at Popham safely, the friendly garrison aiming high, cutting a little of her rigging and sending a cannon ball through her topsail. On she went to London, where her lumber sold for an amount that laid the foundation of a fortune of a famous family of Bath shipbuilders.

[82]

An incident of this voyage is a reminder that the fine art of "hijacking" is by no means a modern maneuver.

The crew, well aware that the ship had no papers and that they could not be reached by the law at home, decided that they should share in the profits of the voyage. Accordingly, they shut up their officers and liberated them only on the promise that each man in the crew should have a bonus of $50 when the cargo was sold in London. They demanded written promises that this would be done. All seemed well, and the crew did not suspect anything untoward when the supercargo was taken sick and set ashore before harbor was reached. But on coming into the docks the ship was met by officers who arrested the crew on a charge of mutiny. They were able to buy their release only upon a surrender of the written promises.

Owners were not always so fortunate. One Bath captain took out a brig and cargo for William King. He sold both ship and cargo, returned home, and kept the proceeds unmolested, as no litigation could reach him.

In the old brick store at Phippsburg Center there were once told tall tales of these days. On the scales were weighed the gold pieces brought back by the *Adoniram* from her voyage to Demerara with a cargo from ports all along the coast, which had been loaded aboard her as she lay on and off south of Monhegan. Here one night there gathered thirty or more friends of the proprietors Hill and Cobb. The *Mary Jane* was loaded and lay at the end of the wharf, armed to defy the Custom House boat or the guns of the fort. In addition to the crew, there were among the thirty men aboard the brig twelve especially hired to get the vessel out of the river. No one of them weighed less than two hundred pounds, and each was disguised beyond recognition by the use of the blacking brush.

To be sure, there were leaks in the embargo, but its enforcement was remarkably effective. The rashness and defiance of the attempts at its nullification illustrate the seriousness of the situation. The scene along the coast of Maine was indeed distressing. The smaller ports of the country suffered most severely. While Portland was by now the sixth shipowning community in the United States, Maine's shipping was not concentrated there. On the contrary, it was widely distributed in many small and independent villages. Every man in the district who had anything to do directly or indirectly with the building, lading, or sailing of ships—carpenters, blacksmiths, lumbermen, sailors, clerks, merchants, teamsters, and farmers—was suddenly deprived of a livelihood. At least 60 per cent of the inhabitants of the seaport towns were unemployed. Soup kettles were set up in the public squares, and even those who a few months before had been living in luxury were forced to share the dole.

The economic loss can never be satisfactorily estimated. For example, the embargo was a knockout blow to Wiscasset's ascendancy. In the year before, its lumber trade had reached its peak. Sea letters had issued at the Custom House to sixty-seven ships. In 1808 but two were issued. Thirty-odd square-rigged vessels, together with smaller craft, lay at anchor in the harbor, their sails unbent, their spars sent down, and inverted tar barrels capping their lower mast heads. These were known as "Jefferson's nightcaps."

Moses Carlton is easily pictured pacing back and forth in front of his beautiful home on High Street, wringing his hands in despair as he looked down on the wealth of the village rotting in the waters below. Bath was caught with sixteen ships, twenty-seven brigs, and a large fleet of schooners and sloops tied out in front of the town. Strung across the broad river from shore to shore was William King's fleet. He had nine vessels, and all but one were loaded to sail. This fleet represented 2,475 tons, and he estimated his loss, exclusive of the interest on the cargoes, at $5,558 a month.

The War Years

Portland's tonnage decreased between 1807 and 1809 by about 10,000 tons. Before the embargo this shipping had been valued at $1,500,000. The sudden check to the profitable employment of this sum resulted in commercial disaster. Within a month after the passage of the act eleven mercantile houses stopped payment. The list of "broken merchants" written on the first blank leaf of Dr. Deane's diary for the year 1807 contains the names of some of the largest Portland shipowners, whose credit until then had been unlimited. The next year the number of failures increased and the business of the town was prostrated. It is said that the failures of 1807, alone, deprived three hundred persons, without counting sailors, of their means of earning a living.

Citizens' mass meetings and town meetings memorialized, petitioned, and offered suggestions to the government. Wells, which at that time included the Town of Kennebunk, claiming to have more square-rigged vessels than any other town in Maine, resolved that it had no confidence in the national government and should turn to the state for redress. The records of almost every seaport town at that period are full of similar strong language. A great anti-embargo demonstration was staged in Portland. This at least served as a safety valve for overheated minds.

An old longboat named the *O-Grab-Me* ("Embargo" in reverse) was loaded on a dray. With sails unbent, running rigging swinging loose, unpainted, and dilapidated, she was dragged stern foremost through the streets by all the dray horses in town hitched tandem. Behind followed a band playing funeral dirges, and bringing up the rear marched all the unemployed of the community. They presented as sad a sight as ever was seen on the streets of Portland. Slowly the procession dragged through the streets and up by the observatory to the battery.

[85]

Here a halt was made and oratory and poetry fitting to the occasion were indulged. Meanwhile the little vessel was undergoing a transformation to represent what might take place if the embargo were lifted. Then the near wreck of a short time before emerged from behind the gun house. She was neatly painted, her sails were bent, and her rigging was trim. She was manned by a nattily dressed crew and navigated merrily down the hill. They launched her from Union wharf amid the cheers of the crowd, which by now had been transformed from a company of mourners into an enthusiastic assembly of merchants, masters, mates, and seamen.

After fourteen months of embargo, the act was repealed the day before Jefferson retired from office. Nonintercourse with the ports of France and England was not lifted for three months, although through a misapprehension President Madison issued his proclamation as early as April. In short order, the Maine fleet was refitted to take its share of the rich profits that were to be had with England and France at war. Every yard was crowded with vessels waiting to be scraped and repaired and refitted for sea. The long-stored products crowded the wharves, and merchants began to make out their orders for imports. Not a few vessels whose owners had their craft loaded and awaiting just such an opportunity cleared port immediately. Every port was a beehive of industry. Asa Clapp of Portland fitted out his *North America* for the Russian trade. She carried out mahogany, logwood, coffee, pepper, indigo, and rum, and brought back iron, hemp, sheeting, Raven's duck, sailcloth, and bristles. The profits were enormous. The little brig *Lee*, owned by Clapp and his partner Matthew "King" Cobb, netted a profit of $80,000 on one voyage.

The War Years

Madison continued his efforts for peace and seemed to be making some headway toward agreement with the belligerents. But the Congress of 1811 contained a group of young men, led by Clay and Calhoun, who brought into it a new spirit. No longer were its decisions to be dominated by the fathers of the Revolution. The rising generation now manifested its power. The young "War Hawks," as they were called, felt that the days were over when it was necessary for the United States to temporize. Political pressure was brought to bear on the reluctant president. In April 1812 a ninety-day embargo was laid. Presumably this was to allow our ships to sail safely to their home harbors. Actually it sent them out to the open seas. On June 18, 1812, Congress declared a state of war to exist with England. Curiously enough, Parliament had revoked her orders in council five days before. The news came too late. It was brought, it is said, by a Wiscasset ship which arrived there on the sixth of August.

Along with the rest of New England, the coast of Maine heard Madison's proclamation with loud expressions of disapproval. It was felt that war was being forced upon them by those who had never seen the sea, let alone sailed a ship. Albeit the cry of the war party had been "Free trade and sailor's rights," it was a solid majority of farmers and traders in the South and West who carried the vote against the sailors and merchants of the Northeast. In the deciding ballot New England stood nineteen to nine for peace. Meetings of citizens convened all through the District to protest.

In Wells, when the sense of the meeting was taken, only 4 voted for war, while 246 stood for peace. In the town's memorial to the president they declared the war to be "unjust, unnecessary and inexpedient." The selectmen of Bath issued a call for a convention of Lincoln County voters. It met in Wiscasset and condemned the government in a most pointed manner. Those of the opposite opinion met to denounce such proceedings as treasonable and to support the government. Partisan politics played its part in all this, and the fact that in the election in 1813 Varnum, who supported the war, received more than a thousand more votes for governor than did Strong, the Federalist candidate, did not lessen the unpopularity of "Mr. Madison's War."

The story of the War of 1812 on the coast of Maine would fill a volume. The tales of the voyages, the dramatic escapes by superior sailing, and the prizes of the privateers—not to mention their own capture and the imprisonment of privateersmen in Dartmoor Prison, the British blockade, and the taking by the British of all the eastern country from the Penobscot to Passamaquoddy—are replete with color and adventure. A century before the day of the U-boat skipper the American privateersman, operating on his own initiative, located the weak point in England's armor—the narrow seas that give access to her main ports. To this, the *Times* in London on February 11, 1815, bears witness as follows:

> The American cruisers daily enter in among our convoys, seize prizes in sight of those that should afford protection, and if pursued "put on their sea-wings" and laugh at the clumsy English pursuers. To what is this owing? Cannot we build ships? . . . It must indeed be encouraging to Mr. Madison to read the logs of his cruisers. If they fight, they are sure to conquer; if they fly, they are sure to escape.

Irrespective of his political opinion, every able-bodied man in the coast towns one way or another went privateering. Our navy, which consisted of only six first-class frigates dating from Federalist days, and about twice that number of smaller vessels, was clearly inadequate. In contrast, England had nearly a thousand ships of war. Hence, a week after the declaration of war, Congress authorized the issuance of letters of marque and reprisal. Every owner of a fast, small vessel began to think of making her into a private cruiser, while those engaged in regular trading voyages lost no time in securing letters of marque in the expectation of the added profits to be had from prize money.

The fleet from Casco Bay consisted of forty-five craft ranging in size from the *Hyder Ally* of 367 tons, which carried a crew of a hundred and mounted sixteen cannon, to the boat *Lark* of 4 tons, with a crew of four men armed with four muskets. With the single objective of speed, keels were quickly laid and hulls built of green timber. Crews were easily signed on among the numerous unemployed seamen and adventurous landsmen. Even if the latter could not reef or steer, they could pull and haul and handle a musket.

One of the first was the *Dart* of South Portland. She was built in five weeks and sailed on her first voyage, only six days over a month after war had been declared. Her fifth prize entitled her to an amusing footnote in maritime history. It was the brig *Dianna*, out of London to Quebec laden with 212 puncheons of rum. It was said to have matured in the casks for many years in the vaults of the London docks, and any mention of "old Dart rum from the original casks" brought a gleam to the eyes of two generations of Portland connoisseurs.

Of these hastily built craft and hurried adventures the story is too often a sad one. Such was the case of the privateer schooner *Gleaner*. At the outset the people of Wells enthusiastically fitted her out with six guns and a crew of fifty and sent her out to make their fortunes. She secured one prize. As she was capturing another an English sloop of war swooped down. Both privateer and prize were taken to Halifax. And the first capture never even reached an American port. Other ventures were never heard from after they cleared the harbor on their first voyage. There are those yellowing letters of great-grandfathers telling of their experiences in the hulks of the Thames, the Old Mill, or Dartmoor Prison.

One of the most successful privateers on the Maine coast was the *Dash*. Of 222 tons burden and pierced for sixteen guns, she was built early in 1813 at Porter's Landing on the Harraseket River in Freeport by Master Brewer for her owners, Seward and Samuel Porter, who were Portland merchants. Save for her last voyage, she was a very lucky ship. In seven cruises, under four skippers—Edward Kelleran, William Cammett, George Bacon, and John Porter—she sent in fifteen prizes. Every one of them made port and was sold as good prize.

Her speed is legendary. Rigged at first as a topsail schooner, it was later discovered that she could carry a greater spread of canvas and her rig was changed to an hermaphrodite brig—that is, square-rigged forward and schooner-rigged aft. With this she carried a ringtail, a light sail bent on a long sliding spar which was fitted to her main boom. This, when hoisted to the gaff as needed, increased the size of her mainsail by one-third. It has been said of her that "She never suffered defeat, never attacked an enemies' ship in vain, was never injured by a hostile shot and knew no equal in speed."

On her last cruise tragedy struck. Having taken leave of his bride of a few months, Captain Porter, aged twenty-four, sailed from Portland in company with the *Champlain*, a new privateer, for a trial of speed. At the end of the first day the *Dash* had her all but hull down. Night came on, and with it a squall. The light of the *Dash* disappeared in the scud. Finding the water shoaling, the *Champlain* altered her course. The *Dash* was never again seen. She is believed to have foundered on George's Bank. With her were lost the Captain, his two brothers, and a crew of sixty able men. She is the subject of Whittier's poem, "The Dead Ship of Harpswell."

Several of the most famous privateers of America were launched from Maine yards although owned in other states. Of these the brig *Grand Turk* was the most famous. She was built by Stephen C. Dutton in the early part of 1812 at Wiscasset and bought by a group of thirty men, most of whom hailed from Salem. Her story is a part of the American tradition. Admittedly the best sailer out of Salem, she was also one of the most successful. She captured over thirty prizes. The *Fox*, launched at Portland by William Moulton and registered in Portsmouth, was the pride of the Piscataqua. With Captain Elihu Brown in command, she had a remarkable success and came to be known as "the million-dollar privateer." One of her richest prizes was the British brig *Belise*. She sent this prize into Saco, and at the sale ship and cargo fetched $205,927.78. This, her fifth cruise, netted her owners $328,731.33. Each seaman's share, according to Captain Brown, was $1,200.

The sea lanes leading from England to Halifax and the St. Lawrence were rich hunting grounds for the privateers of New England and New York. Niles' Register lists some eighty-nine vessels sent into Maine ports during the war. During these years the marshal of the Federal District Court in the District of Maine was a busy man. As early as August 1812, the converted New York pilot boat *Teazer* sent four vessels as prizes into Portland. Of these, two alone were worth $230,000. One Sunday in May 1813, the congregation of Dr. Packard's church in Wiscasset was startled by a gun from Fort Edgecomb announcing the arrival of the Portsmouth privateer *Thomas*. She was escorting a brig and a ship, the latter valued at £70,000. The *Viper* of New York sent in to Camden the ship *Victory* with two other vessels, which sold for $11,500. The Crowninshields' ship *America* is considered to have been the most successful of the Massachusetts privateers. In 1813 she sent into Bath a very rich prize with a full cargo of English dry goods and silks. So valuable was it that to avoid sending this temptation along the coast the owners paid $10,000 to have it hauled overland to Boston.

At first the war bore lightly on Maine, as on all New England. Hopeful that these states might remain neutral, the British blockade was not immediately extended to New England. Her ports were also excepted when the importation of American products into the West Indies was prohibited. During the autumn months of 1812 and through the winters of 1813 and 1814, there was little interruption with trade. The captains of British warships along the coasts allowed vessels to pass and repass, and for a consideration they even acted as convoys for smuggling craft.

This was the case with the British brig *Boxer*. She might never have been found and captured had she not given herself away in a demonstration before the fort at Popham. This was done in order to assist the smuggling schooner *Margaretta* of Bath to get into the mouth of the Kennebec. Fishermen off Half Way Rock heard the guns. They reported the fact to the *Enterprise*, which was then in search of her. There followed the battle of the two brigs off Monhegan, in which both youthful captains lost their lives. They lie buried in adjoining graves in the old Eastern Cemetery in Portland.

When Admiral Cochrane took over the command of the American station from Sir John Warren, the war was prosecuted with vigor. In April 1814 the blockade was extended to the whole of New England. June was a hectic month on the Maine coast. The *Bulwark*, a 74, was sent to harry the shores of the District, destroy all shipping she could reach, and frighten the fishermen from their grounds. On the fourteenth she sent ashore a landing party to the establishment of Captain Thomas Cutts at Biddeford Pool, near the mouth of the Saco River. One of his vessels, which they had chased in from the sea, they burned. The frame of another on the stocks was cut into pieces, and they carried off a third. This they later allowed Cutts to ransom. The next day she appeared off Kennebunk. But here militia quickly mustered, and her people made no attempt to land. On the twentieth she anchored off Seguin and sent her barges up the Sheepscot, occasioning the "great alarm." Here, too, the militia frustrated their plans. Two days later the George's River was visited. From this time forward the blockade was effectively maintained.

WAR ON THE PENOBSCOT

More serious invasions followed. By September all Maine east of the Penobscot had been invaded, conquered, and formally annexed to New Brunswick. Eastport was seized in July. On the first day of September a naval squadron of twenty-five ships under Rear Admiral Griffith sailed into the Penobscot and anchored off Castine, which was quickly abandoned by the American forces. Belfast was taken without bloodshed on the same afternoon. A part of the fleet then sailed thirty miles up the Penobscot to Hampden. Here the United States frigate *Adams* was refitting and repairing the damages received some days before, when she went aground at Isle au Haut. Word having passed that the British were at Castine, the guns of the *Adams* had been quickly landed and arranged for defense. The militia was summoned to give support, but it proved unreliable under fire, and the vessels and the village were in the possession of the enemy within an hour after the fight began.

The British now pushed on to Bangor. Here no resistance was made, as assurances had been given that private property would be respected. None the less, stores and residences were pillaged, and it was only by giving a bond of $30,000 to deliver the vessels on the stocks to Castine before October 30 that they were not burned. The next morning twenty craft in and on both sides of the river were seized. Fourteen were burned and six carried away. The following day the *Decatur*, just in at Hampden with a rich cargo of brandy, wine, oil, and silks was seized, together with the *Kutsoff*. Both were burned. Downriver Frankfort was laid under contribution. Castine was now made a naval base, Machias was soon taken, and the whole territory was held by the British undisturbed to the close of the war.

The fact that "neutral" vessels were allowed to enter any ports of the country, regardless of what nation they came from, brought a great trade to the eastern harbors. Before Eastport was seized, its trade again rose almost to the height of the first months of the long embargo. Sweden was a neutral nation, and it was easy to give a Yankee or "Bluenose" craft a Swedish register. A Bluenose, in the vernacular, hails from New Brunswick. Indian Island and Campobello became great commercial centers. Quantities of English bale goods were received there, stored in a "neutral vessel" until the deck was almost awash, and then towed to Eastport. So rapid were some of these alleged voyages that it was said that the same vessel often made the crossing from Sweden to America twice in one day. Thus was smuggling obstinately carried on. In June 1814 Marshall Thornton deposited in the Cumberland Bank of Portland the sum of $52,345.27, this being the government's share from the seizure and condemnation of one vessel and her cargo.

After the capture of Castine, the neutral trade at Eastport and Lubec came to an end. The easternmost Custom House in the United States was set up on a vessel in the Penobscot River at Hampden. Here, until the ice closed on the river, a great quantity of English goods was brought in under the Swedish

The War Years

flag. Peleg Talman of Bath was accredited as the Swedish consul. In five weeks the amount of duties collected is said to have been $150,000. When the river froze at Hampden the smuggling was carried on across the ice in just as determined a fashion.

Immediately after the capture of Castine the British government established its Custom House and appointed a collector. He received entries of vessels and merchandise until the evacuation of the town in April 1815. Insurance on vessels from Halifax was at this time 20 per cent, but this did not prevent many taking the risk, on account of the large profit involved. Provisions and lumber from the westward were brought here to market and exchanged for English goods at high prices. Fat beeves driven across from the western side of the river made a fair exchange on the eastern side for warm Birmingham blankets. The considerable sum of money collected at Castine, or at least £9,750 of it, was used in 1818 to found Dalhousie College in Halifax.

The blockade had by this time put an end to all coasting activity. In this state of affairs merchants and others had to resort to the slow, creeping transport of ox- or horse-drawn vehicles. These comprised the famous fleet of "mud clippers." The Horse Marine crowded the roads of Maine from the Penobscot on toward Boston, New York, and the South. The newspapers printed reports of its progress in special columns. In the *Kennebunk. Visitor*, this column was headed "Horse Marine Lists." It contained items such as:

Arrived, November 6, at noon two horse cutter "Timothy Pickering" and "Quincy Cannon Ball," Commodore Delande from Portland to Boston. Spoke on her passage sixteen ox schooners from Bath to Portland, cargo, tin plate, all well. Also saw on the Scarborough turnpike a suspicious looking cutter which we escaped by superior sailing.

As the volume of this traffic obviously had a connection with smuggling, the "fleet" was carefully watched by the customs officers. These amusing yet serious reports have many accounts of the boardings and searchings by these officers. The accounts rejoice when the tables are turned on the unpopular inspectors. One story will illustrate. A wagoner, upon being stopped, was asked, "What are you loaded with?" To this he replied, "Quintals of pollock, casks of oil, and dry goods from Eastport." "Drygoods from Eastport!" exclaimed the inspector. "They must be smuggled." The wagoner protested that they were of American make, but the boxes were broken open. They were found to contain, not Yorkshire broadcloth and Irish linen, but dried herrings.

On a cold, clear February night in 1815 there was a brilliant party in the spacious home of Major Moses Carlton in Wiscasset. All the town was in darkness save where light poured from the windows of this hospitable mansion. Suddenly the company was startled by a shriek and the sound of breaking glass as the old slave woman Pendy dropped her tray of whip glasses. They rushed into the hall. A mounted horseman had ridden in through the front doors. He was the messenger bringing to the maritime towns of Maine the welcome news that the war was over.

CHAPTER SIX

The WEST INDIA TRADE

She proved to be the Schr. *Venis* of St. Kitts from St. Kitts
bound to Quebec laden with Rum, Sugar and Molasses.—
The Log of the Privateer Schooner Teazer, August 17, 1812.

> Old horse! Old horse! how came you here?
> From Sacarap to Portland Pier
> I've toted boards for many a year.
> Until worn out by sore abuse
> They salted me down for sailors use.
> The sailors they do me despise,
> They turn me over and damn my eyes,
> Cut off my meat and pick my bones
> And throw me over to Davy Jones.

REGARDLESS OF WHAT was to be a Maine boy's occupation or
profession, an indispensable part of his upbringing was a voyage
or two in the West India trade. In the days when the privateers
of France and England, not to mention the piratical craft
swarming in the Caribbean, might be sighted at any time and
in almost any latitude, this opened up endless vistas of adventure before the young sailor. In *The Hardscrabble* Elijah Kellogg spins a yarn of the building of a sloop by four boys. They
manned her, filled her with ventures, and took her out to Martinique, where, according to Kellogg, "Pluck and principle won
the day" and each came home with "what in those days was
considered a handsome property."

The facts do not belie the fiction. For example, in 1791

Captains Asa Clapp and William McLellan were witnesses to the frightful massacre of the white population of Haiti during the revolution precipitated by Toussaint L'Ouverture. And thereby hangs a tale of the shrewd guile by which a Maine skipper snatched, in the face of disaster, a cargo and a profit.

The insurrection was hardly over when a down-east captain sailed into the port of San Domingo with a cargo of lumber worth $7,000. As soon as he dropped anchor a squad of Toussaint's black soldiers came aboard and took possession. The captain put up no resistance and learned from the sergeant that Toussaint was in camp near by and would be glad to meet any one from the United States, for which country he had a high regard. Now at this time every vessel in foreign trade carried a sea letter calling on all kings, rulers, and potentates to render aid to vessels or crews in distress. They were issued by the governments, and the one carried by the captain was signed by President Washington. The captain told the sergeant that he had a letter from General Washington which he wished to read to his commander.

They went ashore and found the "Black Napoleon" lying in a hammock dressed in full uniform. The announcement that Washington had written him a letter brought him to his feet with a bound, and he ordered the letter read. Thereupon the captain read and the sergeant translated. Immensely pleased by the craftily inserted praise of himself, Toussaint asked what cargo the captain had brought and what he wished to take back. Thereupon he directed that the lumber be discharged and the vessel be loaded cargo for cargo with sugar and coffee. No brig ever had its capacity more fully tested. Every nook and corner was used, and the sailors complained that they had no place to sleep. The profits of this voyage were over $80,000.

★　★　★

The West India Trade

The Bay Colony quite early developed a thriving trade with "the Islands." In 1676 Edward Randolph, the "Surveyor, collector and searcher for New England," reported that Boston should be "esteemed the mart town of the West Indies." On the Maine coast, while there is record of early voyages to the Caribbean, this trade came to its maturity much later. By the middle of the seventeenth century Thomas Cutts was in the Barbados acting as agent for his brothers, receiving their cargoes of Piscataqua fish and lumber and shipping West India goods in return. Later he came to Kittery and carried on an extensive business in this line. Somewhat later The William Pepperells built up and maintained a vigorous trade with the islands.

Even before their settlement was safe from Indian attack the people of York joined together in partnership to build and fit out a vessel to send to the West Indies. By 1745 they had some twenty craft engaged in that trade. At the time that Wells included the present town of Kennebunk, it also had its fleet and varied its trips to the southward with voyages to Halifax and Montreal, where there was a ready market for cattle. This was a profitable but precarious cargo. There is a case on record where one skipper had his entire deckload of thirty-nine head washed overboard the first night out. Colonel Thomas Cutts, a former clerk of the Pepperells in Kittery, came to Saco in 1758, where he soon developed a large business with warehouses and a wharf at Saco Ferry. He is said to have netted a profit of $100,000 on a cargo of molasses which was taken in exchange for one of lumber and which arrived in time to be sold on a high market.

When the people on the neck at Falmouth were engaged in the masting trade, there had sprung up a West India trade of considerable extent. It was carried on principally by Ezekiel Cushing and William Simonton, who had a large and valuable wharf in the cove in South Portland which now bears Simonton's name. Farther on down East the records are of a later date. For example, the first voyage to that part of the world out of Blue Hill was made in 1768. Ellsworth's first vessel, the *Susan and Abigail*, cleared in 1773 on a voyage, which thereafter became an annual affair, to Demerara with a cargo of oak staves and shingles turned out by Captain Isaac Smith's neighbors.

The products of the Islands furnished many of the staples of pioneer life. In 1759, after the fall of Canada, new settlements were established well back from the coast. This increased the demand. Thus merchants in the coast towns not only supplied local needs but became wholesalers for the many little general stores up country, whose signs "W-I Goods" proclaimed them as the depots for rum and treacle. Barter was then the order of the day. The fisherman and the farmer found the merchant an indispensable middleman, whose warehouses and wharves became the center of an ever-growing import and export trade.

Before the Revolution, what with free access to the British islands, plenty of smuggling with the Spanish ports, and trade with the French, American shipowners had been carrying on a most profitable business and were by way of making large fortunes. By the Treaty of Paris, which recognized our independence, the doors of the British West India ports were "slammed in our faces." Parliament told the planters of the islands that they would find their supplies in the Canadian provinces. But the English merchants and the inhabitants of these islands wanted American produce. Yankee captains could supply them more promptly, with better quality, and at lower prices than could their own people in Nova Scotia.

Moreover, the Yankee captain would take in trade West India goods, particularly molasses, which had no ready sale in Europe, or, if need be, he could pay cash. The governors of the islands appointed the collectors and the judges. Backed by them, these officials found many excuses for winking the official eye, and most vessels entering their ports loaded to the scuppers with Maine products went out light. Provided the most important part of the transaction was not omitted and that a five-joe piece crossed an English palm, stress of weather, relief for a starving population, the need for rebuilding after a hurricane, a British charter acquired in Nova Scotia, a Spanish one in Trinidad, or an ancient register dating from before the Revolution, was quite enough. So it was that when Horatio, later Lord, Nelson was sent out in 1786 to enforce the Navigation Acts, he wrote home saying:

> When I arrived in Barbadoes, the Bay was so full of American vessels, lading and unlading without molestation from the customs house officers that there were more American flags than English and had I been set down from the air I should most assuredly have been convinced that I was in an American instead of a British port.

At this time, by virtue of treaties, American vessels had access to the French islands as well as to the Dutch—St. Eustatius, St. Martin, and Curaçao—and the Swedish—St. Bartholomew. The commerce of the island of Cuba was in theory a complete monopoly, but its inhabitants, as well as those of the other Spanish colonies, encouraged smuggling. Thus there was built up an enormous contraband trade which all the fleets of Spain were unable to prevent. It was with this island that the largest amount of the trade from the Maine coast was carried on. Havana in particular offered a ready market for ship timber and . spars for the large number of Spanish men-of-war that were being built there.

The vessels engaged in the West India trade seem surprisingly small today. They comprised large sloops, two-masted schooners, and brigs. For two decades after the Revolution, the average size of a vessel out of the Kennebec was but 129 tons. As this figure includes ships, the majority were much smaller.

Being of moderate draft, they were able to take the more direct route to Cuba across the Great Bahama Bank. Over this route traveled a goodly part of the output of the Maine forests in the shape of masts, spars, boxes, shingles, and staves.

In the early days they were built in forgotten yards all along the shore and on the small rivers from the Kennebec westward to the Piscataqua. Near Smelt Hill and the first falls of the Presumpscot River, which enters into Casco Bay, was a popular location. Here the Merrills, Lunts, Moodys, Batchelders, Knights, Hamiltons, and Smelledges put afloat the full-rigged, hermaphrodite, and jackass brigs which were so popular in the West India trade. At one time nearly a hundred of them hailed from Portland.

These vessels cost no more than fifteen or twenty dollars a ton, since the lumber for them could be cut within a few rods of the building ways. Their floors were of red oak or beech and their tops of pitch pine, Norway pine, spruce, hemlock, or anything that came to hand. Spruce limbs saturated with pitch furnished good treenails. However rough in appearance they might be, they were staunch and lasted well. For example, in 1810 Captain Ezekiel Dyer built himself the brig *Cordelia* at Ferry Village opposite Portland. Thirty-nine years later an item in the Portland *Transcript* announced that she was soon to sail for the West Indies on her ninetieth voyage.

The cargoes they carried were varied. Almost every necessity of life was welcome in islands whose only products were luxuries. There was lumber—sawed lumber and masts, spars, and hewn timbers for the shipyards of Havana. On top of a deckload of lumber and on the decks of other vessels there would often be carried the small, flat-bottomed craft known as "moses boats," which were in great demand in the sugar islands. The planters used them in lightering molasses out of the narrow streams bordering their plantations to the brigs awaiting their cargoes in deep water.

The products of the cooper's trade formed a considerable item. There were shooks with the staves jointed and crozed, hoops shaved, and the headings fitted to put in place. These are terms in the cooper's trade. Shooks are bundles of staves, hoops, and heads, each bundle containing the number sufficient to make up a single hogshead, tierce, cask, or barrel. Boxes knocked down and shipped in bundles are also called shooks. The saving in cargo space is obvious. This aspect of the West India trade has survived into our own time.

Then also there were house frames all ready to put up, oxen and horses for the plow, the sugar and the treadmill, farm produce such as parsnips, potatoes, onions and grain, beef, mutton, pork, pickled fish, soap, candles, and dried codfish in "drums" of from five to eight hundred pounds each. Indeed, the manifests of these vessels read like the inventory of a country store. And what profits they paid! Lumber from the banks of Maine rivers which cost there $8.00 a thousand sold in Havana for $60.00. Beets and parsnips brought $16.00 a barrel in the French islands. Flour sold for $21.00 a barrel, beef for $24.00, and pork for $27.00. How completely this trade absorbed the maritime activity of these early years is shown by the fact that in 1787 seventy-three out of the eighty-nine clearances from Portland were for some port in the West Indies.

With prosperity came the desire for better facilities to take care of this rapidly increasing business. Old wharves and breastworks disappeared. In Portland, Union, Long, and Commercial Wharves pushed far out into the harbor. On these were constructed substantial stores, warehouses, and distilleries. At Kennebunk prodigious efforts were made to improve the harbor with the ill-fated Mousam Canal and thereafter with the more successful piers at the mouth of the Kennebunk River. King's Wharf was built at Bath, and others were constructed at Wiscasset. Up to this time the District had been dependent on Boston for its banking facilities. In 1799 the Portland Bank was chartered, to be followed in 1802 by the Maine Bank. That year also saw the start of the Lincoln and Kennebec Bank at Wiscasset.

Under the name of the Portland Monument Association a company of merchants, headed by Captain Lemuel Moody, in 1807 subscribed for the construction of an observation tower then and since known as "The Observatory." Standing atop of Munjoy Hill and rising two hundred and twenty-seven feet above sea level, it commanded all the approaches by sea. They furnished it with a powerful French telescope. The octagonal brown tower was supported by eight large white-pine posts which rose from a deep foundation of stone eighty-two feet to a sheltered observation deck.

Here Captain Lemuel Moody stood watch from sunrise to sunset. With the glass he could identify a vessel twenty miles off shore. On three flagstaffs—one for ships and barks, another for brigs, and a third for schooners and later for steamers—he set well-known signals which told the town what shipping was in the offing. A foreign vessel was announced by its national flag, and if it was a war vessel, a black ball was set just below. Various pennants told of a ship in distress or a vessel ashore and various other tales. Most valuable was the display of the private house flags of the merchants in town. The setting of these warned them of the arrival of their vessels several hours before they reached harbor.

Here on September 5, 1813, Captain Moody watched the *Enterprise* whip the *Boxer* and recounted the progress of the battle, in the manner of a modern radio commentator, to an expectant crowd at the base of the tower. From this vantage

The West India Trade

REPORT and Manifest of the Cargo, laden at the Port of *Portland*
board the *Snow Harriet* — *John Balson* — master, bound for the port
at *Surinam* — — — *Portland March 2. 1805.*

Marks.	Numbers.	Packages or Articles in Bulk.	Contents or Quantities.	Value at the Port of Exportation.	
				D.	*Ct.*
		Boards — — —	57350 feet — —	573	50
		Shingles — —	102 M — —	204	
		Flour — — —	31 Barrels — —	387	50
		Tallow Candles —	424 lb —	80	38
		dryed Fish —	400 Quintals —	1200	
		Tobacco — —	1123 lb —	78	75
		Soap — —	955½ lb —	95	59
		Beef — —	143 Barrels —	1325	
		Butter — —	2000 lb —	400	
		Clapboards	700	7	10
		Shook Hogsheads	148 —	148	
				4497	78

District of Portland & Falmouth,

I — John Balson — master or commander of the
Snow Harriet — bound from the Port of Portland — to Surinam
do solemnly, sincerely and truly Swear . that the Manifest of the Cargo, on board the said
now delivered by me to the Collector of this District, and subscribed with my name, contains, according to the best of
my knowledge and belief, a full, just and true account of all the Goods, Wares and Merchandize, now actually laden on
board the said Vessel, and of the Value thereof : and if any other Goods, Wares or Merchandize shall be laden or put
on board the said Snow — previous to her sailing from this port, I will immediately report the same
to the said Collector. I do also that I verily believe the duties on all the foreign merchandize
therein specified, have been paid or secured according to law, and that no part thereof is intended to be relanded within the United States, and that if by distress or other unavoidable accident it shall become necessary to reland the same,
I will forthwith make a just and true report thereof to the Collector of the Customs of the District wherein such distress or accident may happen.

Collector's Office, Port of Portland March 2. 1805. *John Balson*
Sworn before

The manifest of the cargo on the snow *Harriet*, Portland to
Surinam, is a typical list of the goods carried out to the
West Indies.

a fleet of two hundred little barks and brigs could be seen sailing out of the harbor on the twenty-ninth of April in 1844. With their white sails glistening in the sun they made, in the words of a contemporary editor, "a fine sight in the offing."

Many of the finest houses in Maine were built in the last decade of the eighteenth and the first of the nineteenth century. There are the beautiful mansions of Wiscasset which reached "the apogee of the Georgian style and the culmination of the colonial and early national architecture." The Nickels, Hodge, Smith, Tucker, Cook, Lee, Wood, and Carlton houses of this town belong to this period. So also does the Hamilton house at South Berwick, the Sewall at York, the Lyman and Robert Lord at Kennebunk, the Thomas Cutts mansion at Saco, the Cobb, Ingraham, Wingate, and Ebenezer Storer houses in Portland, the Cotterill at Damariscotta and the Kavanagh at New Castle. Many attempts have been made to give the credit for the beauty of form and line of these houses to foreign architectural plans. In most instances they were the work in both design and execution of local carpenters and joiners—the very same men who set the frames of their vessels "by the eye." Indeed, no better education in beauty of line could be obtained than by the designing of ships. Ship carpenters framed and erected, ship joiners finished the interiors, and ship carvers, turning from figureheads, trailboards, and stern ornaments, carved with equal facility mantels, stairways, and wainscoting.

★ ★ ★

The news of the Treaty of Ghent, which concluded the three years of "Mr. Madison's War," reached the coast of Maine in midwinter. Many vessels were stripped of their gear and all but their lower masts. Indeed, some were frozen in the ice of the creeks and rivers where they had been hidden away. By April 1816 many little brigs were bearing away on their old courses to the southward. Their masters hoped to find good markets awaiting them, but in this they were disappointed. Very few made saving voyages. Although commerce slowly revived, it did not flourish as it had at the beginning of the century. It was not until some time after the European wars that it became more stable and developed a character all its own. This period from the close of the second war with England until 1840 came to be known to old-timers as the "old West India trade."

The ships and the rigs which were peculiarly adapted to the West India trade have completely disappeared from the seas. They were small craft, on the average around 200 tons, although after 1830 vessels of 300 and over were launched. Drawing but little water, they were able to look into almost any creek or river that emptied into a cove or bay in search of a likely cargo. Being very full-bodied, they could load to advantage. The pros and cons of the various types—not to mention the quarrel-provoking question of their proper designation—have formed a favorite topic of maritime debate wherever those of a sea turn of mind may foregather.

This period is pre-eminently that of the brig—now obsolete for three-quarters of a century. In the building of these Maine had a near monopoly. The full-rigged brig had both masts, main and fore, in three spars and was wholly square-rigged save that on the mainmast was a standing gaff to which was bent a small fore-and-aft sail called the spanker. The snow was much akin to the brig, the difference being that the snow set her spanker on a trysail mast stepped on deck a foot or so abaft the mainmast and secured aloft to the trestletrees of the mast.

These gave way to the hermaphrodite brig. This was a cross between a brig and a schooner, being square-rigged on the foremast and fore-and-aft-rigged on the mainmast. Fewer men were required to handle her, and her economy made her exceedingly popular. A modification of this was that familiarly known as the "jackass brig." This carried one or more square sails on the mainmast. Out of Maine waters the hermaphrodite and particularly the jackass brig was often called a brigantine. But on the coast of Maine the brigantine carried the sails of a brig on her foremast and her mainmast was made in two spars having the rig of a topsail schooner with at least one square main topsail and sometimes a main topgallant sail. This was thought to be a more weatherly rig than the others, for the big fore-and-aft sail was a powerful pusher when close-hauled on the wind.

Then there was the familiar "tops'l schooner," which was widely used though never quite as popular in the District as the brig rigs. Here the masts and sails were those of a fore-and-after, save that on the foremast she carried a topsail and sometimes a topgallant sail, the latter two being square sails. Finally there was the completely forgotten but quite popular "tops'l sloop." One is described by Elijah Kellogg in *The Hardscrabble*. In addition to her mainsail, she carried a full suit of square sails— course, topsail, topgallant sail, and royal. Says the author:

> Her lower mast was rather short in proportion to the top, top-gallant and royal masts. The mainmast was set well aft, and raked a good deal. The bowsprit and jib-boom were long. She had a sprit-sail yard and double martingale. The fore-braces led to the end of the bowsprit, the others to the end of the jib-boom. In bad weather they had preventive-braces that led aft to the rail. She carried fore-topmast staysail, jib and flying-jib.

The number of smart little vessels of all these types and rigs which were owned in the various ports is amazing. Two trips a year was the rule. A vessel would leave the Maine coast in the latter half of December, and arrive at the islands at the end of the three-week Christmas holidays. She would unload, take on a return cargo, and reach home around the last of February. Immediately she would reload and go out on her second voyage,

The West India Trade

reaching port again sometime in the latter part of April. Then they would lay her up over the summer months, during the yellow fever and hurricane season in the islands and the planting and haying season at home. In October the most industrious would go on a coasting voyage.

As time went on the larger merchants established business connections with merchants in the West Indies. This gave assurance of a market and a return cargo and permitted the brigs to sail almost with the regularity of a packet. Others, who comprised the majority, cleared merely to the West Indies with no particular port in view, seeking a market where the best opportunity offered. These voyages did not always bring the warmth, sunshine and delight of the tropics together with enormous profits. A typical experience is that of Captain Theodore Wells in the schooner *Friendship*, bound from Wells to St. Vincents with a cargo of hewed lumber. This his owners had ordered him not to dispose of unless he could get one hundred gallons of molasses for a thousand feet of lumber. He had a short and pleasant voyage down to St. Vincents but found no market there. The captain tells his own tale:

From St. Vincents I sailed for Grenada where not finding a market from thence I left for Trinidad where I was still unable to effect a sale. Proceeding northward I touched at Port Royal in the island of Martinico. Here I failed to find a satisfactory sale. From this port I proceeded to Bastarre in the Island of Guadaloupe where the same disappointment awaited me. I next touched at Nevis but could not dispose of my freight without trusting it in hands of doubtful solvency. From here I sailed for St. Thomas. At this point there was no demand for a cargo like mine. I attempted to reach Porto Rico which was the last island where molasses was to be found excepting Cuba but in this failed because of a fresh blow and thick stormy weather which drove me by it when I ran for Aquin in the Island of St. Domingo and here as elsewhere I found a dull market and no sale.

To cut short this catalogue of frustration, he ran from San Domingo to Aux Cayes, to Jérémie, to Mariguana, and to Port-au-Prince, where he found a large number of vessels that were making losing sales in an overstocked market. Leaving there, he sailed to St. Marks. At last he returned to Jérémie, from whence, after spending twenty-eight days in making a sale and forty more in waiting for his cargo of coffee, he sailed for home, only to lose both his vessel and his cargo when but a few days out.

Neither dull markets nor the reefs of the Bahama Cays were the worst hazards of a West India voyage. There was piracy. During the long years of the American and Napoleonic wars the islands and cays had become infested with pirates of the lowest type. Encouraged by the authorities, they preyed openly on American commerce. In November 1821 eleven pirate vessels were cruising from Maisí on the southeast coast of Cuba. Five worked together as a squadron off Cape San Antonio on the southwest coast and five more east of Matanzas on the north. Between Matanzas and Havana a flotilla of small boats kept constant watch for vessels becalmed in the offing, attacking them as soon as darkness fell. Still another nest of small boats operated at Cape Cruz, the crews living in caves on the shore. The ship news of the period is full of accounts of the atrocious attacks by these gangs of cutthroats who were guided by the maxim, "Dead cats don't mew."

The brig *Dolphin* of Nobleboro was attacked in August 1821 off Cape Antonio, the mate stabbed and the men hoisted up by the neck to compel them to tell where money was concealed. The *Alliance* of Kennebunk fell into the hands of the same gang the next January. The members of the crew were robbed of everything, even their shirts, and were beaten, put into the long-boat, and set adrift. The *Mary Jane*, the *Evergreen*, the *Milo*, the *Dispatch*, and the *Cobbseconte* were given like treatment, the last when only four miles out from Morro Castle, Havana.

The West India Trade

The Portland brig *Mechanic* was burned and the crew murdered. The murder of Captain Clement Perkins of the Kennebunk brig *Belisarius* was particularly horrible. In March 1823, when off Campeche, she was boarded by the crew of a piratical schooner of some forty tons. They were vicious brutes. The captain told them where they could find what money there was on board. Disappointed in not finding it as much as they hoped, they cut off first his right arm, then his left, and finally his leg above the knee. Not satisfied with this cruelty, they filled his mouth with oakum, saturated it with oil, and, setting it on fire, ended his sufferings.

The murder of all but one of the crew of a Maine brig, the story told by this survivor, and the nationwide publicity given to it are said to have brought about a campaign of extermination that all but cleared the Caribbean of these pests. On the twenty-eighth of November, 1824, the brig *Betsey* sailed from Wiscasset with a cargo of lumber for Matanzas. She was under the command of Elias Hilton with two mates, three seamen, and a cook. On a December night, the brig struck a rock off the Double Head Shot Keys. The crew took to the boats, eventually landing on one of the Cuba keys. This they found to be inhabited by five fishermen, the leader of whom the captain recognized as one with whom he had previously traded at Matanzas. Feeling that he could trust him, the captain made arrangements with him to take the party to the island in the morning. This opinion was not shared by the mate. His suspicions were aroused by the secret departure of the fishermen during the night and all but confirmed by his finding evidence of violence in a hidden cove of the key.

As they were leaving the following morning, their vessel was attacked by ten Spaniards in an open boat. Aided by the fishermen, the Spaniards bound them all and carried them to the cove which the mate had discovered the evening before. When they arrived at the head of the cove, they assured their victims that "Americans were very good beef for their knives." Then they began their work of death by decapitating Captain Hilton and murdering all but one of the others in a manner too barbarous to describe. The executioner to whom the second mate, Daniel Collins, had been assigned slipped up. His glancing blow cut the cord with which Collins was bound. Despite his severe wound he was able to escape to the mangrove bushes. Here, creeping in water up to his chin, he reached the edge of the island. Sleeping in the mangroves at night and swimming from key to key by day, tormented by hunger and thirst, the heat, and mosquitoes, he at last reached the island of Cuba.

★   ★   ★

The eighteen-thirties and the roaring forties were days of great activity for the ports of Maine. The railroads had not been built, and the shortest route to the seaboard from northern New Hampshire beyond the White Mountains and from all northern Vermont to Derby Line was through Crawford Notch. There was little money in the new country. Trade was almost entirely by barter. The farmer brought his produce to the seaboard merchant and took "store pay" in return. All this country produce had to be transported to market and exchanged for the flour, salt fish, coffee, rum, and "long sweetening," as molasses was called, which were necessities of life in the pioneer settlements. So in winter the "Vermonters" came down the present Roosevelt trail in long strings of red pungs. On a projecting board stood the driver, clad invariably in a long blue frock, guiding his team over the frozen road. In the pung were his round hogs, his butter, and his lard, together with the large round box which held his provisions—generally huge chunks of cheese and molasses doughnuts.

The whole country was awakening to the economic value

of the back country. In 1825 the Erie Canal was completed, and in Maine various attempts were made to open up the expanding frontier. Lakes and ponds were joined by canals to facilitate the bringing of lumber and other products to a shipping point. From 1820 to 1840 the Maine legislature granted charters for twenty-five such enterprises. The most important was the Cumberland and Oxford Canal. Completed in 1830, it opened up the whole Sebago Lake region with its wide branching system of lakes and ponds. Moving slowly down the twenty miles from White's Bridge in Windham to Portland Harbor, the flat-bottomed boats, *Whirlwind, Major Downing, Honest Quaker, Reindeer,* and others added their cargoes to the holds of the waiting West India brigs.

When a cargo of coffee or molasses came alongside a wharf or when lumber was being loaded aboard, the waterfront resounded with the song of the Negro stevedores. They hoisted the hogsheads from the holds by a tackle (pronounced "taykel") and fall, all the time singing:

> "Everybody he lub something,
> Hoojun—John—a hoojun,
> Song he set the heart a-beating,
> Hoojun—John—a hoojun."

There were no winches in those days. It is said that after they were introduced Negroes disappeared from the northern seaports, for they refused to work with a winch, as with that sort of labor their songs had no place. Adding to the confusion were the busy lumber surveyors who ran from one ox load to another with a shingle for their record in one hand and a rule staff for their scaling in the other. On the wharf, as the cargo came out, stood the gauger checking the hogsheads and boxes against the manifest. Since this document sometimes failed to list all the cargo, there sometimes arose the question as to how

24. — Cargo of the Brig *Freedom*. George Fletcher master from Havannah

October 18. Hugh McCulloch . BF 1 a 37. 37 Hogsheads Molasses 3337 gallons · · · · 417/85
. 1 a 23. 23 Boxes White Clayed Sugar 9623 ...... · · · 276,73
. 1 a 16. 16 Tice Brown Clayed ditto 3442 . 21..... 101,65

Total duties on this cargo: **849.05**

25. — Cargo of the Brig *Columbia*. Simmon Master master from Grenada

October 19. Joseph Moody Esq. {BC 1 a 11/31 } 1st Punc. 2165 Gallons 25 C.ns 538,25
M. 1 a 12, 13 . 2d Rum { 3 . . 1709 · · 25 · · · 333,43
. 1 a 2 . 3d . . 1239 · · 32 · · · 412,48
BC 1 a 16 { 16 Hogsheads Molasses 1734 · · · 3 · · · 57,70

Total duties on this cargo... **619.91**

26. — Cargo of the Brig *Polly*. Robert Smith master from Monsiques and Guadeloupe.

October 28. John Mitchell & Co. {B.P. 1 a 19 19 Puncheon Rum. 2d Punc. 323 Gallons · · 25 Casks 205/15
1 a 26 24 Hogsheads, 3 Tierces, 2 Barrels Brown Sugar, 25196 pounds · · 28 · · · 330,40
1 a 10 8 Barrel & 2 Bags Coffee 1379 formed · · 2t · · · 629,90
1 a 3 3 Jacket Cotton 359 · · 5 · · · 78,95
Robert Smith . 1 a 3 3 Barrels Oranges Cost £1.56 r 17½ p ct. 3 " · · 10/77
32

Total duties on this cargo **1246.09**.

[114]

The usual return cargoes—hogsheads of molasses, boxes and tierces of sugar, puncheons of rum, and some coffee, cotton and oranges—from the West Indies are shown on this Custom House record of duties for three Maine brigs, *Freedom, Columbia* and *Polly*.

this surplus could be landed without detection by the customs officer. It was often solved by the owner taking the inspector home with him to dinner and lingering rather long over the wine. Then a few more hogsheads of molasses or boxes of sugar would be hoisted out and stored in the warehouse without appearing on the tally.

On the inventories of the West India Stores as in the manifests of the West India brigs, rum, coffee, and molasses lead all the rest. After the Revolution rum from Jamaica and the other English islands or from St. Croix and the Dutch ports lost its place in the imports. Before that time old Falmouth had its distillery wharf. With the cost of molasses at thirteen pence per gallon and the cost of distilling it five and a half, Maine merchants were quick to perceive the large profits to be had in manufacturing rum at home. There were seven distilleries at one time in Portland, one in Bath, another in Wiscasset, and Vaughan's great establishment at Hallowell. The amount consumed was surprising. During one winter a country store in Pittston disposed of ninety hogsheads. A boatman on the Cumberland and Oxford Canal reported that during the season he alone delivered three hundred barrels to the towns along his route.

Coffee was the most desired cargo. This was because of its small bulk as against its value. Haiti, which before the insurrection of the blacks had been the richest of the islands, produced much of the fragrant bean. Cuba also was a high producer before the great hurricane of 1844 destroyed her coffee groves. But the islands of the Spanish Main were growing a steadily increasing amount. Brazil, too, was fast attaining the pre-eminence that has made the name of her principal port, Rio, synonymous with coffee. As the years passed, coffee figured less and less in the manifests of the Maine brigs. More and more the cargoes consisted entirely of molasses. In the marine news the romantic names of the Saints of the Leeward and Windward Islands occur with less frequency. They are replaced by a monotonous iteration of Havana, Cardenas or Matanzas in Cuba, and San Juan Guayama in Porto Rico. The brigs built for this trade at Pipe Stave Landing on the Piscataqua by Sarah Orne Jewett's grandfather were known as the Berwick "molasses brigs."

Havana had long been a favorite port for Maine captains. As early as 1826 over one-tenth of the 117,796 tons of shipping which entered this beautiful harbor in that year hailed from Maine. Cuba not only took a great deal of lumber from the state, the best was also demanded. "Large, handsome lumber suitable for the Havana market," so read the orders. In the six years from 1856 to 1861, there went 1,207 cargoes of this staple to this island. As the sugar and molasses trade grew in the later forties and fifties, Cuba turned to the Maine woods for her sugar boxes, molasses hogsheads, and tierces. In 1856 eight vessels sailed from Bath to Havana carrying 12,368 such boxes and 3,102 hogsheads. Portland monopolized the shook trade and became a collecting center for them. During the six years which have been noted above, only 17 of the 1,040 lumber cargoes from here went to any other than Cuban ports. Sugar boxes are claimed to have been first manufactured at Saccarappa. This is the present city of Westbrook on the Presumpscot River. As with the "molasses brigs," the vessels carrying these shooks came to be known as "Saccarappas."

Many small sawmills were busy sawing and fitting the box boards to proper lengths all ready to be set up and nailed on the sugar plantations. The cooper's trade in the manufacture of hogshead and tierce shooks was one of the best paid in the towns near the coast. In 1867 there were 263 such shops in the state. As has been explained, the shook was a package of red-oak staves and heading, numbered and ready to be set up as a hogshead, a tierce, or a cask when needed. This was done by the coopers on the plantations or by State of Maine coopers who went out to the islands for that purpose. They ranged in price from 50 cents to $1.50. Since the going rate was from 30 to 35 cents for the rough stock, a man who could complete four or five sets in a day made a good day's wage for the times.

Molasses was cheap, fetching some fifty cents a gallon at retail. Hence it was consumed in enormous quantities in the country, and particularly in the logging camps. As one writer has put it:

> Foresters float down timber that seamen may build ships and go to the saccharine islands of the south for molasses; for without molasses no lumberman could be happy in the un-sweetened wilderness. Pork lubricates the joints, molasses gives tenacity to his muscles.

A variation in sweetening was the raw brown sugar. This was known to the trade as "muscovado" and was procured by draining the molasses through holes in the bottom of the hogshead after the crystallization of the cane syrup had begun. Another variety was the "clayed" form. This name derived from the fact that the containers were sealed with moist clay. This latter type was shipped mostly from Havana in long wooden boxes, while the muscovado came from Matanzas in hogsheads weighing around a half a ton. White sugar was looked upon as a luxury. Refined of its impurities, it was marketed in a cone or loaf at a price much higher than that of raw sugar.

There were profits to be had in the process of refining. This was perceived by the West India merchants of Portland, one of the first of whom was John Bundy Brown. In partnership with others in 1845 he erected what is said to have been the third sugar house in the United States. By perseverance and constant experimentation he developed a process that produced an excellent quality of granulated sugar. His famous Portland Sugar House was incorporated in 1855. An immense establishment

with warehouses and wharves was erected, and the main re-
finery was eight stories high. With a capital of $400,000 there
were employed two hundred persons. It turned out some 250
barrels of sugar a day and processed 30,000 hogsheads of molasses in a year.

In the sixties the demand of the Brown establishment,
coupled with that of two other sugar houses of good capacity
operating in the city and the market in the vast territory opened
to the west and the east by the Grand Trunk and Maine Central
Railroads, made Portland a molasses port that was a close rival
of New York. In 1860 the national total was 31,000,000 gallons.
New York was in the lead with 8,500,000, and Portland was
second with 5,700,000. In 1868, Portland's peak year of importation, there came into the harbor cargoes totaling 59,510
hogsheads and in addition 10,055 hogsheads and 16,800 boxes of
sugar.

This was the trade and those were the days for the rugged
individualist. In the year 1865 Captain Benjamin Webster contracted for the building of the brig *Emma*. She was built in
ninety days. When the men were in the woods in January cutting her frame, Captain Webster contracted for her cargo with
a Portland West India merchant. On the third of April she
cleared fully loaded and sailed out of Portland Harbor with a
fine northwest wind, reaching Cuba in time to secure a return
cargo.

CHAPTER SEVEN

The SHIPYARDS

Something new and yet expressive of the energies of this country. . . . A river scene with vessels of the period, a saw mill, a lumber yard, a ship on the stocks and a background of forest.

SUCH WAS THE proposal in the year 1802 of Judge Silas Lee, one of the incorporators of the Lincoln and Kennebec Bank, to the stockholders, for a design for the notes of the bank.

The observant saunterer on the beaches and salt-water inlets of Maine will stumble in the most unexpected places upon rows of long timbers pitted by exposure and white with dried salt and barnacles. They mark the birthplace of ships now forgotten and are all that remain of a once busy yard. Indeed, on the upper Sheepscot River there are ancient saw pits in forgotten yards which mark the site of the lost seventeenth-century community known as Sheepscot Farms. Laying these massive timbers was the first step in the preparing of a building yard. They were laid in rows eight to ten feet apart, parallel with the waterside and reaching inshore the length of the proposed vessel. Each log, thirty to forty feet long, was embedded in the soil. With their tops "fared" smooth, they were the "bed logs" upon which the ship rested while she was being built.

The permanent yards were equipped with "breastworks," which were "cribs" constructed at the water's edge of logs filled

[119]

The Maritime History of Maine

with stones and earth. Between these were openings called "slips." Through these passed the ways, which sloped toward the level of tidewater at the proper angle with the shore to take advantage of the deepest water for launching. A favorite site for a yard was handy to a fall of water which would furnish the power needed for a mill to saw the timbers. These "sawmill yards" were numerous on the coast of Maine. In many an instance the very reason for building vessels was to provide a means of transporting lumber from the mill to market.

At the head of the yard or at the sides stood various structures. A long building open at one side like a lean-to provided a place where the men could work in bad weather. In the loft above was a drafting room. In the gable was a clock, and on the roof a bell. Sometimes there was a small shop where ships' wheels were made and another where figureheads and sternboards were carved. In the larger yards the whipsaw pit, ship joiner's shop, blacksmith's shop, oakum shed, and yard office rounded out the establishment. In later days wooden rails and trucks facilitated the moving of heavy material from one part of the yard to another. A boiler house furnished steam for the mill engine and filled the box for steaming planks.

Much of the timber used was bought from neighboring farmers. Cash was paid piece by piece as it was drawn into the yard. The prices seem incredible—30 cents for futtocks, 67 for floor timbers, 50 for naval timbers, and 25 for white ash top timbers. Or there were the ox teams, sometimes as many as two hundred in a day, hauling timber from the towns up country.

Until well into the 1840's native woods were used almost exclusively. The chief exception was southern pine. As early as 1812 there are bills in the King papers covering freight on "pitch pine lumber" from Savannah to Bath, and after 1830 southern pine was often used for planking. White ash was used for oars, buttonwood for windlasses and blocks, elm for keels, hornbeam

[120]

and ironwood for handspikes, hackmatack or juniper for knees, locust for treenails (pronounced "trunnels"), maple for cabin finish, white oak, the toughest of all, for the stem and stern pieces and frames, spruce for spars, knees, and joists, yellow pine for flooring and planking, and white pine—the king of the forest —for masts and larger spars. The Bath and Thomaston yards were exceptions. One hundred workmen from the yards of Bath spent from 1817 to 1821 in Florida and Georgia cutting live oak for the Philadelphia navy yard and thus became acquainted with the value of this timber. As an experiment George Patten and William D. Sewall went to Philadelphia and contracted for a supply of this wood, from which the Pattens in 1838 constructed the ship *Delaware*. From that time on both builders continued its use save as its supply was interrupted during the Civil War. In like manner the Buck family of Bucksport started the little port of Bucksville in South Carolina as a source of supply to New England shipyards of pitch pine and hardwood lumber.

In the days before the yards became few in number and these few concentrated at the larger centers near the open sea, sizable craft were built in what today seem to be impossible places. The records reflect year after year of shipbuilding in the shallow Kennebunk, the narrow channels above the falls of the Sheepscot, and in even more difficult places on the eastern rivers. In the days when transportation posed a difficult problem, it was less expensive to build the craft near the timber supply than to have the timber hauled to a spot convenient for launching. In the tidal rivers locks were built to provide a sufficient depth of water. Rollers would be used to ease the hulls over shallows, and the vessel would be warped slowly down the narrow stream, sometimes taking as many as fifteen tides to get into deep water.

The shipbuilding on the Kennebunk River is illustrative of

this. Here in the nineteenth century there were eight decades of shipbuilding. The yards were located at "Kennebunk Landing"—so called because of the meadows bordering its winding course upon which, since the close of the Indian wars, had been piled the lumber hauled in immense quantities from the inland towns and floated downstream in rafts and gundalows to await shipment to the West Indies. Building was stimulated by the construction of a pier in 1798. This obviated the difficulty caused by a bar at the mouth of the river, of having to load the vessels light to enable them to pass over the bar and then complete their loading outside.

From 1800 to 1880 from six shipyards on this little river there came into being a total of 638 craft comprising 176 ships, 172 brigs, 204 schooners, 50 barks, and 36 miscellaneous craft comprising sloops, barks, boats, and even steam vessels. At low tide the river courses over the upper and lower falls. With a large hull it was sometimes necessary to wait several days for a high run of tide, and even then at "the top of the tide" there was barely enough clearance to get her over the ledges. With the demand for larger vessels increasing, there was posed before the builders a difficult situation. Their answer was a lock to retain the tidewater.

A stock company was formed, and in the spring of 1848 the work was begun. The spot selected was at the lower falls, some three-quarters of a mile above the wharves. Here at the Narrows the contracted channel formed a natural gateway to the river. On either bank massive walls of granite 16 feet high, 4 feet thick, and 140 feet in circuit were built. They faced each other across the stream 42 feet apart. Attached to these were the great gates of squared white pine timbers bolted through and through and equipped with long arms. These acted as balances and gave a purchase with which the gates could be opened and shut. Plank piling, sills, and ballasting were used to make the bed of the river under the gates secure. In 1849 it was completed at a cost of only $5,500.

Even with the help of the lock the warping of a large vessel down the river was an irksome and anxious task. Under the best conditions four tides were required to bring her to the lock. A force of at least twenty-five men stood by on each bank with ropes to warp her to larboard or starboard under the direction of a pilot who knew every turn of the river. Jesse Towne, who did this work, is interestingly described by Margaret J. Thompson in *Captain Nathaniel Thompson and the Ships He Built:*

> He would stand on deck, dancing up and down with excitement and shouting his orders at the top of his lungs at the men on shore. "Pull to the starboard side boys, or copper bottomed ship will go to the bottom! Pull hard, boys! Pull all together! There she goes right into the bank; into the mud; can't get her off; have to wait till the next tide! Heave Ho! See if you can start her again! Splendid ship, boys, all gone to destruction! So much money lost!" Despite it all Jesse always got his vessel down without accident.[1]

When the vessel was to be locked, the water above the gates was usually at a level with that below. The hull would be warped up to within half its length. Then fenders were put in place, bow lines to lead by were run downriver and quarter lines upstream to hold her back, these being reinforced by a great hawser secured to an anchor in the fields. Mishaps, though always feared, were surprisingly few, and during the nineteen years the lock was in use, twenty-nine vessels aggregating 23,080 tons passed through in safety. Twenty cents a ton was the toll charged. The largest was the *Golden Eagle*, 1,273 tons, built at the Titcomb yards in 1852.

Similar instances of ingenious contrivance existed up and down the coast. On the Damariscotta River in 1834 the *Grand*

[1] Charles E. Lauriat Co., Inc., 1937.

Turk, a ship built by J. & W. Madigans, was got through to deep water only with the aid of long strings of oxen. An interesting example is to be had in Lincoln Colcord's note in *Sailing Days on the Penobscot* of a schooner which was built in 1830 at the head of Lake Megunticook five miles inland. In the winter she was hauled across the ice by ox teams and launched into Camden Harbor, being appropriately christened the *Forest*. At Bristol, John Bearce built brigs and schooners of 100 tons or so in his own dooryard. His launchings took place in the winter, when he hauled them fully a mile out onto the ice in the Damariscotta River.

The records of Yarmouth and North Yarmouth reflect a regular practice of building inland and then hauling the vessels to the shore to launch them. There were even devices to steer the ship as it was hauled on sleds over the icy surface of the roads by as many as eighty yoke of oxen. There is of record an account by an eyewitness of one of these almost incredible adventures. He says:

> Several years prior to the war of 1812, two vessels of about seventy tons each were built at North Yarmouth, one near the house of William Titcomb being built by Captain Thaddeus Robbins, the other by Captain Ozias Blanchard on the land where Rufus Sweetser's buildings now stand. These vessels were built in the summer and hauled to the water the winter following.
>
> In January these vessels were ready and as soon as sufficient snow had fallen the owners commenced operations. In order to steer the craft on dry land they rigged out a spar over the taffrail long enough to reach the ground, and when the vessels were in motion they could be easily guided by shoving their sterns either way.
>
> The two vessels were ready about the same time. The one in North Yarmouth was started one Monday in January and hauled to the top of the hill near what is now called Yarmouth Falls. The next day they hooked eighty yoke of oxen on to

the other and started for the sea. All went well until they reached the top of the hill near Captain Thomas Chase's. Here they took off half the team and put them on behind the vessel, to prevent her from going down the hill too fast. They had two mill chains and a seven inch hawser to hold her back with. The bridge at the foot of the hill was very narrow and it required considerable skill to steer her across in safety. When about half way down the hill one of the mill chains broke leaving one string of oxen and the hawser with which to hold her back. No danger was apprehended until within fifty feet of the bridge when the other chain parted throwing all the weight on the hawser.

It now seemed as if the vessel must go off the bridge, but when she reached the structure the vessel's shoe caught one of the stringers of the bridge and she was stopped. The teams in front could not get out of the way quick enough and were all tangled up, the vessel stopping just soon enough to avoid serious damage. Nathaniel Merrill of Cumberland, was the only person injured, he having a leg broken by a falling spar. All hands then took hold of the vessel and she was hauled to the bottom of the hill. The next day the first vessel was placed on the flats and the second day the second one was served likewise.

In those days this work was done gratis, no charge being made for man or team. The owners however treated the men to crackers, cheese, fish, coffee and rum, prepared and served by the women folks, who thus got their share of the general good time.

★   ★   ★

The men who worked at the varied trades which were employed in the building of wooden ships in Maine shipyards deserve especial mention. The work called for the acme of skill of the individual workman. Almost all the labor was done by hand. The carpenter had but few tools besides the broadax, saw, adz, and pod auger. The shipsmith, with the help of his strikers, worked his own iron. On his anvil he forged every spike and bolt, mast cap, and chain link. The painters cut their own varnish and shellac from the gum, blended their own colors, and mixed their own paint. The timbers, though larger than those used in later years, were hoisted by the crude purchases of the day or, more often, were lifted and carried to their places on the shoulders of the workmen. Although all worked together, yet each had his particular skill in which he was pre-eminent. Of this he was very proud. The reputation of being the "second best caulker in Maine" was a title to hand down in the traditions of a family.

A shipbuilder's day was a long one. It was from sunup to sundown before the middle of the nineteenth century, when a ten-hour day was adopted. This meant that in the summer months he was in the yard as early as five o'clock in the morning and did not knock off until seven at night. He had a half hour at six for breakfast and three quarters of an hour for dinner at noon. The change to the ten-hour day caused as much heated discussion as has the forty-hour week in our own time. One old builder remarked he was in favor of it, provided it meant ten hours before dinner and ten hours after.

Judged by modern standards, wages were small. Well into the 1840's skilled craftsmen got but $1.00 a day. There was a sharp rise in the fifties, and the peak in Maine was $3.50. Ordinary workmen or helpers received some 75 cents, while the boy who tended the steam box or turned the wheel in the ropewalk toiled all day for 15 cents. Many of the builders boarded their workmen, and for those who preferred to live at home wholly satisfactory meals were provided at only 8 cents each.

The modern organization of labor was a thing unknown until a very late date. In this connection there was a curious and interesting attempt made at Winterport on the Penobscot River in the midst of the Civil War to embark upon a co-operative venture. Some ten or twelve carpenters and mechanics formed into a company known as the "Bone and Muscle Society" to collaborate in shipbuilding. Construction was started, but a failure to count the cost caused the venture to come to grief and the uncompleted vessel was auctioned off on the block. She was finished and launched by others as the brig *Alpine*.

The really characteristic unit on the Maine Coast was the family. This is well illustrated by the Russell brothers. In 1864 Captain Jacob Winslow, who made the blue "W" of the Winslow fleet known in every deepwater port in the world, persuaded George Russell to leave his home and yard down east in Pembroke and come to Portland to open what became the largest yard in Casco Bay. With him Master George brought his brothers. There was Eben, the joiner, there was Sewell, the planker, there was William, the fastener, and there was Jonas, who did the ceiling. Between them they constructed a goodly part of the early Winslow fleet.

Equally characteristic were the ways of Captain Robert Giving, whose yard was at Middle Bay near Harpswell. Living alone and cooking his own food, he built vessels of as much as 300 tons almost entirely by himself. With the heaviest work he had the help of three or four hands. Every stick of timber he used he picked out himself in the woods.

Strong drink was thought a necessity in the building yards during the first years of the century. On frosty mornings, before work was begun, the men gathered in the shipyard store. There they were served their portion, consisting of a tumbler of rum and two of water. Sometimes "long sweetening" or molasses was added. This mixture was known as blackstrap. This was repeated at eleven in the forenoon and four in the afternoon. Then the welcome cry of "Grog Oh!" often brought the workers together to celebrate some special occasion such as the raising of the stem or sternpost, the hanging of the anchor, or the fastening of the last plank. As the temperance sentiment grew in Maine, yard after yard gave up the custom and the coffee-pot replaced the grog dipper. The Stetson Yard at Camden was one of the first temperance yards, and the immense coffeepot which was substituted for the grog dipper is a prized heirloom in that family.

In many a coastal community it would seem from a study of the shipping lists that almost every inhabitant of the town at some time in his life built a vessel, for there is scarcely a cove on the coast that did not at one time or another contain a building yard. In many families established ways were used for generations. For example, the yards at Porter's Landing in Freeport where the privateer *Dash* was launched were used by the Porters for a generation. Then they passed to the Soules, Rufus and his son Rufus Cushing. The latter, known as "Honorable Rufus," launched over one hundred vessels and is said to have launched his sixty-seventh ship on his sixty-seventh birthday. It is also related of Columbia Perkins Carter of Belfast that after thirty-six years of shipbuilding, his one hundredth ship was on the ways at his death in 1876.

In Wiscasset there were the Johnstons, a family active as builders and merchants with their yards and business buildings at the tip of the Point for over half a century. John, the father, built the vessels. John Junior, known as "Captain Jack," sailed them and directed the foreign business of the firm. The other son, Alexander, took charge of the business at home and was accountant and bookkeeper. They held all their property in common and had but one purse, dividing nothing until just before the death of John Junior at the age of seventy-five. During all this time they kept the same firm name, John Johnston and Sons.

The examples could be many. In Boothbay the Adams family is a famous one in Maine shipbuilding, having been so engaged in four successive generations. In Waldoboro the story of the

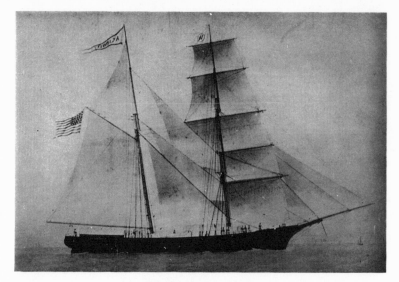

A Hermaphrodite Brig
The *A. G. Jewett* was typical of the old West India trade.
Built at Addison, 1865.

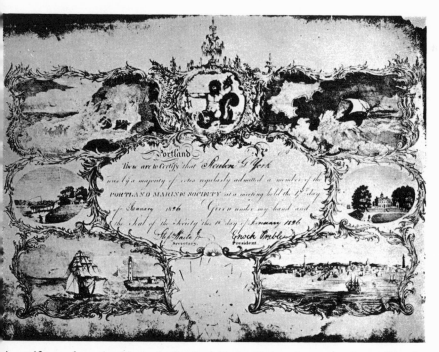

A certificate of membership in the Portland Marine Society, incorporated 1796 "for the promotion of the knowledge of navigation and seamanship." *Courtesy Maine Historical Society.*

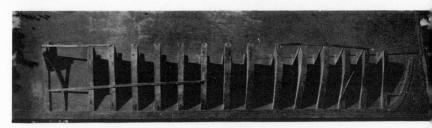

A Hawksnest Model

This model was the one used in the building of the privateer *Dash* at Freeport. Only th
remnants of the fore and aft battens have survived. *Original in B. H. Bartol Library*
Freeport.

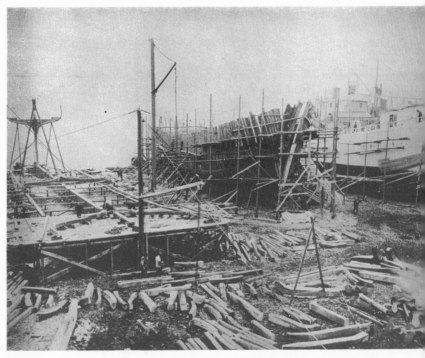

A Maine Coast Shipyard

A view of the Cobb-Butler Yard at Rockland. At the left the sternpost has been erecte
and the process of framing out commenced. In the center this has been completed an
this vessel is in frame. To the right another hull has been planked in and painted and
now ready for the masts to be stepped. *Courtesy Charles S. Morgan.*

yards clusters around a few family names. Henry Kennedy built for thirty-three years; the Storers, father and son, for thirty-four; the Clarks, Joseph and Edwin, forty; the Reeds, fifty-two; and the Welt dynasty, beginning in 1840, launched their last vessel in 1904. Up on the east side of Penobscot Bay at Castine the Buck yard and its successors were more or less active for ninety years, the Ginn yard for nearly eighty, Swasey's for over fifty, and Beazley's for nearly forty years.

A measure of the production of a State of Maine yard may be had in the short experience of Algernon S. Austin in Newcastle on the Damariscotta River from 1846 to 1854. In those eight years he built and sold nine vessels valued at nearly $600,000. His *Black Warrior*, 1889 tons, the largest vessel built in Newcastle, made the run from New York to San Francisco in 114 days in 1858. It is claimed that in the town of Harrington, with a list of 122 vessels, there has been put afloat more tonnage in proportion to its population than at any other place on the Atlantic coast.

The quality of Maine-built vessels was high. As an example there is the ship *Lydia Skolfield*, built in 1860 by George Skolfield at Brunswick in Casco Bay. Thirteen years later she was classed as A-1 with a star. This was the rating she had been given when she left the stocks. Nine years later, when she was twenty-four years old, she rated 1½. This, in the language of the Register, meant that she was "fit for the carriage of all kinds of cargo on all kinds of voyages." When she was re-trunneled, some eighteen hundred treenails were driven into her, and not a particle of rot was discovered in any of the borings.

In size the full-rigged ships from the Maine yards ranged from the *Farmer's Fancy* of but 126 tons, which was built by James Standish probably before 1800 at Warren on the Georges River, to the *Roanoke*, 3,347 tons, launched in 1892. She was the last wooden ship built by the Sewalls in Bath and was exceeded in size only by Donald McKay's masterpiece, the *Great Republic*. The great schooners ran even larger, the *Wyoming*, one of the famous six-masters of the Winslow fleet, measuring 3,730 tons.

★ ★ ★

In the building of ships and in maritime affairs in general the close of the War of 1812 marked the end of an era. Not only were there changes and new conditions at sea, but also the form and rig of American vessels were altered. Many a lesson had been learned, with peril as a tutor, in the roaring days of the neutral trade. Henry Hall's history of shipbuilding in the census report of 1880 gives a not too technical account of this:

> The old high poop decks and quarter galleries disappeared with the lateen and lug sails on brigs, barks and ships; the sharp stem was permanently abandoned; the curving home of the stem above the hawse holes went out of vogue and vessels became longer in proportion to their beam. The round bottoms were much in use but the tendency toward a straight rise of the floor from the keel to a point half way to the outer width of the ship became marked and popular. Hollow water lines fore and aft were introduced; the fore foot of the hull ceased to be cut away so much and the swell of the sides became less marked; the bows became somewhat sharper and were often made flaring above water and the square sprit sail below the bowsprit was given up. American shipbuilders had not learned to give their vessels much sheer, however, and in the majority of them the sheer line was almost straight from stem to stern. [The straight sheer was not a matter of ignorance; the builders were actually following the fashion of the straight-sheered war vessels popular between 1812 and 1840.] Nor had they learned to divide the topsail into an upper and lower sail and American vessels were distinguished by their short lower mast and the immense hoist of the topsail. The broadest beam was still two fifths the length of the hull.

Hemp rigging with broad channels and immense tops to the masts were still retained, but the general arrangement and cut of the head, stay, square and spanker sails at present in fashion were reached.

It has long been a tradition on the coast of Maine that in the yards of the colonial period the general practice was to lay the keel, then set up the stem and sternpost, and finally to fill in the frames between the two, the master builder shaping the hull "by the eye." However, modern authorities are inclined to doubt this. Building by the eye was only practicable when confined to small craft where one or two men could handle the frames, such as pinkies and the like. It would have been extraordinarily difficult with a large vessel. The handling of the heavy frames, raising them and then taking them down again to be refitted, would have involved a waste of labor, time, and even materials.

The early colonial shipbuilders and their successors at the time of the Revolution were highly skilled professionals. They were able to draw plans sufficient—in a shipbuilder's terms—to "prove" the fairing of a ship's lines. The so-called "hawks-nest model"—a frame half-model made of battens—was the natural successor to the plan. It is probably the oldest form of half-model. It could be whittled out of plank without any paper work or drafting tools save a scale or carpenter's rule. In the middle of the eighteenth century a half-model was also carved from a solid block of wood and then this was sawn transversely, i.e., at right angles to the center line, to obtain the shape of the frames.

Sometime in the 1790's the "lift" or water line model came into use. Again the unsubstantiated local tradition is that this type of model was the invention of either Enos Briggs of Salem or Orlando Merrill of Newburyport, two eighteenth-century shipbuilders in Massachusetts. On the coast of Maine hawks-nest models were in use in the design of small fishing craft right through the nineteenth century. The lift model replaced it in the design of large craft about 1820–30. The famous privateer *Dash* of Portland was designed at Freeport by means of a hawks-nest model which is still in existence.

The advantage of the hawks-nest and the lift model was that they permitted an accurate projection of the shape of the vessel's hull from the model to full-size drawings on the mould loft floor. These early models and ship plans were made to scales which were created by dividers to suit the paper or other material used. The scale in the drawings was laid off on the plan so that it looked somewhat like a line of music. Sometime before the Revolution, manufactured scales came into use, and the popular scale for models was one-quarter to three-eighths inch to the foot for large craft. For small craft it was one-half to three-quarters inch to the foot. Three-eighths and three-quarters were particularly handy because the sixteenths on a carpenter's rule then became either two inches or one respectively. Thus no special scale had to be carried.

The art of designing by half-models was no easier than the use of plans save that it took less experience to judge the lines when completed in model form. Usually in each community there were one or two outstanding modelers, and they designed the sloops, schooners, brigs, and ships built in the area. Upon their skill depended a successful blending of the vital qualities of capacity, speed, seaworthiness, and beauty.

Yet errors in building were not unknown. In the case of the *William Wirt*, built by Abner Stetson in 1849 at Damariscotta, the end result was turned to advantage. The error was that her lower deck clamps were placed two feet below where they should have been. This resulted in two feet more head room between decks, but it decreased the more desired capacity of the hold. During the course of the Crimean War she was in an

English port. It was discovered that this unique arrangement made her an ideal transport for horses. In consequence she named her own rates and made a mint of money for her owners.

Once the half-model was completed, the next task, in the jargon of the shipwright, was to "take off and lay down" the lines full size on the mould loft floor. This job was important and it was difficult. In Maine yards it was usually done by the master builder equipped with compass, square, straight edge, chalk line, and battens. Thus when he had taken off and laid down the lines there lay before him on the broad floor of the mould loft a plan in full size of the frames, timbers, backbone, deck beams, stem and sternpost. From these, full-size patterns or moulds were then made in light pine boards. These moulds, also later called templates, the workmen took with them into the woods where the frames would be cut. In the early days the round logs, crotches, and roots which were selected to fit the moulds and from which the timbers and pieces were to be "beaten" or hewed had been brought to the yard and shaped there. But this was not economical, and there soon developed the practice of having the timbers selected, cut, squared, shaped, and numbered in the woods before they were hauled down to the yard by oxen or lumber schooners.

With the arrival of the frames it was time to "stretch" or lay the keel. On the middle of the bed logs there began to rise a long line of blocks superimposed pyramid-like to a height of some four feet. This height was to provide the space within which the carpenters might work underneath the hull. Then on these blocks and with a slope toward the water of about five-eighths of an inch to the foot, there was laid the false keel of water-seasoned elm, to which was firmly bound with wooden dowels or iron bolts, the keel of oak. This was the backbone of the vessel. To it there was next fastened the sternpost of oak and the deadwood.

At this juncture what was called the framing stage came into play. This was a platform as long as the deepest and as broad as the widest frame of the ship, set up crosswise of the keel. It was movable, and to it the frames were now "twitched." Fitted together into the exact shape required by the templates and securely fastened, each frame was now slid down into position on the keel and "shored up" by supporting timbers. This operation was a continuous one, the framing stage moving gradually toward the forward end of the hull as the square frames, which crossed the keel at right angles, and then the stem cants, were set in place. The cants were fastened to the sides of the keel or deadwoods and stood at lesser angles than ninety degrees.

In the early days before sawmills came into use, the frames were beveled after they were set up. This was done with the broadax and adz, and the process was called "dubbing." Since it called for great judgment and skill, it was the prerogative of the older ship carpenters. Later the bevels were marked on the moulds and then these were sawn into the timbers. Then only such light dubbing was done as would be required to fair up the frames when they were assembled. But as late as the end of the eighteenth century only those timbers having great bevel were shaped and beveled before being erected.

When all the frames save the bow cants had been raised, shored up, and held in line by "ribbands" of planks temporarily spiked to their sides, the keelson was bolted in place. This was a great solid structure of wood stretched—that is, laid—just above the keel to give the vessel strength lengthwise and to secure the floors in place. Then came the other "thick stuff"— that is, long timber such as "sister" or side keelsons, bilge stringers, and clamps up to the breast of the bow.

After the long timbers had been put in, the stem was set in place. This called for the finest piece of white oak to be found in the yard. Composed of three pieces or more—stem, apron, and stemson—it was firmly fastened together with dowels to form one piece with the keel. Then with the knightheads, bow cants, and deck beams in place and tightly caulked, the "ceiling" —a term of the trade meaning the inside planking—was secured to the frame with bolts, and the "clamps" upon which the decks were to rest were put in place.

The work now shifted to outside the hull. The men called the dubbers went over the outside of the frames with adzes to fair them up smooth to receive the skin, as the outside planking was called. The plankers were the highest-paid men in the yard. Oftentimes the builder would hire a planker's gang, a craft organization headed by a boss planker, which went from yard to yard doing this work. Only rugged men, as quick with the eye as with the hand, could twist and bend the heavy plank to cover the curves at bow and stern. This was grueling work. To make the plank more pliable its fibers often had to be softened in the steam box. Then would go up the cry, "Hot plank!" which brought men on the run from all over the yard to draw the steaming wood from the box, shoulder it, and rush it up the inclined plane to the brow stage. With the aid of every mechanical purchase available it was forced tight against the frames and permanently secured by the "fasteners," who used treenails which were made of locust wood for below and of oak for above the water line. Spikes and bolts were used only at butts and at plank ends.

Next came the turn of the caulkers. With their irons and longheaded mallets they forced oakum into the seams and then payed them over with melted pitch or tar. The hull was now tested for leaks by "watering up." Though not a common practice, it was often accomplished with the help of the village fire department, which came with its pumper or "hand tub" to fill the space between the planking and the ceiling. After this the spaces between the frames from the saltstops at the water line to the frame heads were filled with rock salt. Often this was a job for the boys of the town. Last of all the outboard joiners smoothed the surface of the hull and prepared it for the painters. This was usually done by first planing with hand planes and then scraping.

The planking took much time. Meanwhile the decks had been laid and caulked, and then the cabin and forecastle built, the hatch coamings laid, the rudder with its gear shipped, pumps, rails, and windlass placed, and even the masts stepped. In the early part of the period, ships had only their lower masts stepped previous to the launching. Later, beginning with small craft, it was found possible to launch larger and larger vessels fully rigged and sparred. Sometimes there was even a cargo on board, so that she sailed direct from the ways on her first voyage. In 1847 Joseph L. Buck of Bucksport launched the schooner *Mentora*, fully rigged, provisioned, and ready to set sail on her maiden voyage as she left the ways. She lasted out forty-three years of service, and today her keel and floor timbers moulder on the flats in front of the village.

The rigging might be done by either the owner, the builder, or the master who was to command. In the latter case he would stay at home over one voyage to oversee the proper outfitting of the ship. Oftentimes the hull would be taken to a larger center and placed in the hands of a firm of ship riggers. Or a crew of riggers came to the local yard and, under the direction of the boss rigger, set up the lower masts, sent up the upper spars and yards, fitted and placed literally miles of cordage, and performed all the innumerable jobs of splicing and worming, parceling and serving, which together with all their intricate knots and splices excited the envy and ambition of the small boys of the town.

The Shipyards

The ship was furnished with one or more suits of sails. These were sometimes made in the yard's own sail loft, but more often in independent lofts. Sailmaking was a craft by itself. It took a skillful man who, with only palm and needle and other hand tools, could fashion some four or five thousand yards of stiff canvas into the properly shaped sails with the stiffness and "belly" to draw well. To each he attached the boltrope around the outer edge and the innumerable reef points, cringles, heartclews and other items. In the early period coppering was seldom done in the home yards, and it was the custom to make one voyage to Europe, where this sheathing could be done more cheaply.

The shipyards developed many allied trades. In the larger towns practically everything that went into their vessels was fabricated. There were the rope walks, "long and low with their windows in a row, like the port holes of a hulk," where the hempen ropes of the ship were spun. An old map of the city of Portland about 1820 shows four of them. The great cables used before chains came into use were laid up with the help of horses to turn the wheel. Near by in their shops the pump and block makers wrought at their trade. For example, for years in Castine, Hatch and Mead were the chain makers and shipsmiths, John Sampson manufactured pumps and blocks, John Dresser conducted a rope walk, and William Chamberlain baked ship bread. At Thomaston village in 1825 there were two sail lofts, two pump and block makers, a mill for picking oakum, a rope walk, a ship carver's shop, and a graving ways.

Boatmakers fashioned the vessel's small boats, often with workmanship so fine that they were objects of great admiration in foreign ports. Anchors, capstans, and windlasses must have been made locally, but the first record we have of a business devoted to them is that of David Crooker of Bath, established in 1840. Another famous firm was the Camden Anchor Works, where were made the famous Alden anchors. It was established in 1866 by Horatio E. and William G. Alden.

One of the most interesting workmen was the ship carver who fashioned the billetheads, figureheads, name boards and scrollwork that adorned bow and stern of many ships and schooners. Almost every yard had its carver, usually a man of considerable skill who in many cases had served an apprentice-ship under an older master from whom he had received a certificate attesting his competency. There was Edbury Hatch in Damariscotta, Emory Jones in Newcastle, and William South-worth of Bath. The skill was sometimes handed down from father to son, as in the case of the Littlefields of Portland and the Seaveys of Bangor. In most instances, of course, the ship carver was also a skilled joiner, and many of the fine houses of such towns as Wiscasset and Thomaston stand as testimonials to his ability.

Carved often from a single block, or from several blocks doweled together, the figurehead was bolted to the stemhead under the bowsprit. Elm or oak was used by some of the earlier carvers, but Maine craftsmen preferred the softer and more workable pumpkin pine. The lines of the figure would be chalked on the block. Then the rough hewing out was generally delegated to the apprentice. The master carver himself finished, painted and decorated the piece and attended to the very particular task of setting it in position on the vessel's bow.

The figurehead sometimes represented the vessel's name by a symbolical figure, bird, or beast. For example, the four-masted bark *Ocean King* launched at Kennebunkport in 1874 carried a magnificent figurehead nine feet high representing King Neptune resplendent with crown, trident, and royal robes carved by the Littlefields in Portland. More often it was a representation of the builder himself, his wife, or his daughter, or even the rotund figure of the managing owner. In the case of one of Richmond's ships, he was complete with top hat, frock coat, walking stick, and a cigar in his mouth.

The scrollwork on which it rested set off the beauty of the figurehead. The stern pieces were also quite elaborate—an eagle with flags, scrollwork with a wreath surmounting a portrait bust, or even a full-length figure such as that of Jenny Lind on the clipper *Nightingale*. The owner might prefer a fiddle or billethead and was often willing to pay liberally for one that was well shaped and elaborately carved. William Southworth received $250 to $400 for a figure. These, with the name board on each side of the prow, gave full scope to the carver's ingenuity and artistic ability.

The day of the launch was a red-letter day. With it nothing could compete save muster day. The village schools had at least a half holiday, the yard was gay with bunting and alive with people who had come down from up country to look on. Laughter and practical jokes, joviality, and general good nature were the order of the day. A successful launching was second only to a happy wedding. But it did not always pan out successfully. There was one launch in Brewer that was long remembered by the participants. This was when the 599-ton ship *James M. Littlefield* was launched fully rigged from the Cooper Yard. Her port anchor was dropped to snub her as she left the ways. This gave her a sharp list. What with the weight of her topmasts and yards and the crowd on her decks sliding to one side, she capsized, throwing everyone into the water. No lives were lost, although a Bangor paper reported "only one Irishman drowned." Some had their superstitions. Hiram Flye at Seal Cove near Bar Harbor would never name his vessels for any living person and always refused to divulge the name he had chosen until the day of the launch.

To the builder, although the launching was all in a day's

work, it required forethought and careful attention to much detail. A master craftsman whom experience had shown to be especially efficient would be put in charge. A ship of 2,000 tons weighed somewhere near 2,500 tons, and it was his task to get this enormous mass of wood and iron into the water safely and smoothly.

Parallel with the bed timbers of the hull and some eight to ten feet out from the sides of the keel, massive timbers were placed at low tide. These were the ways. On top of them were placed other timbers, or slides with flanges to hold them in place. These slides were built up tightly with planks to the bottom of the ship. Beneath the upper tier of this "filling in" and next the ship's bottom there were then inserted, close together, wooden wedges. The purpose of this was that when they were driven home the weight of the ship would be taken off the blocking beneath the keel and she would then rest firmly on her ways. The top of the ways and the bottom of the slides were thoroughly greased with soft soap and beef tallow, plus a thick sprinkling of flaxseed to hold this slippery mixture in place.

About half an hour before the high tide when the vessel was to go off, the most skillful carpenters would go down beneath her bottom. Working from the stern toward the bow in pairs with one on each side, they split out with iron wedges and steel-faced mauls the heavy blocks on which the keel rested. Then an ominous creak resounded. This betokened "the thrill of life along her keel." Warned by the crackle of crushing timber, the workmen leap to safety. There is a rising roar from the crowd. Slowly at first, then gathering momentum, she slides swiftly and smoothly down her ways amid the cheers of the crowd and is waterborne with a young rigger riding the peak of the bowsprit and waving his cap in the air.

In 1854, in the course of a single day at Wiscasset, three large ships slid down the ways. There was the *Mackinaw*, 1,194

The Shipyards

tons, in the Coffin Yard. There was the *Golden Horn* of 1,193 tons burden in the yard of Harriman and Clark. And the Johnstons launched their second *Tamerlane*, 924 tons.

★　★　★

An outside demand for Maine-built ships had begun as early as 1815. And in the generation before this there are numerous instances of Massachusetts men forsaking the shore there to seek their fortunes down East. As early as 1762 Colonel Jonathan Buck from Haverhill on the Merrimac set up the first sawmill and launched the first vessel in Penobscot waters. Before the Revolution George Barstow and Nathaniel Bryant, both from Massachusetts, had begun building at New Castle on the Damariscotta. A little later Samuel Weston and Jonas Standish from Duxbury were building at Warren on the Georges. The town of Robbinston at the mouth of the St. Croix was settled in 1790, and Thomas Vose began building there a decade later. He hailed from Milton. In 1803 Captain Noah Brooks from Scituate was settled in Camden, where he was joined ten years later by Joseph Stetson, who had received his training at the Charlestown Navy Yard and had gone in the winter of 1814 to the shores of Lake Champlain to work on Commodore MacDonough's "green timber fleet."

The reason for this is fairly manifest. Conditions favorable to the building of ships had changed greatly even in Massachusetts. No longer could suitable timber, particularly for the larger vessels now beginning to be sought, be found close at hand. In the District there was white ash for frames, hackmatack and oak for knees, and the towering pine for masts and spars— and all this to be had handy to the building yards. Then, too, labor was cheaper. Men were not entirely dependent upon ship construction. They could profitably spend their slack time in agriculture. In consequence the supply was more stable and

The Maritime History of Maine

vessels could be built on this coast five to fifteen dollars a ton cheaper than elsewhere.

With the peace and the trade which accelerated after the close of the Napoleonic wars marking the end of a forty-year period of wartime conditions and foreign interference, the shipyards on the coast of Maine boomed in the twenties, their production exceeded that of Massachusetts in the thirties, and in the forties it surpassed both New York and Massachusetts and led the United States.

All this was part and parcel of the great boom in the shipping industry which reflected in the three decades from 1830 to 1860 an increase of nearly 800 per cent in the tonnage engaged. The concentration of industry in the larger centers of the country called for mass transportation of raw materials from distant sources and of finished products to faraway markets. Railroads and canals were bringing to the great ports the output of the mills, mines, and fields of the hinterland. The southern cotton crop must be transported to the mills of Lancashire. European emigrants were clamoring for passage to America. Thus there developed a great triangle of profitable commerce. The business of the larger centers was so absorbed in the carrying trade that it was unable to build enough new vessels to meet this increasing demand for tonnage. Even as early as 1815 merchants had been seeking them in the yards north of Cape Cod, and especially from the coast of Maine. The names of the owners on the registers of many a ship of these days are those of well-known merchants of Salem, Boston, and New York.

Even after the boom in shipping caused by the opening of the California trade with the resulting rise in prices, large, well-built cargo vessels could be built in Maine at prices ranging from $45 to $70 a ton. The yards of New York and Boston were crowded to capacity with the high-class vessels—packets, two-decked clippers, and steamboats—while in Maine priority was given to those sturdy freighters of low cost and superior cargo capacity which were so much in demand, especially in the cotton-carrying trade. Much building was done on speculation, the finished vessel being sent to market light under a carpenter's certificate. Because of this custom the total figures of Maine's output may be understated in the official records, since a vessel had its first enrollment in the port of its owners. Much building was also done on contract. Among the pleasant memories in many a shipbuilding community are those of some merchant or captain who came with his family from Boston, New York, Mobile, or New Orleans and spent the summer in town while the vessel for which he had contracted was rising on the stocks in a local yard.

But the Maine product was not only for foreign sale. It is said that in Searsport a vessel was never built on contract for outside parties. All were owned in the town. Moreover, the state was rapidly developing into a shipping community wherein building and operation went hand in hand. As early as 1802 the shipping community in the towns near Wiscasset chartered and located there the Lincoln and Kennebec Bank. The stockholders' list reads like a roster of the shipbuilders of the region. Aside from those resident in Wiscasset—General Abiel Wood, Moses Carlton, and others—there were John Dunlap of Brunswick, Thomas and David Agry of Hallowell, Samuel Howard and Daniel Cony of Augusta, Peter Grant of Gardiner, and William King and Peleg Tallman of Bath. The maritime flavor of this institution has already been noticed. The value of their bills was indicated by the several classes of vessels then in use—sloops, schooners, topsail schooners, brigs, and ships. In 1803 a marine insurance company was also chartered.

The money that in other states was being drawn off into industrialism, railroads, and western speculation, in Maine financed the building and was multiplied by the sailing of ships. There thus came into being fleets which made the owner's name known in all the ports of the world. There were the Pattens of Bath, at one time one of the largest in the United States; the Sewalls, with their broad, flat-bottomed carriers which could pack 2,000 pounds of cotton for each registered ton; the Houghtons, also of Bath; the O'Briens and Wattses of Thomaston; and others who found increasingly profitable employment for their fleets in the charter business of the greater ports. In addition to this there was the constantly growing coastwise trade. This called for a multitude of individually owned schooners, the construction of which kept many a small yard busily engaged.

"Everybody who had a place where a vessel could possibly be built," so runs a contemporary account, "and who knew anything about building one, opened a yard." The writer spoke of the 1840's. The next decade saw the peak. In 1851 there came from State of Maine yards a total tonnage of 75,399 tons. The next year saw this figure raised to 110,047. In 1853 it was 118,916, and in 1854, 168,631. Then with the year 1855 came the peak of 215,904 tons. This was more than a third of the production in all the United States. Maine led all of her sister states.

If the historian is plagued by the paucity of the records of what is believed to be the extensive shipbuilding on the Maine coast in colonial times, their very multiplicity and the size of these records after the establishment of the federal government when the coast was divided into districts with all the paraphernalia of ports of entry and Custom House records, equally defeat his efforts. There are localities where every vestige of shipbuilding has disappeared, such as in the tidal rivers on the western coast—the Mousam, the Kennebunk, the Saco, and even the little Scarborough River.

There are the shores of Casco Bay, with the yards at Stroud-

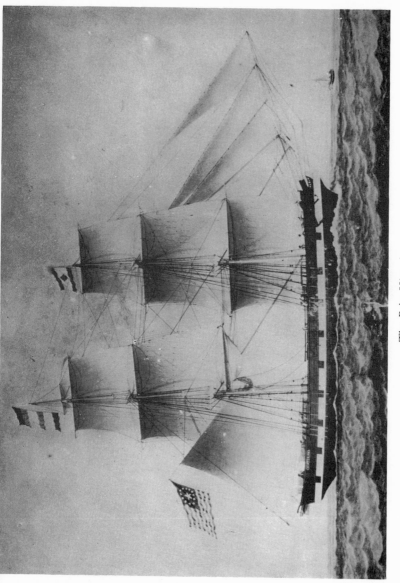

The Brig *Historian*

She was built in Seaville, now Brooklin. This portrait shows her entering the harbor at Marseille.

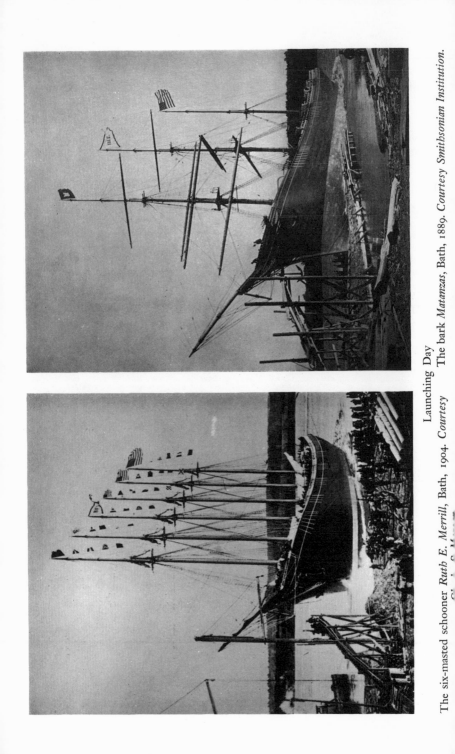

Launching Day

The six-masted schooner *Ruth E. Merrill*, Bath, 1904. *Courtesy*   The bark *Matanzas*, Bath, 1889. *Courtesy Smithsonian Institution.*

water, on Fore River, at South Portland, in the mouth of the Presumpscot, on the foresides of Falmouth and Cumberland, at Yarmouth on the side of Royall's River, at Freeport on the Harraseket, Strouts Point, Brunswick, Pennellville, and Harpswell. Then on the eastward there is Bath, and up the Kennebec —Phippsburg, Bowdoinham and Richmond. The river towns of the Sheepscot, the Damariscotta, the St. George's, and the Medomac all had many yards. These comprise Wiscasset, Alna, New Castle, Nobleboro, Boothbay, Waldoborough, Bristol, Warren, and Thomaston.

The shores of Penobscot Bay saw extensive shipbuilding— there being on the west shore Rockland, Rockport, Camden, Lincolnville, Belfast, Searsport, Sandy Point, Winterport, Hampden, and on up the Penobscot River to Bangor. Then down on the east shore there were Brewer, Orrington, Bucksport, Orland, Castine, Brooksville, Penobscot, and the fishermen's ports of Great Deer Island, Crotch Island, Isle au Haut, Swan's Island, Sedgwick, and Brooklyn.

Finally there is the coast east of the Penobscot, which was especially the home of the small schooner. Of the 1,990 vessels registered in the District of Machias, 1,550 were fore-and-afters. There are the towns on the shores of Frenchman's Bay— Hancock, Franklin, Sullivan, Sorrento, and Gouldsboro. As always, the rivers play their part—the Union with Ellsworth, the Narraguagas with Millbridge and Cherryfield, the Harrington with the little town of that name. Here in 1856 the yards gave work to eighteen master builders, and there were as many as eight vessels on the stocks at one time. Between the bays of Harrington and Machias, which is a distance of but twenty miles, there are nine rivers which gave access to rich forests of spruce and pine. From then on Jonesport, Machias, Cutler, East Machias, Eastport, Pembroke, Robbinston lead on to Calais at the mouth of the St. Croix River.

From the Piscataqua with its long record of naval and governmental construction away down east to the St. Croix, from which region there came legions of lumber schooners, river after river and place after place can furnish a full-bodied chronicle of the yards and the ships and the men who built them throughout the nineteenth century.

CHAPTER EIGHT

SHIPBUILDING *on the* KENNEBEC

"Of all the northern quarters of the Union, Maine is that which will increase the fastest and the Kennebec will have the greatest share of this increase."—*The American Encyclopedia, 1808.*

A COMPLETE ACCOUNT of shipbuilding on the Maine Coast calls for a volume in itself. Indeed, its history on the shores of the Kennebec cannot be recounted in its entirety in a single chapter. Nonetheless a chronological story of Bath and its environs does reveal a true cross section of the development of the building of the wooden ship in Maine, its climax, and its decline. The pattern here traced is revelatory—here and there at different times and in a differing tempo and scale—of that to be seen on the shores of Casco Bay and on the western coast to the Piscataqua and to the eastward at Wiscasset, New Castle, Waldoboro, Thomaston, on the shores of Penobscot Bay, and on the rivers farther down east to Machias and Eastport.

As New England migrants spread from the seaboard inland along the streams in the years following the Revolution, the valley of the Kennebec was a region of great expectations. It is a significant fact that Arnold's route to Quebec followed the Kennebec up to the "Great Carrying Place" thirty miles north of Norridgewock falls. Then and later the landowners and settlers on its banks felt in their bones that the river was the natural outlet from Canada to the sea. They had visions of a time when there would be a great trade route from the northern portions of New Hampshire, Vermont, Montreal, and Quebec down along the Kennebec to the sea.

Even before the war Dummer Sewall of Bath, Reuben Colburn of Pittston, and others had projected the Coos trail from Hallowell to Erol, New Hampshire. This provided a shorter route to tidewater than the Connecticut River. Charles Vaughan of Boston, the most enthusiastic of the promoters, spared neither money nor effort. He designed Hallowell to be the chief shipping port on the upper river, and here he built a prodigious brewery, a distillery, and a flour mill. Then some four miles below Bath on the east bank at Jones' Eddy he constructed wharves, docks, and storehouses in the expectation of a great export trade. His high hopes were never realized. He had been too optimistic in his building operations, and with his financial failure dreams of a riverborne commerce faded away. Rather it was shipbuilding that lay ahead.

Following the colonial period there was little encouragement for shipping in the decade after the close of the Revolution. Only fifty vessels with a total tonnage of 4,724 were registered at the Bath custom house. These consisted mostly of large sloops and small schooners, with a sprinkling of hermaphrodite brigs. The average size was only 89½ tons. There was but one ship, the *Atlantic*, built by Jonathan Davis at Bath. At Pittston were the active yards of Thomas Agry, the patriarch builder of the upper Kennebec. Nearby in 1788 William and James Springer launched the first of their large fleet. Two years before, Elihu Getchell had put afloat the first vessel in Bowdoinham. Even at this early date Bath had eight builders—Joshua Shaw, Joshua Raynes, Ring and Mitchell, John Clark, Jonathan Davis, A. Howland, and David Trufant. Upstream at

Shipbuilding on the Kennebec

Hallowell Isaac Pillsbury, Captain Isaac Smith, and Ebenezer Mayo were building.

In the decade following the setting up of the federal government in 1789, shipbuilding was greatly stimulated by the adoption by Congress of its wise policy of protection for the infant merchant marine. All along the Kennebec it increased nearly sixfold. The average size was now 135 tons, more than double that of the preceding decade. Thirty-five ships instead of one now appear on the register. The largest, leaving aside Dr. Tupper's timber ship, the *Experiment*, was Jonathan Davis' *Kingston* of 408 tons.

Shrewd men had foreseen that the portion of the west bank known as the Long Reach, with its deep harbor and broad water front, would put Bath in the lead. At this time Pittston had the largest yards above the Chops. Thomas Agry had died, but his sons, John and Thomas, and their brother-in-law, Thomas Oakman, carried on the business. In 1795 the Springers had moved across the river to Bowman's Point in what was then Hallowell and is now Farmingdale. In a part of the town of Topsham which is now Bowdoinham, Robert Patten was building. He was the uncle of the Pattens who later did so much to establish the character of the Bath ships. Names to be long familiar in the lists now begin to appear—J. Drummond and Mark L. Hill of Phippsburg, then Georgetown, Stephen Sewall, the founder of the famous Bath firm, John M. Moody, Charles Clapp, Samuel Davis, John Peterson, Peleg Tallman, and William King. It is interesting to note that with but one exception all of these men built for their own use.

Interesting careers were carved out. William King and Peleg Tallman may stand as examples. Eleven years before he built his first vessel in Bath, William King had come into that town barefoot. He had driven a pair of steers, his share of his father's estate, from Scarboro forty miles down the coast.

Going on to Topsham, he found work in a sawmill. Soon he owned half a saw, then the whole mill. Next a store, and within six years he was building his own vessels and shipping his own lumber. Moving down to Bath, he dominated the life of the town for half a century. He organized its first bank, represented it in the General Court, led the fight in the state for separation from Massachusetts, and became the first governor of Maine.

By way of contrast with King, who got his start and rose to power as a lumberman and merchant, Peleg Tallman came up by way of the sea. Born in Rhode Island, he served his apprenticeship on various privateers and lost an arm in the fight between the frigate *Trumbull* and the *Wasp*. He found a friend in Dr. Sylvester Gardiner and first came to the Kennebec as the master of one of his ships. He married a daughter of John Clark, one of the pioneer shipbuilders, and made his home in Bath and Woolwich. Tallman, together with King and the Wiscasset shipbuilders, Abiel Wood, Jr., and Moses Carlton, formed the "great quartette" in the business and politics of the time and the region. He became shipbuilder, merchant, real estate operator, and bank president, with interests as far afield as Boston and Newburyport. Successful in all that he undertook, in Deacon Perkins' view "he must be one of the elect he was so prosperous."

Despite the interference with our merchant marine on the high seas by the Barbary corsairs, French privateers, and English press gangs and ashore by two periods of embargo, the first ten years of the century were prosperous on the Kennebec. Three hundred and eighteen vessels totaling 51,438 tons and averaging 165 tons each passed out by Seguin to share in a peculiarly lucrative trade. While the Napoleonic wars were devastating Europe, despite British orders in council and the Berlin and Milan decrees, the Yankee masters did a thriving business with the warring nations. William King's ship *Reunion* paid her initial cost three times over in as many round trips to England. The lumber which cost $8.00 a thousand on the banks of the Kennebec, selling in the West Indies for $60.00, coupled with a corresponding profit on the cargo home, was the source of the shipping wealth of the region.

The first attempt to enter the cotton-carrying trade in 1802 was an event of marked importance. Bath had almost a monopoly in this trade for nearly eighty years. It even influenced the build of her vessels. The first vessel to go from the state of Maine was the ship *Androscoggin*, owned by William King and under the command of Captain Nathaniel Harding. Upon asking General King where New Orleans was, the Captain received only the vague information that it was somewhere in the Gulf of Mexico. Fortunately he found an old Spanish chart by which he was able to make his way up the Mississippi.

The rigs of the vessels changed during this decade. Brigs and ships began to predominate and the number of sloops to dwindle. Bath's 103 craft are typical. They comprised 43 brigs, 38 ships, 18 schooners and but 4 sloops. In total building Hallowell was next to Bath, launching 38. The Agry brothers built in this town for a part of the period, as did Stephen Hinckley and Peter Grant. Georgetown, which then included Phippsburg, followed with 36. The next was Topsham with 26, then Bowdoinham with 16, Pittston 15, Waterville 7, Augusta 7, and Vassalborough 2.

With the recovery after the Embargo in the one year 1810, Bath alone launched 16 vessels totaling 3,784 tons. This was a record that stood for twenty years. The second decade of the century opened with great promise. In 1811, 45 vessels were sent to sea and in 1812, 23, but in 1813 only 3—two schooners and a brig—were launched into the river. Then the war abruptly closed the yards. With peace came revival, and in 1815 the fleet numbered up to 45, but as a whole these ten years reflect a loss

as compared with the preceding decade. In 1814 James Mc-
Clellan built the ship *Cleopatra*, which was the first vessel above
500 tons to be launched on the river. The average vessel was
smaller, being but 130 tons. While the total output was only
two ships less than in the preceding decade, the total tonnage
showed a decrease of over 10,000 tons.

New builders now began to appear all along the river. The
Bradstreets had begun the long career of their family. In Phippsburg, the Morrisons were building at Dromore Bay, and in
Georgetown Benjamin Riggs had opened his yard at Robinhood
Cove. George Houdlette and the Alleys were building at Dres-
den. Richmond, then a part of Bowdoinham, had launched the
first of her large fleet, the *Portumnus*, with Barzilla White as
builder. The largest yard in Bowdoinham, that of Thomas
Harward, was opened in 1817. The new village at Cathance
Landing, so convenient for the lumbermen of Bowdoin and the
back country, was growing rapidly. Josiah Colby and James
Rogers had been building there since early in the century, and
in 1817 George Henry joined them. Even Vassalborough and
Waterville built two vessels each, one of them a ship of 290 tons.

The year 1820 marks an important date in the history of
the Maine coast. Then it was that the country from the Piscataqua to the St. Croix ceased to be the District and became the
State of Maine. In his searching about for a *quid pro quo*, Henry
Clay, the architect of the Missouri Compromise, found it in
William King's long campaign for the separation of Maine from
Massachusetts. This was a period of transition in the state as
well as in the nation. The struggle was on between "wharf and
waterfall," between manufacturers and merchants, and between
a high tariff, sought by the former, and free trade, upon which
the shipping interests thrived. All this was reflected in the Kennebec yards.

The panic of 1819 saw a falling off in building, and in 1820, aside from a few small brigs and schooners, but one small ship of less than 300 tons was built. In fact, there were only 21 ships among the 330 vessels launched during this decade, and the total tonnage was only 53,247. Thus the average size was but 160 tons. In the mid-twenties, England announced the opening of her closed West India ports. On the strength of this, 101 vessels slid down the Kennebec ways in 1825 and 1826. Then the door closed tight again in December of the latter year. This caused a great decrease in building and hard times along the river. Bath carpenters and joiners sought work in New Brunswick but found so little there that on returning home they were glad to have occasional work at fifty or seventy-five cents a day, working from daylight to dark and taking store pay. Then in 1828 came another heavy blow in the passage of the "tariff of abominations," which doubled the duty on molasses. Building on the river all but ceased during the next two years. One can well understand the rejoicing in 1830, when by treaty the British West Indies were once again opened to American ships.

Despite the rough seas of this ten years, many of the largest firms were launched at this time. George F. and John Patten, who had begun their long career in Topsham in 1821, built their first vessel in Bath, the brig *Jasper*. Five years before, Levi Houghton had put afloat his first, the brig *Bolton*, and in 1823 William D. Sewall launched the brig *Dianne*. Samuel Veazie was the largest builder at Topsham, constructing six vessels there. John Agry built the first bark, the *Caroline*, on the river at Hallowell in 1828.

In the South, cotton production more than doubled between 1820 and 1830. Four-fifths of the crop went across the Atlantic, and ships were needed to carry it. The yards on the Kennebec furnished a goodly proportion of those ships. During the first three years of the thirties the yards hummed with unprecedented activity, and 139 vessels, 38 of them full-rigged ships, left the ways. The size increased rapidly to meet the demands of the cotton trade, and the output for the whole decade was 304 vessels with a total tonnage of 69,559, reflecting an average size of 222 tons. The *Florence* of Hallowell, measuring 449 tons, was considered a monster in 1831, but two years later T. D. Robinson passed the 500-ton mark with the *New England*, and in 1840 the Patten's *Monmouth* of 728 tons was built. By this time a distinct type had been evolved with square sterns, bluff bows, and kettle bottoms. They were by no means things of beauty, but they could stow cotton bales to great advantage and brought home handsome returns from the penny cotton freights of the thirties.

But the boom was short. Overoptimism and unwarranted credit brought their inevitable result. In 1837 the banks suspended specie payments and the panic was on. It took five years before the nation began to recover, but New England banks resumed specie payments in 1840. As times improved, the Kennebec yards reached a new high in the 1840's with a total of 369 vessels measuring 118,732 tons, an increased average of 321. Of these, 125 were full-rigged ships. Brigs had to a large extent been replaced by barks ranging from 300 to 450 tons. This rig rapidly became popular, especially in the upriver yards at Bowdoinham, Richmond, Gardiner, Pittston, and Augusta. During the thirties only 14 had been launched, while during these ten years 75 were built.

In 1841 President William Henry Harrison visited Bath and marveled at the enormous bulk of a ship then on the stocks in the Clark and Sewall yard. It was the *Rappahannock* of 1,133 tons. When launched and for several years thereafter, she was the largest ship in the world. She was only surpassed in Bath eight years later, when Trufant and Drummond put afloat their 1,200-ton *Saratoga*. It is said that the *Rappahannock* was too large to be profitable in the cotton trade and that freights dropped a quarter of a cent a pound whenever she appeared in New Orleans.

Although the next decade would see higher figures in the total tonnage and the number of ships built, there were probably a greater number of active yards on the Kennebec in the forties than at any other time in its history. The list is an impressive one. Bath had at least seventeen builders who produced 84 full-rigged ships and 29 smaller vessels. Richmond, which had pushed ahead rapidly, came next. There the busy yards of T. J. Southard, William Patten, W. H. Sturdivant and M. S. Hagar and others launched 37 vessels. At Phippsburg the family yards of the Morrisons, Olivers, and Morses put off 26. Pittston was still active, building 25. Benjamin Follansby and his son Benjamin, who had come from Salisbury, Massachusetts, to build at Smithtown, and the Stevens yards at the present Randolph, were large builders. In Bowdoinham, the Harwards on the Kennebec and William Purington and St. Vincent Given at Cathance Landing accounted for 21. The same number were also launched at the yards of Richard Clay, William Bradstreet, and Samuel C. Grant in Gardiner. Augusta added 22 to the list, Woolwich 13, Topsham 11, Hallowell and Georgetown each 5, Arrowsic 4, and Dresden 3.

The sudden leap of Richmond into a leading place second only to Bath and to first place above the Chops was in large measure due to one man whose energy and business acumen were extraordinary. This was Thomas J. Southard. Born in Boothbay, he had come to Richmond as a young man. While he worked at the trade of shipsmith, he studied drafting and construction to such good purpose that when only twenty-eight he launched his first schooner, the *Texas*. This he followed with a group of small coasters evidently designed for the southern trade. They bore the names of cities of that section— *Savannah, Richmond, Wilmington,* and others. Gradually he

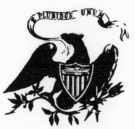

(FORM. N. 36)

BILL OF HEALTH

CONSULAR AGENCY OF THE UNITED STATES OF AMERICA

AT TRAPANI

I, *Leonardo Marino* Consular Agent of the United States at Trapani, do hereby certify that the Amer.ᵗ Brig called the "*Don Jacinto*" of Portland burthen per register — 465⁵/₁₀₀ tons. commanded by T. W. Hanima navigated by Ten men, and having on board one passenger & the Captain's wife leaves this port of Trapani in per pratique, bound for *Bucksport (Me.)*

I certify that good health is enjoyed in this town and the adjacent country, without any suspicion of plague, cholera, or contagious distemper whatsoever.

In witness whereof we have hereunto set our hand and seal of office at Trapani this *fifth* day of *October*

Leonardo Marino
U. S. Consular Agent

This Bill of Health for the Portland brig *Don Jacinto* shows the captain's wife as the one passenger aboard from Trapani, Sicily, for Bucksport.

expanded, building brigs, barks, and finally large ships which had an enviable reputation for reliability of construction and trimness of line.

His industry was prodigious. Besides supervising the work in his yards, he ran a dry and West Indies goods store which did a business of $50,000 a year, was the village postmaster, managed a drugstore, operated a planing mill and a grist mill, became the leading promoter of the Southard Cotton Mill and built several business blocks in his town. He also served as an active director of various railroads, telegraph companies, towage corporations, and banks. His eighty-eight years were full indeed. His fleet bore at the masthead the Southard house flag displaying an anvil as its device.

Thus we come to the fifties. The building of the full-rigged wooden ship now reached its climax. From the days of small things at the turn of the century it had advanced slowly up through the twenties, speeded up under the stimulation of the cotton trade in the thirties, pushed on powerfully in the forties, and now reached its culmination in the fifties. There was to follow the tragedy of war in the sixties and then the Indian summer of the seventies. With the eighties and nineties came the decline and fall. Thus the 1850's will be remembered as the golden age of the wooden ship.

Trade conditions conspired to make it so. Favorable treaties with various nations turned a large proportion of their commerce to American bottoms. The discovery of gold in California caused passengers and goods to be carried to the west coast. In turn the China trade and the opportunities "Out East" presented a challenge, since Pacific Coast lumber furnished a cargo westward, while silk, rice, hemp, and the riches of the Orient made the homeward-bound passage profitable. Years of experience and study had developed builders who knew their trade, together with masters and crews who could sail their ships.

The State of Maine surpassed all the other states in building, and from the Kennebec there came in this period 476 vessels averaging 680 tons to a vessel and totaling 324,888 tons. This was a record not to be surpassed during the era of the wooden ship.

This was pre-eminently the decade of the square-rigger. After 1860 the tall ships ceased to crowd the registers. But in the fifties they all but eclipsed every other rig. Of the 232 vessels sent from the ways in Bath, 210 were ships. Of the 82 launched at Richmond, 60 were square-rigged. Out of Bowdoinham's 22, 18 were full-rigged, and Hallowell, building the same number, had 12. Farmingdale built 16, of which 11 were ships. Pittston, just across the river, equaled this record. Phippsburg had an even larger porportion—12 out of 14, Georgetown 6 out of 10, Woolwich 3 out of 4, and Augusta 2 out of 5. If the 6 ships built at Brunswick and registered at Bath are eliminated out of a total of 418, approximately three-quarters of them crossed their yards on all three masts.

It was also the era of the clipper ship. Very few Maine ships appear in the registers as clippers. Only one, the *Flying Dragon*, built by Trufant and Drummond in 1853, made the run from New York to San Francisco in less than one hundred days. She made it in ninety-seven. The technical requirements of the register aside, not a few fast ships sailed out of the Kennebec.

The ships of Trufant and Drummond, who were early in the field, rendered good accounts of themselves. They were the *Monsoon, Emerald Isle, Viking, Flying Dragon,* and *Windward.* In Richmond in 1853 T. J. Southard launched the *Gauntlet.* She was registered as of 2,031 tons and for many years held the record as the largest vessel built in Maine. A year later Southard built the *Wizard King,* which made a fine record in the Australian service. In this same town of Richmond, Patten and Sturdivant built the *Peerless* and the *Pride of America* and

Shipbuilding on the Kennebec

G. H. Ferrin launched the *Wild Wave*, destined to founder on a coral reef in the Pacific. Other ships that made their mark were the *Carrier Pigeon* and *Undaunted*, built by Hall, Snow and Co. of Bath, the *Miss Mag*, by Grant of Farmingdale, the *Dashaway*, by J. Rideout of Hallowell, and the *White Falcon*, by William Stevens at Pittston. It has been claimed by some Bath shipbuilders that the *Pocahontas*, built by the Houghtons in 1855, has the best claim to the title. She was classed by Lloyds as a "half clipper," having very fine lines and a record for speed as well as carrying a good cargo. Her proper place may be between the last of the "clippers" and the first of the "down-easters."

In 1857 came financial panic and disaster. Many yards closed down, never to open again save perhaps for a short revival during the hectic days of the first World War. In Hallowell, for example, the yards which had been all but dormant during the forties and had been stirred into active output by the enterprise of Rufus K. Page and Henry Reed closed that town's long maritime history with the ship *Sarah Judkins* in 1856. At Topsham the building of a few small brigs and schooners continued, but the building of ships there ended with the launching by Adam Lemont of the *May Queen* in 1853. With the removal of Joseph Berry to Bowdoinham in 1856 after he built the *Henry C. Booker*, Georgetown was retired from the lists. Woolwich's last was the *Charles C. Duncan* in 1857 and Augusta's the brig *Madeira* in 1856. After 1857 but three were launched in Pittston. Gardiner passed from the picture in 1851 after losing her busiest yards at Bowman's Point by the incorporation of Farmingdale and the construction of a railroad over the site of the old yards. In fact, it may be said that after the fifties building on the Kennebec was practically limited to five towns—Bath and Phippsburg on the lower river and Bowdoinham, Richmond, and Farmingdale above the Chops.

Then the shadow of war passed over the ships and yards. In 1861 but eleven vessels were built, and of these, seven were small schooners and sloops. The fleets forced out of the cotton trade found other voyages, especially "around the Horn." For cargo they sought and found California wheat, guano from the Peruvian islands, and rice and the other products of the East.

Considering the large amount of tonnage that hailed from the Kennebec ports, the vessels taken by Confederate cruisers were remarkably few. The owners in Bath suffered the heaviest losses—nine large ships. During the decade 310 craft were launched, but the total tonnage had materially shrunk. It was but 163,539, an average per vessel of only 527 tons. This was 160 less than the tall ships of the ten years before. The European trade had become so hazardous and coastwise commerce so much more profitable that many builders began the construction of smaller hulls and to rig them fore-and-aft. So rigged they were better adapted to the coastal lanes. Indeed, 102 out of the 246 ships from the Bath yards were fore-and-aft-rigged, and in the whole district over one-third were schooners.

The period from 1871 to 1880 showed an increase in building over the tragic days of the war. None the less the effect of that conflict was evident in depression and change. The grass was growing in many yards, and only those in Bath, Richmond, and Phippsburg were at all busy. The output was less than that of the fifties by nearly 10,000 tons. The total built in the district was 379. Of these all but 26 were launched at Bath. The tonnage aggregated 225,046, an average of 594. By now the schooners are greatly in the majority and the list of craft enrolled is longer than that of those registered. The fore-and-aft rig is rapidly pushing forward in popularity and importance.

However, there came a definite revival of the tall ship in the years from 1873 to 1877. The type which had come to be known as the down-easter was reaching the acme of its development as the California wheat trade provided wide scope for its operations. In 1873 the E. and A. Sewalls launched the *Granger*, the first of their fine grain ships. There followed her down the ways within the next three years companions, the *Harvester*, the *Thresher*, and the *Reaper*. Despite the decrease in the number of ships built—about twelve a year—their tonnage was rapidly increasing. Some of the good-sized ones of the time were the *St. Paul*, 1,893 tons, by Chapman and Flint of Bath; the *Haggarstown*, 1,903 tons, and the *Yorktown*, 1,955 tons, by James M. Haggar of Richmond; the *M. P. Grace*, 1,928 tons, by John McDonald of Bath; the *Thomas B. Reed*, 1,988 tons, from the Sewall yard; and Allen and Hitchcock's *St. Mark* of 1,973 tons. The largest of the decade was the *Eureka*, launched by the veteran Richmond builder, Thomas J. Southard. She was of 2,101 tons burden.

In the first three years of the eighties the building of the square-rigger continued on a steady level. The bumper western wheat harvest of 1882 brought an Indian summer of prosperity to the grain carriers and a boom in the building of down-easters. Although shipbuilding on the Kennebec as a whole would never surpass its record figures of the fifties, the total from the Bath yards was greater than in any preceding decade. The figure of 233,398 tons exceeded that of from 1851 to 1860 by more than 50,000 tons. In the peak year, 1882, 59 vessels were launched there compared with 39 in 1854. But the demand for the wooden square-rigger was now on the decline, and of the 52 built in Bath in this decade, 34 were launched in the first three years. The slump began in 1884, and during 1886, 1887, and 1888 not a vessel of this type left the ways.

The type of vessel best adapted to the demands of the American merchant marine was being rapidly altered. The tall wooden ship was passing, and that rapidly. In 1882 the San Francisco grain fleet had employed 169 American ships. Five years later it contained but 32. All this was induced by a variety of causes. Foreign competition—British, Norwegian, French, and Italian—was pressing, and after 1884 the main output of the yards was rigged fore-and-aft. This was the type which was better adapted to the alongshore voyage and to the east coast to west coast trade, in which our carriers could participate with less competition and greater profit.

The contrast is set in clear relief by the fact that in Bath during the decade ending in 1860 there had been built 199 ships and only 12 schooners. But in the decade ending a generation later in 1890 the schooners numbered 255 as against 52 ships. The advance in size of these schooners is also notable. The average tonnage of the fore-and-after in the fifties was only 61 tons. In the eighties this had increased to 514, and individual vessels had attained a size comparable with that of the ships of the period. The *Augustus Hunt*, launched by B. W. and H. F. Morse in 1882, measured 1,141 tons, and in 1889 the *Tecumseh*, built by G. C. Moses & Co., reached 1,658 tons.

By this time the great ice business of the Kennebec had developed to enormous proportions. The banks of the river were lined with acres of ice houses—many of them on the sites occupied three decades before by busy building yards. In the summer a large fleet of schooners, as well as outmoded ships and barks, carried the ice to southern ports from which they brought back coal or southern pine timber. The Knickerbocker Towage Company came to have a virtual monopoly of this trade. Their ocean-going tugs, which were built by the Morses, with long strings of these vessels astern, were a picturesque sight as they wound down the river and along the coast. In 1889 the Morses began to construct immense sea-going barges. The first of these, the *Independent*, of 2,254 tons, was the forerunner of a great fleet. They later became the chief product of the Bath yards, 164 being built in the next thirty years.

Shipbuilding on the Kennebec

Since the *Hotspur* and the *Willie Rosenfeld* had left the ways in 1885 no full-rigged ship had been built in Maine. When Arthur Sewall and Company announced its intention to construct four very large wooden ships, the wishful thinkers hailed them as forerunners of a fleet which would restore to the American merchant marine its former prestige. The first was the *Rappahannock*. Launched in January 1890 with a registered tonnage of 3,053, she was a three-masted, three-skysail-yard ship crossing double topgallants and spreading, when under full sail, fourteen thousand yards of canvas. Her companions the *Shenandoah*, *Susquehanna*, and *Roanoke* were four-masted barks. For them a new name, shipentine, was invented, but the term failed to stick.

The second of these big ships, the *Shenandoah*, was launched in November of the same year, 1890. In point of capacity—3,258 tons—she was the largest sailing ship ever built up to that time. The fourth four-masted square-rigger constructed in this country, her cost was $175,000, and her spread of canvas could be measured in acres. Despite her size and the predictions of critics, she was seaworthy in every respect—"sailed like a pilot boat and handled well in any weather." Over eight thousand people gathered to see her launched. Pride in her was so great that the United States government placed her picture on the registers of all American ships and on the licenses of their masters. The *Susquehanna*, which was launched in the following September, was smaller by some 630 tons. She was considered to have the prettiest lines and to be the best sailer of the lot.

The last of the four, the *Roanoke*, was the last wooden ship to be built by the Sewalls. With the exception of the *Great Republic*, she was the largest wooden ship ever built in an American yard. Launched in 1892, her registered tonnage was 3,347, but on a draft of 27 feet she could stow away 2,000 tons more. The lower yards were 95 feet long, and her foremast truck was 180 feet from the deck. The keel was in two tiers of 16-inch white oak, her garboards were 8 inches thick, and her ceiling in the lower hold 14 inches. Into her construction went 1,250,000 feet of yellow pine, 24,000 cubic feet of oak, 98,000 treenails and 550 hackmatack knees. One of her builders, Samuel S. Sewall, claimed that with her his firm had reached the limit to which wood could be used in shipbuilding. Thereafter the Sewalls turned from wood. On February 3, 1894, they launched the first steel sailing ship to be built in America, the mighty four-masted bark *Dirigo*. She was the forerunner of a famous fleet of steel adequately described by the pen of Mark Hennessy.

In the nineties the schooners both at Bath and in the yards of the Bowkers at Phippsburg had become the most important in the wooden-ships register. They had increased in size by leaps and bounds. Three-master craft that had been pointed to with pride in the early nineties were soon outmoded by those with four and five masts and in 1900 by a six-master, the *Eleanor A. Percy*, measuring 3,400 tons and launched by Percy & Small. The latter, the Deering Company, and other builders turned off larger and larger craft until the Bath schooner reached her ultimate development in 1909 with the *Wyoming*, of 3,730 tons, the largest wooden fore-and-after ever built.

The decade of the nineties saw 190 merchant vessels with an aggregate of 199,300 tons turned out in Bath. Among these were 11 ships, 4 barks, 75 schooners, an equal number of barges, and 26 steamers. In the ten years from 1901 to 1910 but 4 ships were built, 74 schooners and 43 barges. So large had the individual tonnage become that the 143 vessels measured by the Custom House were 164,467 tons. In the next decade under the stimulation of the war 105 vessels—schooners, barges, and steamers—were produced with a total tonnage of 165,261.

The individual builders who contributed their share to the massive total of 2,000,000 tons of shipping launched from the banks of the Kennebec have been listed by Colonel Owen in his *History of Bath.* There were 238 in that city alone. Families of builders passed their skills and traditions from generation to generation—Agrys, Springers, Southards, Pendletons, Morrisons, Bowkers, Sewalls, Pattens, and Houghtons. Through eighty years from 1823 to 1903 the Sewall family launched 150 vessels, for the most part ships, all on their own account and known around the world. Next north from their yard was that of Johnson Rideout. He was personally the master builder of 72 vessels aggregating over 20,000 tons. South of the Sewall yard was that of the Patten family. Their house flag, a blue fouled anchor on a square white ground, marked at one time their fleet of 65 vessels, which was then said to be the largest in the United States.

Shipbuilding in America began near the mouth of the Kennebec within the present town of Phippsburg by the launching in 1607, under the direction of Digby of London, of the "pretty pinnace Virginia." It is an interesting coincidence that in the same town nearly three centuries later the last wooden full-rigged ship should have slid from the ways. This took place on the fourteenth of July, 1893, when the *Aryan* was launched from the yard of C. V. Minot at Phippsburg Center. She was a remarkably fine specimen of her class. Registering 1,939 tons and crossing three skysail yards, with trim lines and glistening white hull—"her brasswork like gold and her wood-work like snow"—she represented the best in Maine shipbuilding in the era of the wooden ship.

CHAPTER NINE

The STATE *of* MAINE
CLIPPERS

A bully ship and a bully crew,
   Doo-da, Doo-da.
A bully mate and a captain too,
   Doo-da, Doo-da-day.
Then blow, ye winds, Hi-oh, for Californy O!
There's plenty of gold, so I've been told
   On the banks of the Sacramento.
      —Joanna Colcord, *Songs of American Sailormen* [1]

"Clean, long, smooth as a smelt. Sharp arching head. Thin, hollow bow; convex sides; light round and graceful stern. A genuine East Indiaman or Californian. Aloft, large built, iron-banded lower masts; taut tapering smaller masts, long proportioned spars from lower to skysail yards. Above board, she towers up with strong fibrous arms spreading a cloud of canvas to the gale." This was what the mariner of the fifties had in mind when he spoke of clippers.—Carl C. Cutler—*Greyhounds of the Sea.* [2]

ANY ATTEMPT to sort out the clippers from among the sharp-built ships of the 1850's is likely to provoke controversy. Lloyd's had a rigid classification in which a given ship received in the register a rating of "C," "S," "M," or "F." The magic letter C, of course, stood for clipper. The S meant sharp ship, the M, medium ship, and finally the full-bodied ship received the rat-

[1] W. W. Norton & Company, Inc., 1938.
[2] G. P. Putnam's Sons. Copyright 1930 by Carl C. Cutler.

ing F. Quite apart from these rigid ratings, if an ordinary merchantman had the good luck to make a more than average
voyage, she and the magic talisman "clipper" came together
and clung to each other like droplets of quicksilver. In this
perhaps the advertising talent of her owners played its part.
Then again even an old apple-bowed hooker that "beat her head
three times against a billow and then fell off and sailed around
it" is likely to turn up in the sympathetic chronicle of some
member of her owner's or skipper's family as a "clipper ship."

And so casting close definition and technical classification
aside, we choose to tell the tale of the fast, sharp ships of the
fifties—some ninety of which were built and launched on
the coast of Maine from 1850 to 1856. Commencing in the late
forties, the clipper era lasted little more than a decade and came
to an end in the financial debacle of 1857. The urge which
impelled designers, builders, and owners—the entire shipping
fraternity—was speed, more speed, and then still more speed.
This desire received a powerful stimulus in the year 1849 with
an episodic adventure which belongs to any account of the
days of the clipper ships.

On a spring day in 1848 a powerfully built man bolted into
the old Plaza in the little town of San Francisco. His shaggy
hair was wind-blown and his flashy clothes were stained with
the dust of travel. His black eyes flashed as he shook an old
horse-radish bottle energetically up and down. In it were several good-sized yellow lumps. With a bull-throated bellow,
he yelled:

"Gold! Gold! Gold! From the American River."

The bystanders recognized him at once as Sam Brennan of
Saco, Maine, the manager of Captain John Sutter's store at his
fort near Sacramento.

During the year ending April 1, 1848, but two ships, one
bark, and a brig had come into San Francisco from Atlantic

ports. During 1849 there took place the gigantic migration which changed that city from a drowsy Mexican trading station into one of the busiest seaports of the world. There cleared for the Golden Gate from the eastern harbors some 775 vessels. Almost every port on the Atlantic seaboard was represented in this fleet. In the Maine newspapers the news had been published in late September, 1848. In this famous migration of the forty-niners, Bath led off with 19 vessels, Portland and Bangor each sent 13, Eastport 10, Belfast 3, Saco and Thomaston 2 each, and other smaller towns 1 each. This made a total of 67 sail. These argosies of the forty-niners were not the tall clippers so soon to be launched. All but one were brigs and barks, and the one ship, the *Andrew Scott,* was of only 318 tons burden.

The first band of gold seekers to sail direct from Maine to California set forth from Belfast. The owners of the bark *Suliot,* just off the ways in January, 1849, announced that she would sail for San Francisco so soon as a company of forty passengers was obtained. Fifty soon applied for passage. A mixed company it was and typical of those to come. There were fifteen mechanics, eleven lumbermen, five merchants, four farmers, three surveyors, two mariners, a chemist, a printer, a dentist, an apothecary, a hatter, a lawyer, and three who signed on as "gentlemen."

The freight brought in for shipment was equally quaint and varied. Some idea of the multitude of different articles may be gathered from the fact that the *Suliot's* manifest was fifteen feet in length. The merchants sorted over their stocks and sent out as ventures every imaginable kind of merchandise—dry goods, groceries, clothing, shoes, and medicine. Some of the passengers carried small frame houses knocked down and ready to be set up when they arrived. In order to fill the hold to a height suitable for the construction of cabins and staterooms, a large lot of hemlock boards was put aboard, they being the readiest thing at hand.

The sailing caused all manner of excitement along the Penobscot. On Saturday night a great banquet was held with Governor Anderson presiding. The speakers pictured the glorious future of California and its opportunities for development and unbounded wealth when it should be pervaded with the enterprise and thrift of New England. Sailing day, January 30, was bitter cold, but an enthusiastic crowd gathered to see the company off. After a voyage of 171 days they arrived in the following July at San Francisco. There the hemlock boards proved to be the most profitable venture of all. Bought in Belfast at $10 a thousand, they sold in San Francisco for $300.

Many forty-niners joined up with such men as William L. Hanscom, a member of the Piscataqua family of shipbuilders who built the schooner *Mary M. Wood* and sailed her round the Horn. Another favorite way to go to the gold fields was by the organization of a mining company. The Portland and California Mining Company was one of these co-operative enterprises. There were thirty-five shares, thirty-four held by men and one by two boys who were counted as one man. They chartered the little brig *Ruth*, of only 146 tons, under the command of Captain Jabez Stevens. The cargo, which had been bought by the company as a speculation, consisted of lumber and fitted house frames. Then there was a bountiful supply of provisions and tools to be used in mining. It was the custom of many of the mining companies to attend church in a body to listen to a sermon preached for their benefit on the Sunday before the voyage began. The favorite text, it is said, was Genesis 2:12—"and the gold of that land is good." The services in this instance were held on Long Wharf, whence the *Ruth* was to sail at midday on the eighth of September. There the

[169]

Rev. William T. Dwight made an address appropriate to the occasion. Just at noon the *Ruth* slipped away from the wharf.

On the second of October the bark *I. A. Thompson* sailed from Bath with forty-nine passengers from Augusta, Hallowell, Sidney, Vassalborough, and Skowhegan. It was a gala day in Bath. Just before the *Thompson* cast off, the T. D. Robinson yards launched the ship *Old England*, and the Moses yard, the ship *New England*. As she slipped away down the Reach the *Thompson* fired a salute. It was answered by the brig *Anna C. Maine*, which was scheduled to follow her to California the next day. The price of passage was $150 to $200. A clergyman, the Rev. Amariah Kallock, was carried free and paid his way by preaching to the passengers. Daily prayers were also held after breakfast. The *Thompson* made her passage to San Francisco in 128 days from Bath to find over three hundred vessels crowding the harbor. This fleet was later augmented by the brig *Margaret*, which had sailed from Portland on October 12.

Not all these little brigs and barks of 300 tons burden and less had good luck in rounding Cape Horn. The *Condor*, commanded by Captain Long, sailing from Portland on the twentieth of August, was so buffeted by gales that she spent thirty-five days in getting around. Some tried to sail through the Strait of Magellan, with even less success. This route is especially treacherous, running from the Atlantic to the Pacific against the prevailing westerly gales. The more prudent captains who knew the hazards of this course carried abundant stores. But many underestimated their needs and suffered extremities of hardship and even failure. No tragedy was more terrible than that which befell the *Abby Barker*, a bark hailing from Yarmouth in Casco Bay.

Timothy Pratt was the eldest son of Master David Pratt, the first shipbuilder in old North Yarmouth. Like most of his family, he "had salt in his blood" and began early to follow the sca. In 1848 his home burned, and when rumors of the great discovery in California reached the East, he decided to go there with his whole family. He took one of his father's vessels, the *Abby Barker*, a bark of 259 tons, and loaded her with house frames. His eldest son, Timothy Augustus, a student in Bowdoin College and a poet of some promise, went as his first mate, and his next son Enos as second mate. With his wife and his twin boys, William and Henry, then about eleven, he sailed out of Royall's River full of hope.

To save time the *Abby Barker* attempted to pass the Strait of Magellan and spent the next eighty harrowing days in those terrible waters. Beset by fierce currents, she fought against the westerly gales and "willewaws" and could find no anchorages on the sheer rock coast of that inhospitable region. To add to the discomfort and anxiety, the *Abby Barker* ran short of provisions and water. But at last she passed out by Cape Pillar and entered the Pacific. Then there was further trouble. Soon after they had reached good water and were sailing up the west coast, the captain, worn out by the anxiety and the long struggle, suddenly fell dead on the deck.

Timothy Augustus, the eldest son, now took command. He succeeded in bringing the bark into Sacramento Bay. Here cholera broke out. The crew, taking all they could lay their hands on, deserted the ship. Augustus soon became sick and died. Enos and William, one of the twins, followed. The mother, either from the disease or broken-hearted by the loss of her family, next succumbed. This left only the surviving twin, Henry, of eleven years. All that the family at home had to tell them of these tragic days was an unfinished letter commenced by Augustus. In it he wrote, "Already the ravages of the dread disease are upon us."

Captain Talbot of Freeport happened to put into Sacramento. Recognizing the *Abby Barker*, he went on board, to find to his horror the dead bodies of William and Mrs. Pratt. Burying the dead, he took Henry with him. Two years later— for his voyage was a long one—Captain Talbot brought the lad back home to Yarmouth.

The experience of the only full-rigged ship to carry "forty-niners" around the Horn, the little *Andrew Scott*, was typical of the times. She had been financed by a group of Portland men who had heard that lumber was selling in San Francisco at $400 a thousand. Upon her arrival in May 1850, it was found that the bottom had dropped out of the lumber market. Her master, William Leavitt, was able to turn another item to account.

He had taken with him aboard the *Scott* a small two-masted sailboat, the *Naumkeag*. She had cost him $180. He sold her for $2,000. And the reason was this: Between San Francisco and Sacramento freight rates ran from $60 to $120 a ton. The demand for small, smart sailing craft was great. The purchasers of the *Naumkeag* cleared from $600 to $1,000 a week.

This small episode, coupled with the *Scott's* missing of the high lumber market, is the key to the clipper era. Indeed, with the term there goes as often as not its counterpart, the California clipper, and again the Australia and China tea clippers. The *Scott's* passage out had run in excess of 160 days. Had she been able to do it in 110 or better her cargo of lumber might have made its high market.

A desire for speed had been latent in the blood of every master builder worth his salt. With the rush for California gold and profits, swift passages became the profitable consideration and his opportunity to show what he could do had arrived. Owners ceased to be their own shippers. They found the greatest profit in rendering service to the merchant, whose success in turn lay in getting his goods to market in the shortest possible time. This was the reason for the sixty- and eighty-dollar freights. Capacity counted but little. Speed was the prime requisite, and to this end builders carved their models.

Although Maine had led the United States in the building of ships since the early forties, her builders were late in feeling this urge for speed. Their construction of sharp-built ships began in 1850, and the bulk of it was achieved in the four years from 1851 to 1854. By 1856 the demand for fast ships had evaporated as quickly as it had come. The greatest production was in four yards. There was Fernald and Pettigrew of Kittery, whose most famous ship out of eight, the 1,610-ton *Typhoon*, was long known as the "Portsmouth Flyer." At Bath there was Trufant and Drummond, who put over six, among them the *Flying Dragon*, which held the record on the Maine Coast for the run to San Francisco. She did it in 1857 in 97 days. Five came from the yards of Metcalf and Norris at Damariscotta, among them the first one, the *Alert*, launched in 1850. In Penobscot waters from Deacon George Thomas' yard at Rockland there came indubitably Maine's most famous ship, *Red Jacket*, together with three others. In this colorful period many other yards from the Piscataqua to the St. Croix launched one or more fast ships.

The output of the Maine yards in 1850 totaled 326 vessels. Only three of these could, in the light of their later performance, be called clippers. The first was the *Alert*, launched in November, and rushed to New York. From there, flying Crocker and Warren's blue and yellow house flag, she sailed under Captain Francis Bursley on December 29 for San Francisco.

She was followed out of New York two weeks later by the *Grey Feather*, built at Eastport by C. S. Husten. She sailed into the ranks of the record-breakers under two down-east captains: first, when Captain Daniel McLaughlin, a native of Grand

Manan, in 1854 made the run from Melbourne to Calcutta in her in 36 days; and second, when Captain Bartlett Mayo of Hampden covered the 14,000 miles from New York to Australia in 84 days. This latter run, which was considered a record for ships of limited size, would be a credit to any. The *Grey Feather*, while listed in the registers as "full modeled" and of only 586 tons register, had lines approaching those of the out-and-out clippers.

The output in 1851 was but little larger. Of the 254 built, but 9 could be called clippers. At Rockland, George Thomas launched the little bark *Springbok*, a miniature forerunner of his famous *Red Jacket*. Trufant and Drummond began their notable fleet at Bath with the *Monsoon*. Alfred Butler at South Portland sent off Casco Bay's most notable contribution to the fleet, the beautifully named *Snow Squall*. Two others, authentic Maine-built clippers built on the east bank of the Piscataqua, were registered at Portsmouth, owing to a confounding of state and customs district lines. On Badger's Island at Kittery, Fernald and Pettigrew launched their *Typhoon*, and up river at Green Acre in the town of Eliot, Samuel Hanscom built the beautiful and romantic *Nightingale*. The last three deserve a careful scrutiny.

The *Snow Squall* was said to have cost $30,000. She was purchased when just off the stocks by Charles R. Green & Co. of New York. For thirteen years she held an enviable place among the smaller clippers. Even when she was twelve years old, she showed her heels to the Confederate cruiser *Tuscaloosa*. Her life was spent mainly in the China tea trade. Under the command of Captain Ira Bursley, a famous shipmaster of the packet and clipper era, she made the Australian voyage from New York to Melbourne in 79 days. In 1856, making a short detour in the coffee trade, she made a fine run from New York to Rio de Janeiro in 28 days. Returning in 34, she completed a round trip, including detention, equal to any made. Three years later she sailed a close race over the China course with the *Romance of the Seas*, one of Donald McKay's big clippers, a thousand tons larger than the *Snow Squall*, and reached Sandy Hook two days ahead of her.

Fully rigged with skysail yards aloft and all colors flying, the *Typhoon* slipped down the ways in February 1851. Owned by D. & A. Kingsland of New York and commanded by Captain Charles H. Salter, she made the passage from Portsmouth to Liverpool during the month of March in 13 days and 10 hours from wharf to dock, a feat unequaled up to that time. It was this voyage, her first, which gave her the sobriquet "Portsmouth Flyer." She was the maritime sensation of the year, being not only the first American clipper but also the largest merchant ship ever seen in Liverpool.

Back on this side of the Atlantic she sailed for California in August, taking part in one of the keenest and most interesting races ever sailed. Her competitors were the *Raven* and the *Sea Witch*. Sometimes one was ahead, sometimes another, and sometimes over the long course they fought it out tack by tack. The little *Raven* won. She slipped through the Golden Gate 105 days out from Boston, while the time of the *Typhoon* was 106. A later passage of the *Typhoon* from Calcutta to the Cape of Good Hope in 37 days was never beaten, and it was equaled only by the *Witch of the Wave*, which had been built the same year as the *Typhoon* in the George Raynes yard on the Portsmouth side of the Piscataqua.

One of the most beautiful of the extreme clippers was the *Nightingale*. Named for Jenny Lind, whose likeness she carried beneath her prow as her figurehead, she represented all that was lovely and exciting on the high seas in the glamorous fifties. From that fair day in June, 1851, when she slipped from the ways in Samuel Hanscom's yard under the hill at Greenacre, South Eliot, until she disappeared beneath the waves she had skimmed for nearly half a century, hers was a long life of adventure. She led off in a race to the Australian gold fields. She won the English tea races. Sold, she became a slaver and acquired "the taint of a musky ship." In the rebellion she saw service as a vessel of war. And again and again as a California clipper she rounded the Horn until she foundered in 1893.

The clipper builders never scrimped in their work. But Samuel Hanscom determined to surpass them all in prodigality. For his model he turned to his nephew Isaiah Hanscom, who was later to become chief of the Bureau of Construction in Washington. He designed her on the lines of a yacht. She was intended not for the Cape Horn trade but rather to carry passengers, who could well afford to pay for luxury, to the World's Fair in London. Also Hanscom was ambitious to put his handiwork on exhibition in the Thames as the model American clipper. To this end she was fitted out between decks with luxurious saloons and staterooms which were finished with carved and gilded moldings and panels and furnished with upholstery and hangings of figured brocade. Inboard and outboard all was richness and beauty. Besides the portrait bust on the bow, the stern was ornamented with the figure of Jenny Lind reclining with a nightingale perched on her finger. On stern, bow, and quarter the name *Nightingale* shone in a contrast of blue and gold.

All of this cost a deal of money, and she was launched heavily mortgaged and sent to Boston for sale. She was first bid in by ship brokers, to whom Sampson and Tappan were glad to pay $75,000 for her. She long sailed under the house flag of that firm—white over blue with a red ball in the center. So proud and confident were her owners that they offered to match the *Nightingale* against any British or American ship for a race to China and back for a stake of £10,000. The challenge was never accepted.

In the fall of 1851 came the word that gold had been discovered in Australia. The days of forty-nine were repeated. Although she had been advertised for the London run, the call was so insistent that the *Nightingale* joined the rush for the gold fields. The first to get away, she sailed from Boston on the eighteenth of October. This first voyage of 90 days to Melbourne, however, gave little promise of the fast passages she was later to make. For examples there are her runs—in 1853 from Portsmouth, England, to Shanghai against the northeast monsoon in 106 days; in 1854 from New York to Melbourne in 75 days; and the next year from Shanghai to London in 91 days.

In 1860 she was sold and became a slaver. When under the command of Captain Francis Bowen, the notorious "Prince of the Slavers," and flying the American colors she was captured by the U. S. sloop-of-war *Saratoga*. After her cargo of 961 blacks had been liberated at Monrovia, she was sold to the government. She was armed and served during the Civil War with the Gulf Blockading Squadron as a supply and coal ship. At its close she was again sold and under various owners sailed in the California and China trades until 1876, when she went under Norwegian colors. Rigged as a bark but keeping her old name, she came to her end in the North Atlantic lumber trade. In 1893, when forty-two years old, she was abandoned at sea on a voyage from Liverpool to Halifax.

In 1852 the Maine yards launched some twenty fast ships. They were considerably larger than their predecessors. One, the *Defiance*, registered 1,690 tons, and six others exceeded 1,000 tons. Built by Deacon George Thomas in his Rockland yard from plans drawn by Boston's twenty-five-year-old genius of maritime design, Samuel Hartt Pook, the *Defiance* was the most extreme type of clipper. Her concave sides, with ends longer and sharper than those of the *Flying Cloud*, made her a supremely beautiful ship. Sensing the deficiencies of the earlier clippers as cargo carriers and taking a hint from the flat-floored Western Ocean packets, young Pook evolved a type which was almost universally adopted by later builders. On her voyage in ballast from Rockland to New York the *Defiance* logged twenty nautical miles an hour. Two Maine ships launched this year became record-makers. The *Rattler*, also from the Thomas yard, when twenty-six years old and known as the Costa Rican ship *Martha*, made an unsurpassed voyage in 28 days from Callao to San Francisco heads, and the *Red Rover*, built by Fernald and Pettigrew at Kittery in 1855, made the voyage to San Francisco in 110 days and equaled it again the next year.

In 1853 the high-water mark was reached in both the building and the sailing of clippers. Enthusiasm was at its height, freights were still good, and few eyes detected on the horizon the ominous signs of commercial depression. It is estimated that nearly half the number and more than half the tonnage of the clipper fleet was built this year. "Everybody who had capital to invest wanted one or at least shares in one," writes Captain Arthur Clark. The Maine yards which specialized in sharp ships built thirty-three, twenty-four of which were over a thousand tons. Some of the best-known vessels of the fleet were put afloat. Among them were the only five from Maine which made the voyage from Boston or New York to California in less than 110 days. These were the *Flying Dragon, Dashing Wave, Spitfire, Viking,* and *Oracle.*

Of the Maine-built California clippers the fastest was the *Flying Dragon*, built by Trufant and Drummond at Bath. Sailing from Boston under Captain Judah P. Baker of Brewster, on the twenty-first of July it took her 31 days to fight her way around the Horn into the Pacific. In the struggle she sprung her bowsprit and main yard and lost her jibboom. The grim battle off the Horn proved too much for the forty-six-year-old captain, who died before reaching San Francisco. This grueling voyage had taken 148 days. But better luck followed. Not counting that voyage, her average time for five successive years over this 15,000-mile course is 112 3/5 days. Moreover, the *Flying Dragon* is the only vessel from Maine during the days of the clipper ships to make a run of less than 100 days. In 1857 she did it in 97. In 1860 she sailed from Sydney, Australia, to Hampton Roads in 75 days. This is a record passage between these ports.

A close second to the *Flying Dragon* was the *Spitfire*. She was an extreme clipper launched in September 1853 by James Arey and Sons at Frankfort and commanded by John Arey. Sailing from Boston on the twenty-seventh of October, she put in to Rio de Janeiro the last week in November, where she remained twenty days. Here four men were discharged for incompetence. Elkanah Crowell, the mate, is credited with the saying that he "wished no man in his crew who could not jump over the foreyard before breakfast." These he must have had, for despite being baffled for fifteen days by gales off the Horn, the *Spitfire* arrived in San Francisco only 120 days out of Boston. This made her actual sailing time a few hours less than 100 days. The voyage around from Rio in 65 days is said never to have been beaten by any loaded vessel except the *Witchcraft*, and then only by three days. The *Spitfire's* best record was made in 1860, when she sailed a dead heat over the California course with the *Black Hawk*. They both arrived in 107 days.

This time was equaled by the voyage of Fernald and Pettigrew's *Dashing Wave* when sailing from Boston on New Year's Day, 1858. It is a tribute to this Kittery firm's fine workmanship and material that the *Wave* was the last of the clippers in active service. Like so many of the wooden ships, she spent the last of her days as a barge in the fishery business on the west coast. When sixty years old, in 1920, she was examined and her hull found to be in sound condition. She was lost the same year.

Metcalf and Norris of Damariscotta, the pioneer clipper builders of Maine, put afloat their most famous vessel this summer. The *Flying Scud* was of good size, 1,713 tons, and extremely sharp, calculated for speed. So quickly did she pass down the river after her launch that her officers could not believe it possible. They thought their chronometers must be out of order. Soon after her arrival in New York she was purchased by R. W. Cameron for his Australian Pioneer Line, for which he was using the advertising slogan, "Sixty days to Melbourne," and under Captain Warren H. Bearce she sailed on the ninth of September. In the Gulf Stream she was struck by lightning, which magnetized the cargo of iron in the after hold. This affected the compasses, and the needles whirled so rapidly as to make them useless. For a long time they could only be used by placing them on a board extending out from the port side. Despite this and despite the fact that she was so overloaded that her scuppers were nearly awash and she was trimmed by the head two feet, making her very crank, she made the passage in seventy-six days.

A notation in her log on November 6 stated that on that day she ran 449 nautical miles. If this fact could be substantiated, it would credit the *Scud* with the best day's run ever logged by a clipper. It is greatly to be regretted that the log book is not now available. The possibility of a mistake in the reckoning of Captain Bearce—although highly improbable in the opinion of those who knew the man—leaves Maine's claim to this record forever a matter of dispute. Her later performance is good evidence of her speed. To her credit is a passage of 19 days and 20 hours from New York to Marseilles and also one from the same port to Bombay in 81 days. The latter was a record at the time and was thereafter beaten by only a few days.

On the last day of November, 1853, Trufant and Drummond launched their second fast ship of the year, the *Viking*, built for George Hussey of New Bedford and bearing as her figure-head a northland warrior in full armor. Her best run to California was 108 days in 1858. The *Oracle*, the sole contribution to the clipper fleet by Chapman and Flint of Thomaston, made herself a place among the faster ships this year by a passage in 109 days.

At this juncture it seems appropriate to set forth the days run to San Francisco by fast Maine ships. With the yard from which they were launched and the year of their launching, they are as follows:

Flying Dragon	Trufant and Drummond, 1853	97 days
Typhoon	Fernald and Pettigrew, 1851	106 days
Spitfire	James Arey & Sons, 1853	107 days
Dashing Wave	Fernald and Pettigrew, 1853	107 days
Viking	Trufant and Drummond, 1853	108 days
Red Rover	Fernald and Pettigrew, 1852	110 days
Midnight	Fernald and Pettigrew, 1854	111 days
Euterpe	Horace Merriam, 1854	112 days
Talisman	Metcalf and Norris, 1854	112 days
Live Yankee	Horace Merriam, 1853	114 days
Golden Rule	William Hitchcock & Co.	114 days
Nonpareil	George Donham, 1853	115 days
Mary Robinson	Trufant and Drummond, 1854	115 days
Golden Racer	Mortons, 1852	117 days
Anglo Saxon	Francis H. Rhoades, 1852	118 days
Flying Eagle	William Hitchcock & Co.	118 days

Another well-known run—from dock to dock, across the Atlantic to Liverpool, the *Typhoon* sailing from Portsmouth and the *Red Jacket* from New York—reflects the following:

Typhoon	Fernald and Pettigrew, 1851	13 days, 10 hours
Red Jacket	George Thomas, 1853	13 days, 1 hour, 25 minutes

The fast ships will always be best known by their records. For swiftness they were built, and their proper story is of how well they fulfilled their purpose. Some have an interest beyond the beauty of their lines, the list of their passages from port to port, and their best day's run. Two of those launched in 1853 have a prominence that does not rest on knots and miles, but on their stories, which are a part of the romance of the sea. Such are the *Wild Rover* and the *Wild Wave*.

The medium clipper *Wild Rover* was built by Austin and Hall at Damariscotta. She was long the property of Alpheus Hardy and Co. of Boston. In 1863, laden with lumber, she sailed out of Shanghai with a young Japanese hidden in her locked storeroom. He was the first of his nation to seek an education in the United States. In Boston he found a firm friend in the owner, Alpheus Hardy, by whom he was educated at Amherst College and Andover Theological Seminary. When he returned to Japan in 1874 he founded Doshisha College at Kioto and became its president. His own name combined with that of his benefactor is world-famous—Joseph Hardy Neesima.

The *Wild Wave* was a medium clipper. She was built this year by G. H. Ferrin of Richmond. In 1856 she made the run from Callao to Plymouth in 70 days, a record never beaten. The pluck and ingenuity of her captain when she was wrecked two years later made her story one of the classic epics of the sea. Josiah N. Knowles of Eastham, one of the most brilliant of the Cape Cod shipmasters, was in command. In March 1858 she was bound from San Francisco to Valparaiso with a crew of thirty, ten passengers, and two chests containing $18,000 in gold coin. Charts of the South Seas were then very inaccurate. At about one o'clock in the morning of March 5, the lookout saw breakers under the lee bow. Her people were unaware that there was land any nearer than twenty miles away. The *Wild Wave* attempted to come about but missed stays and, wearing, she

struck an uncharted coral reef. Within five minutes she had lost
her masts, bilged, and was among breakers so violent that they
tore the copper from her sides and bottom and tossed it up on
deck.

At daybreak it was found that she had struck a circular reef
about two miles from a little coral atoll called Oeno. The island
was nothing but a strip of sand half a mile wide. The crew and
passengers were able to get ashore and land much of the provisions and livestock aboard the ship. Shelters were then built,
using the sails of the ship. A dug well gave them water, and
fish, sea birds, and their eggs were to be had in abundance.
After about a week the captain with the mate, five men, and
the two chests of treasure put to sea in an attempt to reach the
settlement of the mutineers of the *Bounty* on Pitcairn Island.

This lay eighty miles to the south. After a hazardous three
days' voyage they succeeded in reaching Pitcairn. On account
of the surf they could not land in Bounty Bay and soon after
getting ashore on another part of the island their boat was stove
beyond repair. They salvaged the treasure, which was brought
ashore and buried. Great was their disappointment to find that
the island was uninhabited, the whole community having removed to Norfolk Island. There was plenty of food. Fruit grew
abundantly, and there were chickens, sheep, and goats which
had been left behind.

A boat had to be built. A diligent search turned up some
discarded axes and other tools, and they set to work. They
fashioned a schooner 30 feet long and of 8-foot beam. She was
the result of immense labor and real Yankee ingenuity. Some of
the small houses were burned and the nails which they contained
were salvaged. This supply fell far short, and in many places
wooden pegs had to do. Everything imaginable was used. An
old anvil served as an anchor, a copper kettle as a stove, and
their flag was made from the red hangings of the church pulpit,

a cast-off white shirt, and a pair of blue overalls. Old rope was picked up, reduced to oakum, and spun again on an improvised wheel. The schooner was named the *John Adams* after one of the Bounty mutineers. She was finally put afloat and the treasure chests loaded in. Leaving three whose hearts had failed them on the island, they again set sail.

This time they had planned to go to Tahiti, but head winds increasing into a gale forced them to change course and head for the Marquesas. For eleven days they tossed about, suffering terribly from seasickness. At Resolution Bay they dared not land, the natives appearing hostile. They pushed on to Muka Hiva, where, to their joy, they found the U.S.S. *Vandalia*. The schooner they had built at Pitcairn was quickly sold to a missionary for $250, and the *Vandalia*, picking up the party on Oeno and the three men at Pitcairn, took them all to Tahiti. Those left on Oeno had constructed a large boat from the wreckage of the *Wild Wave*, but when finished it was so heavy they could not get it into the water. Their health had been remarkably good. Only one of the whole party had died.

On the second of November, 1853, in the presence of an immense crowd, some of whom had come from New York and Philadelphia to witness the event, there was launched at Rockland, the largest, the fastest, and one of the handsomest of the Maine fleet—the extreme clipper *Red Jacket*, of 2,306 tons. Designed by Samuel Hartt Pook, built by George Thomas, and commanded by Captain Asa Eldridge, she combined skills all but unsurpassable. Trim and sharp, the delicate beauty of her graceful lines, arched stem and exquisitely modeled stern were matched by her finely proportioned spars and standing rigging. Her figurehead was a life-sized likeness of the Seneca chief whose name she bore, while on her light, round stern, surrounded by heavy gilt scrollwork, was a bust of the same

Indian warrior. To the end of her long life she was considered one of the more beautiful of the larger clippers.

No expense had been spared in furnishing her inboard and outboard with the best. The after cabin was finished in rose-wood mahogany, satin, and zebra wood which was set off by black walnut and gilt work. Exclusive of the officers' quarters, with the forward cabin there were fourteen staterooms. And the forward house accommodated a crew of sixty-two men. A week after launching she was towed to New York, where she received her masts and spars, was rigged and her sails bent. Then on January 10 she sailed for Liverpool.

It was a memorable voyage with every sort of handicap. Uncoppered, with an indifferent crew, with hail, rain, or snow on almost every day of her run, the *Red Jacket* arrived on January twenty-third. Her elapsed time from dock to dock was 13 days, 1 hour and 25 minutes. This is a record that still stands for sailing ships. For six consecutive days her runs averaged over 343 miles, and on the ninth day out the crew "spliced the main brace." This was to celebrate a twenty-four-hour run of 413 nautical miles. Although Donald McKay's *Lightning* was to surpass this by 23 miles about two months later, it has been beaten on only two other voyages in the history of sailing ships, unless the claim of the *Flying Scud* to 449 can be established.

The *Red Jacket* created much excitement in Liverpool. Her arrival was dramatic. At least a day before she was expected by her greatest admirers, a steamer coming in announced that she was just behind. A crowd went down to Point Linus to greet her. Two tugs succeeded in getting lines aboard her but were unable to draw them taut. The great ship swept on up the Mersey with every stitch of canvas drawing in the brisk northwest wind, fairly flying toward her pier.

Then Captain Eldridge accomplished a feat not often attempted. The *Red Jacket* came about, threw her yards aback, and laid herself up to the pierhead with a precision that brought appreciative shouts from the spectators.

She never returned to America under the stars and stripes. The White Star Line immediately chartered her for the round trip to Melbourne. So pleased were they with her record—5 months and 4 days, with a spurt from the Cape to Melbourne in 19 days that was never equaled—that they were anxious to keep her in their fleet even at a cost of £30,000.

In 1854 the urge for speed began to lessen. Sobered by rising costs, falling freights, and long waits in port, owners and builders realized that the mad and merry days of these swift sharp ships were numbered. Trade conditions on the west coast had become stabilized, and it mattered little whether the voyage was made in 90 or 110 days. Conservative merchants began once more to think in terms of freight money, and many of the proudest of the tall ships were forced to find a cargo at the dusty Peruvian guano islands, at the southern cotton ports, or even in the wretched coolie and "black ivory" trades. Their days had been glamorous, but after all, afloat or ashore, it is a workaday world.

Maine builders were not slow in sensing this. During this year only fifteen ships were built that could be classed as clippers, and nearly all of these were of medium model and considerably less tonnage than their predecessors. George Thomas made no contribution to the fleet, for he had removed to Quincy, Massachusetts. Horace Merriam still built in Rockland. Although his *Live Yankee* of 1853 had shown up badly in comparison with the *Red Jacket*, his *Euterpe* sailed into the fleet of the record-makers. Fernald and Pettigrew put afloat the *Midnight;* Trufant and Drummond, still optimistic, launched the *Mary Robinson* and the *Windward*, two beautifully modeled and sparred ships, and Metcalf and Norris sent off the *Talisman*. Of these the *Euterpe* made a record that stood for many years by running from Calcutta to the Cape in 39 days and thence to London, the whole voyage taking only 85 days. She was the first ship to enter the new Victoria Docks, none of the others being big enough to accommodate her 1,975 tons. The *Talisman*, the last clipper to be built by the pioneers, Metcalf and Norris, made her builders proud when in 1859 she led the *Great Republic* home from San Francisco by 4 days.

Of the new builders the most ambitious was Captain Nathaniel Blanchard. After having one vessel burned at great loss before she was launched, he built at the Thomas Knight yard at South Portland a beautiful and lofty vessel to which he appropriately gave the name *Phoenix*. She was very heavily sparred. Besides crossing skysail yards on all three masts, she carried the rather unusual moon-sails on her fore and mizzen. In 1859 she sailed what is considered by not a few authorities the best transatlantic voyage. Crossing from Savannah to Cork Harbor, she made the run in 14 days and 9 hours. When distance is considered, her admirers claim this equals a 13-day run from New York to Liverpool. Curiously enough, in 1860 she too came to her end in a fire.

By 1856 shipbuilding in the United States had reached its apogee with Maine leading all the states. Yet of the 215,904 tons built in the state in 1855, less than 5,000 was in sharp ships. They number five. There was the *Criterion*, by Hitchcock of Damariscotta, the *Midnight*, by Fernald and Pettigrew of Kittery, the *Dictator*, by Cox of Robbinston, the *Stephen Crowell*, by Burgess and Clark of Warren, and the *Young Mechanic*— built from a model whittled out by his son—by Rhoades of Rockland. Five only were registered in 1856. The full fury of economic depression in 1857 wrote finis to the construction of Maine-built clippers.

CHAPTER TEN

The CONFEDERATE
COMMERCE RAIDERS

"Sheets and halyards were let go by the run and the huge cloud of canvas seemed to shrink and shrivel up as the vessel was rounded to with folded wings like a crippled bird."

"It was about ten o'clock at night when the first gleam of light burst from the cabin hatch. Few, few on board can forget the spectacle. A ship set on fire at sea! It would seem that man was almost warring against his maker! Her helpless condition, the red flames licking the rigging as they climbed aloft, the sparks and pieces of burning rope taken by the wind and flying far to leeward, the ghastly glare thrown on the dark sea as far as the eye could reach and the death-like stillness of the scene—all these combined to place the *Golden Rocket* on the tablet of our memories forever."— Raphael Semmes, *The Cruise of the Alabama and Sumter*, 1864.

THE PEAK OF shipbuilding on the coast of Maine was reached within two years after the crest of the clippers. In 1855 there was constructed in the State of Maine 215,904 tons of shipping. This was a third of the total production throughout the United States. But discordant notes were sounding.

Cargoes were hard to secure, freights were low, and the demand for new ships had begun to decline rapidly. Even in the peak year of 1855 Maine-built vessels sold for twenty-five per cent less than twelve months previous. Since 1853 the apprehensive had feared and warned of approaching commercial disaster. In the fall of 1857 the storm broke in full fury. For the next eight years there faced the shipping interests of the country first the ravages of a severe economic depression and then—civil war. These conditions earmarked and coincided with, but did not cause, the decline of the American merchant marine. In short, depression and the toll of shipping taken by the Confederate raiders merely hastened the complicated process of the ultimate substitution of steam for sail.

Never since the days of the long embargo had American ports presented so depressing a picture. The beautiful, tall ships were rotting at their anchorages, sails unbent, in charge of keepers. These were the ships which night and day had loaded cargoes for California that they might hurry to sea with no delay. Freights which had been urged upon them at sixty dollars a ton were now hard to procure at ten. In foreign ports they lay idle, waiting for employment which would at least pay their way home. All this was reflected in the Maine yards.

In the mania for building vessels these yards had set afloat since 1852 nearly eight hundred thousand (793,411) tons. Now there was little use for these vessels. In the five years from 1855 to 1859 building declined from 215,904 to 40,905 tons. This was more than 80 per cent. In Bath in 1857, 220 families received aid, whereas two years before only 93 had been on relief. These were tragic times indeed! Then came the Civil War.

In the years before the War the seaport towns of Maine were caught in a tangle of conflicting interests. Abolition was no academic matter. It was a difficult political question complicated by social and commercial considerations. Forty prosperous years of cotton carrying had woven strong ties between the shipmasters and builders of the state and merchants of the southern cotton ports. Indeed, it is said that "though so widely separated on the map Bath and New Orleans were closer neighbors than Washington and Richmond." Families had intermarried. Custom House registers showed many southern names in the list of owners of Maine ships. The vessels themselves often bore the names of prominent merchants of New Orleans, Mobile, and Charleston on their name boards. Northern houses had agents and in some cases branches in the cities of the South. It is small wonder that as the war clouds gathered there was bitterness of heart and the sadness of conflicting loyalties.

However, relatively few ships hailed from the southern ports. Although the United States held second place among the commercial nations of the world, only one-tenth of her tonnage belonged in the seceding states. In Maine alone there was owned nearly twice as much shipping as in the entire South. Nearly a fifth of the American merchant marine was owned in Maine. Even before the commencement of hostilities the leaders of the Confederacy planned to make war at once on the commerce carriers of the North. They well knew that there they might strike heavy blows with but little fear of retaliation in kind.

Sumter fell on the thirteenth of April, 1861. Four days later President Jefferson Davis issued his famous proclamation inviting applications for letters of marque and reprisal. Immediately individuals, communities, and stock companies bestirred themselves to put privateers afloat. A score of tugs, steamers, fishing schooners, pilot boats, old slavers, and other small craft were fitted out. Their armament, though small, was a match for any unprotected vessel which they might meet. For nearly six months until the northern blockade became effective, they harassed and destroyed vessels all along the Atlantic coast from the Gulf as far north as Cape Ann.

One of the larger and more efficient of these raiders was the *Calhoun*, a steamer of 1,058 tons burden. She had been fitted out by a syndicate in New Orleans and rushed out of the Mississippi in the first weeks of May to watch the passes. On the twelfth of that month near the mouth of the river she made her first capture—the Machias-built brig *State of Maine*, valued at $33,000—which was sent back to New Orleans and confiscated. Six days later the Bath ship *Milan*, owned by the Houghtons, with a cargo of $20,000 worth of salt, met a like fate. On the same day the Rockland barkentine *Ocean Eagle*, loaded with over three thousand casks of lime, was added to the list. Then on the twenty-first another Bath ship, the Patten's *Ariel*, was sent in. The owners of the *Calhoun* had in ten days enriched themselves by nearly $150,000 at the expense of Maine shipowners. On the twenty-sixth of May nineteen northern vessels lay at New Orleans as prizes of the Confederacy. Among them six hailed from Maine.

On the Atlantic coast the privateers also met with success. With their capture of nineteen or more Maine vessels their names—*Lady Davis*, *Savannah*, *Jeff Davis*, *Winslow*, *York*, *Dixie*, and *Sally*—became an anathema in the ports of the state. Some raiders lay hidden in the inlets along the Carolinas. When an unsuspecting merchantman was sighted, they would sally out, strike, and scuttle back to cover. Others, like the *Jeff Davis*, cruised the coast from Florida to New England. Unsuspecting and unprepared, the northern ships were easily seized. For example, when the little *Lady Davis* hailed the schooner *A. B. Thompson* of Brunswick, she was thought to be a tug seeking a tow until she bobbed up under the schooner's stern and demanded her surrender in the name of the Confederate government.

The *Savannah*, the first privateer to receive a commission from the Confederacy, had a short career. Her only capture was the brig *Joseph* of Rockland, which was taken less than twenty-four hours after she had sailed out of Charleston harbor.

She accompanied the *Joseph* almost into the port of Georgetown, S. C. Turning back on her cruise, she sighted what she
thought was another merchantman a little north of the Hole in
the Wall. Flushed with success, Captain Baker crowded on all
sail to intercept her. When within a mile of his prey and too
late to turn back, he found to his dismay that he had run afoul
of the U. S. brig *Perry*. The *Savannah* was easily taken and sent
in to New York. Great crowds gathered to see the "pirate"
anchored off the Battery with the stars and bars flying beneath
the stars and stripes. The members of her crew were charged
with piracy and sent to the Tombs. A similar fate awaited the
crew of the *Jeff Davis*, taken a little later. There then ensued a
prolonged debate over the status of privateersmen.

In respect to privateering, the wheel of fortune had made a
full turn. When the Civil War came on there were many men
still active on the Maine Coast who had gone privateering in
the War of 1812. For example, William Cammett, one of the
masters of the *Dash*, was now inspector of customs in Portland
by appointment of President Lincoln. Because of the country's
experience in the earlier war, the United States had refused to
adhere to the Declaration of 1856, which all but abolished the
practice among European nations. This time, however, the shoe
was on the other foot.

Now it was the Rebel privateers who were sent out with
the traditional commission to "sink, burn and destroy." In 1863
Congress authorized the issuance of letters of marque, but the
power was not to be used unless the Confederates should be
successful in commissioning privateers in European ports. Indeed, these privateers commissioned in southern ports were the
last the world has seen. No privateers were used in the Spanish-
American or in either World War, and the Constitutional provision for the issuance of letters of marque and reprisal has
become, for all practical purposes, a dead letter.

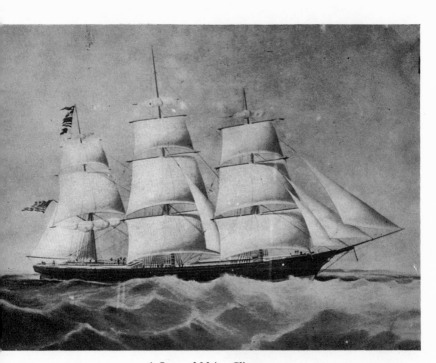

A State of Maine Clipper
he *Red Jacket*, built in 1853 by George
Thomas at Rockland.

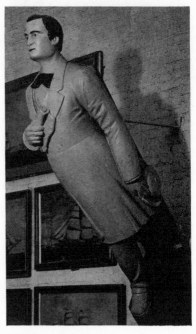

igurehead from the ship *George R. Skolfield*,
uilt at Brunswick, 1885. Carved by Emery
ones. *Courtesy The Mariners' Museum, New-
ort News, Va.*

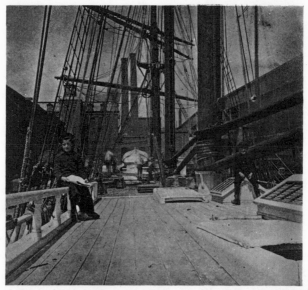

Deck view of the barkentine *Clara E. McGilvery*. The boy and girl are Lincoln and Joanna, the children of Lincoln A. Colcord, her master. *Courtesy Penobscot Marine Museum.*

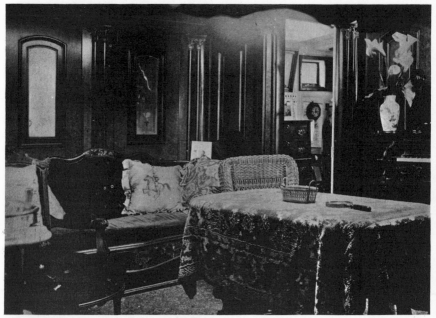

The bark *Guy C. Goss*. The starboard side of the main cabin is shown. The captain's stateroom is to be seen through the door. The finish was of bird's-eye maple, satinwood, and mahogany, and the capitals of the pilasters were in gold leaf. *Courtesy Penobscot Marine Museum.*

The Confederate Commerce Raiders

The brig *Jeff Davis* was the boldest of the Confederate privateers. She had formerly been a notorious slaver, the *Echo*, which had been captured and condemned in 1858. Fitted out by the city of Charleston, she sailed the last week in June. Before she was wrecked on the Florida coast six weeks later, she is estimated to have taken northern vessels to the value of $225,000. Off Nantucket on the ninth of July she overhauled the ship *Mary Goodell* of Searsport. The *Goodell* drew eighteen feet of water, and it was out of the question to get her over the bars into any southern port. So taking six seamen, provisions, and water out of her, she was released after putting aboard twelve prisoners. Shorthanded and unable to continue her voyage, the *Goodell* put into Portland, where she refitted. This ninth of June was an unlucky day for Searsport, as the *Davis* found a second prize from that town. The brig *Mary E. Thompson* was stripped of provisions and supplies, another group of prisoners was transferred, and she made her way into Newport, Rhode Island.

The *Jeff Davis* was now within a hundred miles of Nantucket Shoals. Great excitement prevailed in the New England ports. Fleets of revenue cutters, cruisers, and gunboats were sent out from Boston and New York in search of her. The *Davis* turned southward and escaped. Before she was wrecked attempting to cross St. Augustine bar, she added four more Maine vessels to her list—the brig *William McGilvery* of Prospect, the schooner *Windward* of Stockton, the brig *Santa Clara* of Eastport, and the ship *John Carver* of Bath.

The *B. T. Martin* of Bristol, the largest full-rigged brig out of Boston, was captured by the privateer *York* on the twenty-third of July off Cape Hatteras. The *Martin* attempted to run away, but the *York* outsailed her, put aboard a prize crew and then attempted to run her in. As she was running down the coast to reach Hatteras Inlet she was sighted by the U.S.S.

Savannah. To avoid capture the crew ran her ashore. As she lay aground she was shelled by the U.S.S. *Union* and destroyed. The same day the *Dixie*, a privateer out of Charleston, took the bark *Glen* of Freeport laden with coal for Fort Jefferson on the Tortugas. The old *Glen* ended her life in flames. The schooner *Mary Alice* of Machias and the brig *Itaska* of Bangor were taken by the privateer *Winslow* about the first of August.

The last of the privateers of 1861 was the brig *Sallie*, which ran the blockade out of Charleston on the tenth of October. In twenty days she took, among others, four Maine brigs, the *Grenada*, built at Cape Elizabeth, the *Betsey Ames* of Wells, the *Elsinore* of Bangor, and the *B. K. Eaton* of Searsport. The name of the *Betsey Ames* was changed to *Lolla* and she was pressed into service as a blockade runner. She was captured as she attempted to run the blockade by the U.S.S. *Quaker City*. Taken to Boston, she was recognized by her owners, although she had been altered from a half- to a full-rigged brig.

Other privateers appeared during the war, but their careers were short. Among these was the *Retribution*, a schooner fitted out in Cape Fear River, which cruised along the coast of Cuba, taking and destroying the Bucksport brig *J. P. Ellicott* and the Pembroke-built bark *Emily Fisher*. The crew of the *Ellicott* performed an exploit reminiscent of the days of the Napoleonic wars. They retook the bark from her captors and successfully navigated her to her port of destination.

Early in the war the Confederate government initiated a program which was to have dire results on northern and Maine shipping. In addition to the issuance of letters of marque to the privately owned vessels traditionally known as privateers, there were commissioned regularly armed naval vessels, procured for the most part in England. The first of these Confederate cruisers was the *Sumter*. She was a 500-ton steamer which had previously plied between Havana and New Orleans. She was fitted out in May 1861 and placed under the command of Captain Raphael Semmes.

Semmes was a romantic and colorful figure. Born in Maryland, he had received his training as a naval officer in the old navy before the establishment of Annapolis, when officers trained as midshipmen at sea. He had seen active service in the Mexican War. In the course of his career, he had acquired some knowledge of the law. These acquisitions were coupled with a vivid imagination and an undoubted gift with the pen. The result is a curious rendition of his experiences as one of the world's most efficient commerce raiders which is a blend of vituperation, legal controversy, and scientific discussion, interspersed with truly remarkable pen pictures of the sailing ships of the day and their destruction in flames.

The *Sumter* evaded the blockading fleet at the mouth of the Mississippi on the last day of July. During her six months' cruise, she took fifteen prizes. Nine of these were Maine vessels. Fifteen miles off the Isle of Pines, on the third of July, she found her first victim. This was the Bangor ship *Golden Rocket*, a fine craft off the ways in Brewer three years before and, according to the statement of her owners, worth $51,000. Unarmed, unsuspecting, and taken in by Semmes' utilization of the traditional trick of displaying English colors at his cruiser's peak, the *Rocket* was easily taken. In his career of destruction, Semmes was to apply the torch to many a goodly merchantman and leave in his wake many a flaming hull. The burning of this, his first capture, stirred him deeply. In his account, he exults that she hailed from the "Black Republican, Yankee State of Maine." Then he goes on:

> Suddenly, one of the crew exclaimed, "There is the flame! She is on fire!" The decks of this Maine-built ship were of pine, calked with old-fashioned oakum, and paid with pitch; the woodwork of the cabin was like so much tinder, having

been seasoned by many voyages to the tropics, and the fore-castle was stowed with paints and oils. The consequence was, that the flame was not long in kindling, but leaped, full-grown, into the air, in a very few minutes after its first glimmer had been seen. The boarding officer, to do his work more effectually, had applied the torch simultaneously in three places, the cabin, the mainhold, and the forecastle; and now the devouring flames rushed up these three apertures, with a fury which nothing could resist.

The burning ship with the *Sumter's* boat in the act of shoving off from her side; the *Sumter* herself, with her grim, black sides, lying in repose like some great sea monster, gloating upon the spectacle, and the sleeping sea, for there was scarcely a ripple upon the water, were all brilliantly lighted. The indraught into the burning ship's holds, and cabins, added every moment new fury to the flames, and now they could be heard roaring like the fires of a hundred furnaces, in full blast. The prize ship had been laid to, with her main topsail to the mast, and all her light sails, though clewed up, were flying loose about the yards.

The forked tongues of the devouring element, leaping into the rigging, newly tarred, ran rapidly up the shrouds, first into the tops, then to the topmast-heads, thence to the top-gallant, and royal mast-heads, and in a moment more to the trucks; and whilst this rapid ascent of the main current of fire was going on, other currents had run out upon the yards and ignited all the sails. A top-gallant sail, all on fire, would now fly off from the yard, and sailing leisurely in the direction of the light breeze that was fanning rather than blowing, break into bright, and sparkling patches of flame, and settle, or rather silt into the sea. The yard would then follow, and not being wholly submerged by its descent into the sea, would retain a portion of its flame, and continue to burn, as a floating brand for some minutes.

At one time, the intricate net-work of the cordage of the burning ship was traced, as with a pencil of fire, upon the black sky beyond, the many threads of flame twisting and writhing, like so many serpents that had received their death wounds. The mizzen-mast now went by the board, then the foremast, and in a few minutes afterward, the great main-mast tottered, reeled, and fell over the ship's side into the sea, making a noise like that of the sturdy oak of the forests when it falls by the stroke of the axeman.

By the light of this flambeau, upon the lonely and silent sea, lighted of the passions of bad men who should have been our brothers, the *Sumter*, having aroused herself from her dream of vengeance, and run up her boats, moved forward on her course.

By the light of the burning ship the *Sumter* moved on in search of other prey. The next day she came up with two brigantines, the *Cuba* of Millbridge and the *Machias* of Machias, bound from Trinidad to London laden with molasses and sugar. Taking them in tow she headed for Cienfuegos. On the way the *Cuba* parted her hawser and a prize crew was put aboard. A few days later the original officers and crew, who had remained aboard, were able to overpower them and bring the brigantine safely into New York. When the *Sumter* arrived off Cienfuegos it was too late to enter the harbor, and the *Machias* was ordered to lay to until morning. The *Sumter* went off in pursuit of two brigs which had just come out. They were speedily taken and proved to be the Falmouth-built *Ben Dunning* and the *Albert Ames* of Dennysville. In the morning, with three more prizes, and guided by the same pilot who had brought out the *Dunning* and *Ames*, the *Sumter* steamed into the harbor. It was Semmes' intention to test the attitude of the Spanish government toward the Confederacy. He found that despite his legal arguments Spain did not intend to lose her best customer by favoring the South. The general in command ordered all the prizes restored to their owners.

It was September before another Maine vessel was taken. This time it was the brig *Joseph Park*, built at Stockton and known among seamen as "Captain Park's yacht." On her were newspapers telling of the battle of Manassas Junction, the first Bull Run. The merriment of the *Sumter*'s crew was heightened by Captain Brigg's entry on the first day's log. "We have a tight, fast vessel and we don't care for Jeff Davis." The brig was burned. This was also the fate of the schooner *Arcade* of Hampden, taken on the twenty-sixth of November. Her master, Captain Alexander P. Smith, had a handsome telescope which had been presented to him for gallant work saving lives at sea. In a gracious gesture it was returned to him by Captain Semmes. Two more Maine vessels, the ship *Montmorency* of Bath and the *Investigator*, built at Searsport, were searched. But since their cargoes were neutral they were released on a ransom bond. In January 1862, the *Sumter* reached Gibraltar. Here she was laid up and finally sold.

At this time a vessel then known only as "No. 290" was being built for the Confederate service at the Lairds' yard in Birkenhead, opposite Liverpool. On the twenty-eighth of July, 1862, she slipped out of the Mersey headed for the Azores. There, after receiving her armament, which was shipped to the Azores in two British ships, and her crew, largely British, and stores, she was put into commission by Raphael Semmes. Directly she made prizes of twelve of the whaling fleet off Fayal.

Early in October the *Alabama* was on the Newfoundland Banks in the direct path of the grain ships from the eastern ports to Europe. Here, in a little over two weeks, sixteen captures were made. The first vessel from Maine to be taken was the bark *Lamplighter*, built at Calais, which was burned on the fifteenth. She was loaded with tobacco for Gibraltar and represented a loss of $117,600. As she plunged in flames head foremost to the bottom a savory cloud lingered over the sea. This, Semmes wrote later, "almost made her destroyers regret their work."

For eight days the *Alabama* was out of luck, tempest-tossed and without a prize. On the afternoon of the twenty-first the cry of "Sail ho!" came from the lookout. A large ship was sighted running under a press of canvas "cracking on" with her royals and fore topmast studding sails set in a wind that was blowing half a gale. Dashing along before the wind, she soon came directly across the path of the *Alabama*. A shot across her bow and all was changed.

> Sheets and halyards were let go by the run and the huge cloud of canvas seemed to shrink and shrivel up as the vessel was rounded to with folded wings like a crippled bird.

The ship proved to be the *Lafayette*, one of the finest from the Soule yard in Freeport. She was bound from New York to Belfast with grain. Though her cargo was certified as being the property of neutrals and was covered with British consular seals, which hitherto had been respected, Semmes raised the question of her neutrality. "The prize court of the Confederacy now sat in Semmes' cabin and all questions of law or fact were settled by the captain's decision."

On board the *Lafayette* had been found New York papers in which his recent acts had been condemned as piracy. This may have influenced him to give some show of legality to his decision. He took until ten that night to decide. In his journal he wrote out in detail the grounds of his decision. This custom he continued throughout his career. The end result was the same. A boat was sent to the ship to bring off the personal effects of the crew. Then the mattresses were pulled from the bunks, soaked in oil, and fired. Captain Semmes, realizing from the newspapers which had been found that his location was known, turned the prow of the *Alabama* southward. At midnight the *Lafayette*—the beautiful white bird of the afternoon—was but a dim glare on the distant horizon.

Five days later the bark *Loretta* of Damariscotta was overhauled and burned in the latitude of New York. Her crew was allowed only ten minutes in which to abandon ship. The following day the *Baron de Castine* of Castine, on her way from Bangor to Cardenas with lumber, was seized. Since she was old and of little value, Semmes released her on a ransom bond and sent her into New York as a cartel with forty-five prisoners whom he had taken from the *Lafayette, Loretta,* and *Cranshaw.*

The *Alabama* took no more Maine vessels until the next year. After coaling and refitting in Kingston, Jamaica, she ran north to where the vessels coming from the East Indies or the Pacific would cross the thirtieth parallel. Semmes hoped to reap a rich harvest where these trade routes met. Here on the twenty-seventh of February he detained the Pittston-built ship *Washington* and the *Bethia Thayer* of Thomaston. Since their cargoes of guano belonged to the Peruvian government, they were bonded and released. No plea to neutrality could be set up for the cargo of white pine lumber in the ship *John A. Parks* of Hallowell for Montevideo, and she was burned.

Semmes now sailed south to cruise the Brazilian coast. Just after crossing the line he took the Rockland ship *Louisa Hatch.* She was laden with Cardiff coal. This was an invaluable find for the *Alabama,* and the cargo was promptly seized and condemned. An attempt was made to transfer the coal at sea, but it proved impracticable and the *Hatch* was towed to Fernando de Noronha. At this island, "in the wayside of the commerce of the world, sighted by more ships and visited by fewer than any spot on earth," the precious fuel was filled into the *Alabama's* bunkers. The *Hatch* was then taken to sea and burned. Her crew were left on the island, from which, after a stay of ten days, they made a rough and stormy trip in an open boat to Pernambuco.

On the twenty-sixth of April the *Dorcas Prince,* built at Yarmouth, but owned by the Griswolds of New York, was burned with her cargo of coal intended for the United States ships of war in the East Indies. On May second the *Sea Lark*, built at Trescott, met a similar fate. Her value, including cargo, was estimated at $550,000. A letter was found aboard which read, "We hope you will arrive safely and in good season, but we think you will find business rather flat in Liverpool as American ships are under a cloud, owing to dangers from pirates, more politely styled privateers which our kind friends in England are willing should slip out of their ports to prey upon our commerce."

The word "pirate" was a red flag to Semmes. The members of the *Sea Lark's* crew were treated with unusual severity, being thrown into irons and landed in Bahia nine days later in a destitute state. The ship, *Jabez Snow* of Bucksport, was taken on the twenty-ninth of May, and four days later the Damariscotta-built ship *Talisman*, one of the Maine-built clippers. On the day before the Fourth of July, just as the *Alabama* turned eastward to the Cape of Good Hope, the ship *Anna T. Schmitt* met the usual fate. At the Cape, Semmes boarded the bark *Martha Wenzel*, built at East Deering, but finding her within the three-mile limit he was obliged to give her up.

Thence the cruise across the Indian Ocean to the Straits of Sunda, over the China Sea and returning by way of Singapore, the Malabar Coast, and the Mozambique Channel was disappointing. Although a few had very narrow escapes, only one Maine vessel, the ship *Emma Jane* of Bath, was taken. She was burned and the crew put ashore at a small town seventy-five miles south of Cochin. They reached there in native boats and came home by way of Bombay. Rounding the Cape to the westward, the *Alabama* finally entered the port of Cherbourg, France, on June 11, 1864.

At this time the *Kearsarge* was in the near-by port of Flushing. She was a State of Maine product, having been built at the Kittery Navy Yard. Within a few days she stood off Cherbourg. A challenge was sent and accepted. On Sunday, the twenty-first of June, 1864, the *Alabama's* career of destruction came to an end. She was sunk by the guns of the *Kearsarge*.

Hers was a remarkable cruise of commerce raiding. In twenty-two months 386 vessels had been boarded. Semmes took 2,000 prisoners. Out of 71 northern ships he made 6 into cartels, bonded 10, made a tender of 1, sold 1, and sank 1. To the remaining 52 he applied the torch. And of these, 11 were State of Maine vessels. Nor was this all of the destruction by the Confederate cruisers. Some idea of the large-scale damage to the shipping interest of the nation may be had from an examination of their other depredations among Maine fleets. It makes an imposing catalogue of disaster.

The *Tallahassee* was a captured blockade runner which was refitted as a cruiser. She took the following Maine vessels:

James Littlefield, ship—Brewer
Glenavon, bark—Thomaston
P. C. Alexander, bark—Harpswell
A. Richards, brig—Columbia Falls
Atlantic, brig—Machiasport
Carrie Estelle, brig—Cutler
Billow, brig—Gardiner
Carroll, schooner—Machias
Spokane, schooner—Tremont
Restless, schooner—Boothbay
Etta Carolina, schooner—South Bristol
Magnolia, schooner—Friendship
Pearl, schooner—Friendship
Josiah Achorn, schooner—Rockland
Roan, schooner—Harrington
A. J. Bird, schooner—Rockland
E. F. Lewis, schooner—Portland

The Confederate Commerce Raiders

The *Chickamauga* was also a captured blockade runner refitted as a cruiser. Her trophies were but two:

> *Mark L. Potter,* bark—Brewer
> *Emma L. Hall,*　　—Millbridge

The regular armed cruiser *Georgia* ran out of Dunbarton, Scotland. She accounted for:

> *Dictator,* ship—Robbinston
> *Constitution,* ship—Bath

The regular armed cruiser *Shenandoah* operating from Melbourne, Australia, took:

> *Alina,* bark—Searsport
> *Delphine,* bark—Bangor

The *Florida,* also a regular armed cruiser, sallied forth from Liverpool in March 1862. Her toll in Maine vessels comprised:

> *Estelle,* bark—Millbridge
> *M. J. Colcord,* bark—Prospect
> *Greenland,* bark—Brunswick
> *Anglo Saxon,* bark—Rockland
> *Corris Ann,* brig—Machiasport

In almost every instance the tale was the same. The fleeing vessel was brought to with a shot, her people were taken out, and the torch was applied. In the case of the bark *Delphine,* taken in the middle of the Indian Ocean, the wife of Captain William G. Nichols of Searsport demonstrated the stuff of which Maine seafaring women are made. With perfect self-possession she directed the transfer of herself, her six-year-old son, and the steward's wife from the *Delphine* to the deck of the *Shenandoah* in a bos'n's chair on a whip from the yard arm. Nor did she forget to bring along her canary bird in its cage.

The cruise of the *Florida* in the spring of 1863 had an interesting sequel in Casco Bay. On May 6 she took the Baltimore brig *Clarence*. With a crew of twenty men and armed with a single howitzer, she was sent north under Lieut. Charles W. Read on a roving commission. Off Hatteras she took the Blue Hill-built bark *Whistling Wind*, and several days later she was off Mt. Desert Rock. Here Read took the bark *Tacony*, and since she was a faster vessel than the *Clarence*, he transferred his flag to her. With the *Tacony* he made ten prizes. The last of these was the Southport fishing schooner *Archer*, taken off Cape Sable. He converted her into a cruiser and burned the *Tacony*.

Lieutenant Read's orders were to run into seaport towns and cities with little defense, burn the shipping in the harbor, destroy the building yards, and work all the havoc possible. He had knowledge that two "double ended gun boats" had just been completed in Portland, and he hoped that he might be able to cut out either the New York or the Boston steamer. Therefore he stood westward toward this harbor. On the morning of June 26 two Falmouth fishermen, Albert Bibber and Elbridge Titcomb, were in their fishing sloop the *Village* hauling their trawls about eight miles off Damariscove Island. They were hailed by what appeared to be another fishing schooner and asked for news. Thinking the *Archer* had on board a crew of drunken fishermen on a frolic, they talked freely and piloted the schooner into Portland harbor. She came to anchor at sunset near Pomeroy's Rock off Fish Point.

It had been Read's intention to seize the New York steamer *Chesapeake* and the revenue cutter *Caleb Cushing*, which was lying in the harbor preparatory to going out in search of the *Tacony*. Being doubtful of his ability to get the steamer out of the harbor, he abandoned this project. He concentrated on a plan to cut out the *Caleb Cushing*. After getting from under the forts he meant to return and burn the shipping. Chance aided the Confederates. The commander of the cutter had just died, and many of the men were ashore for the funeral. Only a lieutenant and twenty men were aboard. They were quickly overpowered and imprisoned in the hold. The wind being light and the tide running in, the cutter and schooner were towed from the harbor, passing out by Hussey's Sound. It was half-past seven the next morning before the *Cushing* was discovered to be missing.

Two men of character and force, Captain Jacob McLellan, mayor of Portland, and Jedediah Jewett, the collector of the port, organized the pursuit. The Boston and New York steamers were fitted out and were soon under way, accompanied by the tug *Tiger* and other small steamers. In the light air the cutter and the schooner could not escape. Surrounded by their pursuers, a few ineffective shots were exchanged. The *Cushing* was set on fire and blew up.

★　★　★

Apart from privateers and refitted blockade runners, all of the Confederate cruisers except the *Sumter*—the *Alabama, Florida, Georgia* and *Shenandoah*—had come, it will be noticed, out of British ports. This state of affairs, and particularly the circumstances under which the *Alabama* got to sea, produced a result which forms a concluding note to the depredations of these commerce raiders.

Early in the struggle English neutrality had been proclaimed. In May 1862 a vessel which had been built at Lairds and was obviously intended as a man-of-war was launched. In late June, Charles Francis Adams, the American minister, warned the proper authorities that No. 290 was intended for use against the United States and asked that she be detained.

Some proof was demanded. He supplied the proof. The

papers were shunted from one office to another. On July 29, the law officers having given their opinion that the vessel should be detained, such an order was issued. It came too late. There were Confederate ears close to the ground, and the bird had flown the day before.

Adams pressed the issue, and in 1871 a treaty was made whereby the matter was to be submitted to arbitration. An impartial international commission found that in the cases of the *Alabama*, the *Florida*, and the *Shenandoah*, the proper officers had been lacking in diligence. An award of $15,500,000 was made. To the Maine coast the business was reminiscent of the French spoliation claims—with this difference: the *Alabama* claims were paid.

CHAPTER ELEVEN

The DOWN-EASTERS

The part of the Maine shipbuilders and designers in the history of American sailing ships has never received full recognition. The so-called "down-easters" that followed the clipper were almost wholly the work of these men. *Some of these vessels were, without doubt, the highest development of the sailing ship;* combining speed, handiness, cargo-capacity and low operating costs to a degree never obtained in any earlier square rigger.—Howard I. Chapelle, *The History of American Sailing Ships.*[1]

One by one the few remaining sailing ships are disappearing. They drop away, and are heard of no more. With them goes much that is worthy and incalculable. It passes like a high squall sinking beyond the horizon, wind and sea, motion and color, romance and inspiration, a whole range of human endeavor, all vanishing to leeward with the tall ship in their midst. . . . The sailing ship stood for a sociological achievement of the highest order. She stood for a means whereby men were brought to their fullest development. She stood for a profession which only merit could indure. She stood for real efficiency of spirit and character. She stood for things the world cannot afford to lose.—Lincoln Colcord, Introduction to *Songs of American Sailormen.*[2]

A WORD ABOUT this phrase "down east." It is as pure American as apple pie. Beyond the confines of New England the benighted user of the phrase has reference to New England. He is wrong. In Connecticut, in response to a query, the thumb will be jerked over the left shoulder toward Massachusetts. In Boston

[1] W. W. Norton & Company, Inc., 1935.
[2] W. W. Norton & Company, Inc., 1938.

it means Maine. But in Maine it is always a bit farther off. If you are in Casco Bay, Penobscot Bay is down east and Eastport and the maritime provinces are away down east. Thus one's arrival in this never-never land is always postponed. This usage has been traced in print to as early as the 1820's. To it there is an important exception.

In the maritime world of two generations ago "down-easter" was a term of fixed and no uncertain meaning. It conveyed a picture par excellence of a full-rigged wooden ship or a bark with her canvas spread in the wind, designed, built and launched in a shipyard on the coast of Maine, and more often than not commanded by a Maine captain.

The down-easter and the clipper, besides their points of contrast, have much in common. It was California gold which had heightened the demand for the clippers. Now it was the California wheat which called forth the down-easter. The career of the beautiful but expensive clipper, like the gold rush, was short and romantic. The clipper ship era lasted but thirteen years—from 1846 to 1859. That of the down-easter extended the era of the wooden ship by at least a quarter century. The maritime history of Massachusetts flowered with the clippers; to Maine there came the Indian summer of the down-easter.

Once the discovery had been made that the sun-drenched valleys of California could produce wheat so hard and dry that it would stand the 14,000-mile voyage around the Horn and arrive in the European ports in prime condition, the development of her agriculture was phenomenal. Its mathematics, if not its romance, rivaled the gold rush of forty-nine. In 1860 but 1,087 tons of wheat and 58,926 barrels of flour had been exported from San Francisco. Ten years later these figures had risen to 243,199 tons of grain and 352,969 barrels of flour. The rapidity of this growth may be gauged from the fact that while in 1865 the value of the grain exported amounted to $1,750,494, it had

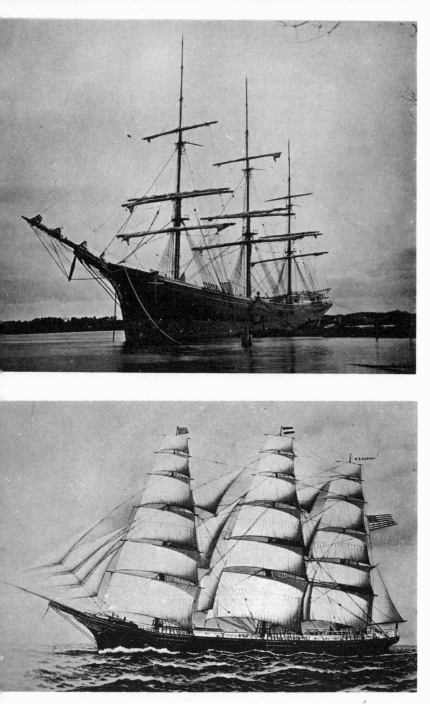

The Down-Easters

The *Henry B. Hyde*, Bath, 1884 (above). *Courtesy Smithsonian Institution.*
The *E. B. Sutton*, Bath, 1881 (below). *Courtesy Peabody Museum of Salem.*

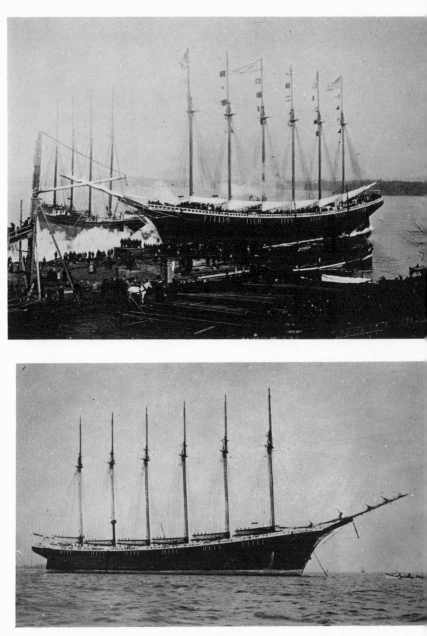

The Great Schooners

The ways smoke as a six-master is launched (above). *Courtesy Howard I. Chapelle.*
The schooner *Wyoming*, 3,730 tons, Bath, 1909, the largest wooden fore-and-after
ever built (below). *Courtesy Howard I. Chapelle.*

increased *the next year* to $6,717,825. This was nearly 400 per cent! In the bumper harvest of 1882, 559 ships carried out 1,128,031 tons of wheat and barley and 919,898 barrels of flour. By this time wheat raising had spread all over the North Pacific coast from San Pedro in the south to Vancouver in the north. As one enthusiastic chronicler has remarked: "The bay and water front of San Francisco, the forest shaded waters of Puget Sound and the tideway of the Columbia River were crowded with magnificent sailing ships loading the golden grain."

This, then, was the trade that, just after the disastrous years of the Civil War, opened a new and perhaps the most important chapter in the history of the Maine-built wooden ship. The center of wooden shipbuilding had moved away from New York. During the next two decades Maine was almost without a rival. The voyage from San Francisco to the ports of Europe was one of the longest and most trying known to sea-borne commerce. Also a cargo of grain is a severe test of the strength and endurance of a sailing vessel. Maine builders met this challenge. Out of their century and more of experience and skill they developed the down-easter. Probably no vessels were ever turned out in America, if we except the clippers of Donald McKay, that are more alive in people's imagination and are pointed to with more pride by the descendants of their builders. Spurred to their best by pride and competition, stung by the discrimination of the English Lloyd's against the wooden ship, and backed by years of study and experience, the builders made the product of the yards, particularly from 1875 to 1883, the pride of Maine.

There was the *A. J. Fuller*, with a main yard ninety feet long and spreading twenty-five "kites" to the wind. She was owned by the Flints of Bath and planned by their famous builder, John McDonald. There was the handsome three-sky-sail-yarder, *Tacoma* of Goss and Sawyer, William Roger's beautiful *Abner Coburn*, and McDonald's masterpiece, the *Henry B. Hyde*. She is generally acknowledged to be the finest three-masted sailing ship built under the Stars and Stripes since the clippers, and her only rival is the *A. G. Ropes* of T. F. Chapman. In 1883 Goss and Sawyer put afloat the *Benjamin F. Packard*, which, being exceedingly well built, outlasted her contemporaries. She was long hailed by the emotional as "the last of the clippers." Phippsburg and the yards of C. V. Minot contributed three worthy representatives to the fleet—the *James Drummond*, built in 1880, the *Berlin* in 1882, and the fine top-gallant-yarder *St. Charles* the following year. The *Drummond* made a passage from New York to Astoria in 105 days, which gave her an enviable reputation for speed. T. J. Southard closed his long career and also the building of ships at Richmond when he launched the *Commodore T. H. Allen*, 2,271 tons, in the spring of 1884.

There were many yards up and down the coast from which the down-easters were launched. It was no uncertain compliment to the skill of Eben Haggett of Damariscotta as a builder that he was chosen by a company of Searsport captains to build the *Elizabeth*. This ship and also his *State of Maine* and *Josephus* were fine examples of this class.

It was a staunch fleet of down-easters which made the port of Thomaston a well-known hail at this time. They came from the yards of Samuel Watts and Edward O'Brien. It is claimed that Thomaston at one time had 100 deep-sea captains. Of these, 25 bore the name of Watts and many were masters of Captain Samuel's 31 full-rigged ships which were notable as large carriers. They also made remarkable passages for such full-bodied models. Particular attention was given to furnishing comfortable quarters for the officers and crew.

Edward O'Brien was of the type typical. After 1858 he owned every timberhead in his vessels, his last ship being the only exception, for he gave a sixteenth of her to an intimate friend. He frequently owned the cargoes they carried, and for years he was his own insurer. His ships were strong and staunch —good, solidly built freight carriers, lightly sparred but of large tonnage capacity. They were known as soon as sighted on every ocean by their old-fashioned high line, destitute of paint but well scraped and varnished, which ran from stem to stern six planks below the deck line. Many were built of white oak. He is said to have been among the first of the Maine builders to use this timber, which he cut from his own tract in Virginia. For years his efficient master builder was Herman Beriner. At the time of his death he owned over 20,000 tons of shipping and had on the stocks the third *Edward O'Brien*—the "big Edward."

Some unusual vessels of this period came from the yards of the Carleton Norwood Company in Rockport. In September 1877 they launched the ship *Wandering Jew*. Her distinguishing feature was a flush deck with neither poop nor quarter deck, there being but one other similar full-rigged vessel in the United States. Her passage from Hong Kong to San Francisco in 33 days has been equaled but never beaten. The *Robert I. Belknap*, built in 1884, was conspicuous because of her three sets of top-gallant and three skysail yards. It is said that no other American ship was so rigged. In 1885 they put afloat their largest square-rigger—she was the Penobscot's largest as well—the *Frederick Billings* of 2,497 tons. She followed Donald McKay's *Great Republic* and Nathaniel Thompson's *Ocean King* as the third four-masted ship to be built in this country. She was literally a tall ship with her main truck 180 feet above deck.

Up at the head of Penobscot Bay is another town—Searsport —which is famed for its association with Cape Horners and blue-water captains. Here at the head of the harbor Captain William McGilvery with his master builder Marlboro Packard set afloat some of the finest examples of the down-eastern fleet, notably the *Oneida*, *John C. Potter*, *William McGilvery*, *Clara E. Mc-Gilvery*, and the *Premier*. The largest vessel launched at Searsport, the *William H. Conner* of 1,496 tons, came in 1877 from the neighboring Carver yard. In the same year up the river at Brewer, which long had close association with Searsport, the 1,393-ton *Llewellyn J. Morse* began her fifty years of adventurous life at the Oakes yard. She did duty as a Cape Horner, Pacific trader, salmon packer, and in 1925 as a member of the "Motion Picture Fleet." With her bulwarks pierced for wooden cannon and piles of wooden balls on her decks, she was the *Constitution* in the picture *Old Ironsides*.

The launch of such a vessel was a great event. In September 1878, the Cushing and Briggs yard in Freeport put afloat the *John A. Briggs*. This launching of Freeport's largest ship was a red-letter day. As great a number of people gathered to see her floated as ever witnessed a launch in Casco Bay. From the surrounding countryside they came in all manner of conveyances, from carriages to oxcarts. The Maine Central Railroad ran a special train, and two or three island steamers brought crowds from Portland and the Foresides, while the river was white with sailboats from Harpswell, Brunswick, and the Islands. The papers estimated that over seven thousand people were present. The governor of the state, Alonzo Garcelon, was there—also James A. Garfield, who was scheduled for a campaign speech in Yarmouth later in the day. Never having seen a launch, he drove over to see the *Briggs* take the water.

★   ★   ★

In appearance the down-easters resembled the full clippers of the fifties but more nearly, it has been remarked, the last and sharp-modeled packets. Their lines were neither as sharp nor as hollow as the clippers, while to increase their cargo capacity they had little dead rise. The term "dead rise" connotes the angle at which the bottom rises outboard from the keel and means specifically the rise given in inches for each foot from the keel. Hence the down-easter, as compared with the clipper, had a flatter floor. The trim lines of the plain bows and counters of the clippers were retained. This eye-appealing contour was accentuated by running the bowsprit into the sheer (that is, the upward curving line of the deck) instead of on top of it.

Sturdiness of frame was a major requisite. White-oak ribs with planking and ceiling of thick pitch-pine plank produced an almost solid hull, often 16 to 20 inches thick. Keel and keel-sons were massive sticks of pitch pine. On the *John Rosenfeld*, built by the Sewalls in 1884, these formed 12 feet of solid timber. Knees of native hackmatack braced the deck beams, and copper or yellow metal bolts were used to fasten her throughout, save in some cases where iron was used above the ballast load line. Some hulls were further strengthened by being braced diagonally with iron straps.

On deck the white-painted houses gave excellent accommodations for crew and officers. The forward house contained, besides the crew's quarters, the carpenter's shop and galley. Aft was the captain's cabin with a dining saloon flanked on either side by staterooms. Here also were the captain's bathroom, steward's pantry, chartroom, and storeroom. Farther aft was the large wheelhouse. Here in the forward part were the wheel, compasses, bell, and log line, while the after part contained the massive rudder head and tiller and the pigeonhole case for the signal flags, life buoys, foghorn, and so forth. Carvel-built long boats rested on top of the houses, lashed to their skids, while whaleboats of beautiful workmanship hung from the davits on either quarter.

Aloft these ships were not so heavily sparred as the clippers, but they could spread plenty of canvas to give them speed. The masts, generally of wood, were built up of three pitch-pine logs rounded and banded with six iron hoops painted black, white, or red. Many had three skysails and a few crossed double top-gallant yards, while one or two boasted a moon sail—the only sails higher than the skysails. Studding sails had all but disappeared with the clippers, and Sewall's *Indiana* was the only Maine ship that carried "stunsail" booms in the nineties. With the flowing lines of her hull accentuated with black paint and little or no ornamentation, her masts and spars of natural wood scraped, varnished, and squared as with a tape line, her deck houses of shining white and the deck holystoned and oiled so as to equal them in whiteness, and without a line out of place from stem to stern, no yacht was ever neater and more ship-shape than a State of Maine down-easter in her prime. These are the great ships that live on the canvases of Charles R. Patterson and other famous marine painters.

To keep such a ship sailing and shining required a captain and mates who could enforce such a fierce discipline that for the crew a voyage with them would be far from a summer holiday. This called for the stronger and not always the loveliest traits of character in an officer. There is no doubt that the stories which abound in sea fiction of "bully" captains and "bucko" mates who had little regard for the lives and limbs of the crews are not all exaggeration. "Belaying pin soup" and "knuckle dusters" played their part in the navigation of these big ships. Of the crew Basil Lubbock has written:

> It was always easy to tell an old Cape Horner by his wonderful aptitude in ship cleaning, in the use of sand and canvas, holystones, bible and prayer books and other back-breaking instruments of toil such as the deck bear, though he was often an indifferent marlin-spike seaman.

It was an accepted principle that to maintain such discipline and carry on the ship's work an officer had to be rough, strong, and "able to lick his weight in wildcats." It is not to be wondered at that with the almost unlimited power they had over their men while the ship was at sea some went too far, gave a good ship a bad name, and furnished a lurid tale for the pages of the Red Record. These highly colored stories may be matched with many that did not receive such great publicity. There is the case of the *Frank Pendleton*. When the crew went over the side in port, they lined up on the wharf and gave three rousing cheers for the ship, three for Captain William Green Nichols, and three more for the officers. Lubbock's conclusion is well put, that the Maine officer "was no Nancy and was far from suffering fools gladly, neither would he put up with the incompetent nor the slacker but was a prime sailorman whose equal it would be hard to find."

Since the earlier days great changes had taken place in the make-up of the crews. The old law of 1817 which required that two-thirds of the crew of an American vessel should be American citizens had long been a dead letter. Few Americans could have been found in the forecastles of either the clippers or the down-easters. For the Yankee lad who had the nerve and the pluck to begin at the bottom and work his way up, his rise was rapid. For various reasons this career had ceased to be attractive, and masters were forced to have recourse to shipping agencies and boardinghouse keepers to fill up their crew lists. With this system of crimping and shanghaiing the percentage of foreigners and incompetents increased.

The complement of the *A. G. Ropes* is a fair illustration of the make-up of such a crew. Of the thirty-four souls aboard only the family of Captain Rivers, the mate, and the sailmaker were American. The second mate was a Swede, the third mate Scotch, the boatswain Irish, and the carpenter Danish. The steward was a German and the cook Irish. The balance of the list was of all sorts, including even a Maltese. Of the seventeen so-called able-bodied seamen, but four could do a job of rigging.

When Captain M. A. Woodside had command of the *Charles E. Moody,* he had with him eight white sailors and fifteen Japanese. Very queer specimens were often brought aboard by the crimps. Three of the crew furnished the *St. Stephen* at San Francisco in 1877 were cowboys who had never seen salt water until the week before. The Bath ship *St. Paul* had a Baptist minister turned over to her, and the *Henry B. Hyde* once found herself outside New York with a crew of Bowery pugilists and roughs. There was not a single sailor among them.

If Maine was not supreme in the forecastles of the down-easters, she most certainly was in their cabins. Figures are not available for the total number of Maine shipmasters of this period, but one town, Searsport, in 1889 had 77. It is estimated that these men comprised 10 per cent of all the masters of American sailing ships. Of these, 33 commanded Cape Horners. As has been noted, Thomaston, it is claimed, was the "home of a hundred captains," 25 of whom belonged to one family. Many tales of these ship captains have been preserved which reveal their qualities of leadership, their resourceful skill, and their intimate knowledge of men and the sea.

When the *May Flint* ran into a cyclone and had her fore and main topmasts and her mizzen topgallant mast carried away, Captain E. D. P. Nickels of Searsport declined all offers of assistance. After a strenuous two weeks in 'mid-ocean, he repaired and refitted his spars and was able to work his ship home to New York under its own sail. Of similar tenor was the achievement of Captain William H. Blanchard of the same town. When his bark, the *Herbert Black,* had her rudder carried away in the South Atlantic, he rigged a jury rudder and improvised steering gear. Not only did he round the Horn with this rig, but after calling at several ports on the west coast returned east to New York without further repairs.

Rounding the Horn is the setting for many a yarn. One of

the longest and toughest fights was that of Captain Richard Quick of Bath in the *Edward Sewall*. Beset by gales of sleet and snow, he was off the Horn for sixty-seven days. During this time the *Sewall* traveled fifty-four different courses, zigzagging, circling, and crossing her own tracks no less than twenty-five times and running thereby 23,407 miles. As a result her voyage from Philadelphia took 293 days. An equally harrowing experience was that of the *Benjamin F. Packard*. Her running gear froze in the blocks, and for fifteen days this made it impossible to work the ship in those dangerous waters.

Few ships have collided with an iceberg and returned to tell the tale. Owing to the skill of her captain, A. C. Larrabee, the *San Joaquin*, built in Freeport, was one. Striking an enormous berg reported to be nine miles in length, she was partially dismasted, her bow was badly stove, and the ship was firmly grounded on the ice. There she remained until the following morning, when, by carrying a line to another part of the berg, the crew succeeded in heaving her off. She returned under jury rig to Portland, her home port.

There is the remarkable exploit of Captain Josiah Mitchell of Freeport. When his ship, the *Hornet*, was burned in the doldrums off the west coast of South America, he safely carried fourteen of his men in a small open boat four thousand miles to the Hawaiian Islands. This voyage of forty-three days and eight hours is the longest of its kind on record. It exceeds the famous open-boat voyage of the survivors of the *Bounty* mutiny. Of like resourcefulness was Rockland-born Captain Isaac W. Keller. When the *Elizabeth Kimball* was wrecked on lonely Easter Island, he and his crew built a ten-ton schooner out of material salvaged from the wreck. In it they reached Tahiti, 2,550 miles distant, after a voyage of twenty-four days.

On one Cape Horn voyage Captain Rasmus B. Anderson of Thomaston in the *Alaska* met the peril of fire and explosion in a cargo of coal by running his ship aground, scuttling and sinking her in Orange Bay. Then with the fire extinguished, he pumped her out and refloated her with little material damage. There were perils from collision, as when the Thomaston-built *Andrew Johnson* was struck and cut halfway through by an English ship. In two minutes she sank, carrying down with her seventeen of the crew, while Captain J. H. Kelleran and eleven others saved themselves by jumping aboard the other ship. There was the peril of the shifting of cargo, as in the *Eureka* of Richmond, which was thrown on her beam ends. By Captain J. O. Woodworth's use of oil and the almost super-human labors of her crew she was righted and completed her voyage. Peril also came from so unexpected a source as the poison gas from decaying wheat, which brought death to some and near blindness to others of the crew of the *H. S. Gregory* of Thomaston. Of such are the rough-hewn tales of the sea that illustrate the dangers of the long California voyage of the down-easters and the character of their masters.

★　★　★

The down-easter was by no means confined to the California grain trade. There were the voyages "Out East" and on the "West Coast." A word of explanation is due here. To the blue-water sailor "Out East" signified the Australian, East Indian, and Chinese ports of call. And the "West Coast" did not have its contemporary meaning. Rather it meant the west coast of South America, where cargoes of Chilean nitrate were to be had, and copper and the guano from the deposits on the Peruvian Islands.

The old China trade had received a fillip in 1849, when the repeal of the British Navigation Acts opened to outsiders the carrying trade between China and London. This enabled the Maine-built clippers to unload in San Francisco as quickly as possible and then cross the Pacific to China to pick up a cargo of tea for the British market. Out of Cutler's list of 139 such voyages by American vessels from 1850 to 1861, there were twelve Maine-built ships sailing principally from Shanghai. In 1853 the Pembroke-built clipper bark *Comet* took part in one of the closest and most exciting derbies over the China course. In company with such fast vessels as the full clippers *Samuel Russell*, *W. B. Palmer*, and *Wild Pigeon*, the *Comet* arrived in Boston only three days after the winner, the *Samuel Russell*, had come in to New York.

There were ships which operated in a manner akin to the tramp steamer of recent times. A good example is to be had in the voyages of the *Helios*, a forerunner of the down-easters. She was a ship of just under 700 tons, built in Yarmouth and commanded by Captain Benjamin Webster. Just after the Civil War broke out she cleared from Baltimore laden with copper ore. Feeling her way out of Chesapeake Bay, where all aids to navigation had been removed by the Confederates, she made Liverpool in nineteen days. Here a ready market was found for the copper and a cargo of salt was taken on for Wyborg, Finland. There she picked up deals, that is, heavy timber, for Bordeaux. Here she chartered for San Francisco, earning a freight of $15,000 in gold. Since gold was at a premium, the ship netted $30,000. In San Francisco the *Helios* took on wheat, flour, and oats for Melbourne and made the passage in forty-two days.

In Australia, to accommodate a complement of Chinese passengers at fifteen dollars a head, a galley was built on deck and berths set up between decks. Discharging these in Hong Kong, she took aboard a full cargo as well as another large group of Chinese who wished passage to California. Then followed a second round trip to China. Business slackened, and she went to Kodiak Island for ice. On her return she found a third cargo for Hong Kong waiting. In Hong Kong word was received that Semmes was in the Pacific in the *Alabama* and had coaled at Singapore. From December to March no American ship left the harbor. These three months were always recalled by every captain there as a vacation of rare enjoyment. All were royally entertained at the consulate and by the mandarins. One of the features was a trip to Tokio in a Russian corvette. In March 1864 the *Alabama* was reported to have rounded the Cape on her way to France. The *Helios* returned to San Francisco, and there she was sold.

There were few cargoes from Maine. Maine lumber could not compete with that of the rapidly developing Northwest. The most distinctive cargo shipped from the state was Kennebec ice, carried to Calcutta, Bombay, and Batavia by the *C. C. Chapman*, *Fannie Tucker*, and *Cheeseboro*. After the Civil War the ships came more and more to load in the larger ports of New York, Philadelphia, and Boston. Typical freights to the Orient were coal or case oil supplemented with "general cargo." The enumeration of this would involve a copy of the customs list. Within its scope it included everything from a locomotive on deck and a complete sugar mill in the hold to wheelbarrows, ready-made clothing, baby carriages, and Yankee notions.

Of more interest were the return cargoes. There was raw sugar from the Hawaiian Islands or the East Indies, hemp from Manila, rice from India, silks, matting, and sulphur from Japan, tea and, not infrequently, coolies from China, and flax, tallow, kauri gum from Australia. Many ships remained away from their home ports for long periods. They found freights and did practically packet service between the eastern ports. For ten years the *Valley Forge* of Farmingdale was not out of eastern waters, plying all this time between China and Sumatra and the ports of the Inland Sea. The Brewer-built *Phineas Pendleton* was in an American port only once in nineteen years.

The Down-Easters

On the West Coast some of the earliest ships to go around the Horn had brought back rich ladings of copper ore from the mines of Chile. Maine's contact with the copper and nitrate trade with the West Coast had a pioneer in Augustus Hemmingway. Although born in Salem and one of Boston's most influential merchants, he got his start trading along the coastal towns of Maine. After he had branched out into the West India and South American trade, he found many of his cargoes in Machias. Here he had a sawmill to which he floated down logs from his own township. There he loaded his schooners with lumber for Cuba, where he owned a plantation and sugar mill, and for round the Horn to Valparaiso, where he had warehouses and stores. In addition to lumber his outgoing cargoes were made up of everything salable on the West Coast—sugar, soap, candles, kerosene, sewing machines, and cabinet organs —the stock of a true Yankee trader. For the voyage home his ships were loaded with copper ore, nitrate of soda, wool, hides, and goatskins. Many of his vessels were built under the supervision of William Hemmingway, his Maine representative, at Machias, Addison, Whiting, Harrington, and other Washington County towns.

But it was the guano dug from the Peruvian islands and the nitrate mined in the great salt desert of Tarapaca that furnished paying voyages in the days when the cotton-carrying business was declining, the San Francisco trade had dwindled, or the grain crop was a failure. Guano is a Peruvian word. It means manure. The Humbolt or Peruvian Current which flows along the west coast of South America is more crowded with fish than any other water. These provide abundant food for millions of sea birds. Their droppings on the rocky points and islands of this arid coast, where no rain falls to wash them away, had accumulated for ages. These deposits had risen to heights of forty to eighty feet. The most important were those of the Chinchas—three small islands a few miles off the Peruvian coast. It was estimated that in 1865 here alone were more than 20,000 shiploads of 2,000 tons each. In the boom days of this trade it was not uncommon to see two hundred square-riggers lying in the protected anchorage between the north and central islands awaiting cargoes.

Admittedly guano was no ideal cargo. At first it was looked down upon as a dirty trade, hardly fitted for any but second-class vessels. After 1850 it developed on so stupendous a scale that a contemporary writer in *Hunt's Merchants Magazine* argued that the guano deposits of the Chincha Islands were intrinsically more valuable than the gold mines of California. It is a fact that between 1851 and 1872 10,000,000 tons of this fertilizer, to a value of $20,000,000 to $30,000,000 a year, was brought from the Pacific to enrich the fields of the Atlantic seaboard, England, and Holland. A goodly proportion of this was carried in the holds of Maine vessels.

The guano was dug by Chinese coolies together with a few peons or criminals from Peru. For these unfortunates the system was one of absolute slavery, the worst and most cruel in the world. Under the blistering sun and all but naked, be he strong or weak, each must dig and wheel to the "manqueras," or large enclosures at the edge of the cliffs, at least five tons of the dust each day. At the lower end of these manqueras were long canvas pipes or "chutes" through which the guano was poured into the launches for conveyance to the waiting ships. Often it was dropped directly into the hatchways of vessels moored to buoys below. So bold was the shore that with its yards cock-billed (that is, set aslant the masts) and all but rolling out its royal masts in the strong Pacific swell, a vessel might in this way load its cargo. The guano was as fine as flour. Loosed by the force of the fall of 150 feet, strong ammonia fumes and stifling yellow dust penetrated into every nook and corner. The three or four days "under the chutes" were one of the most uncomfortable experiences of a seaman's life.

This export trade was a Peruvian government monopoly. Licenses were issued to shipmasters which permitted them to load a certain amount. The vast sums of money pouring into the Peruvian treasury excited the cupidity of adventurers and politicians and became the cause of frequent revolutions. In one of these the Kennebunk ship, *Lizzie Thompson*, was in the middle in an incident which resulted in international complications and threatened war.

A General Vivanco had seized the islands and custom houses and was administering the guano trade at a great profit to himself. In perfect good faith, Captain Horace Wilson had obtained a license from him to load a thousand tons. When about a quarter of the cargo was in, a Peruvian gunboat arrived. The captain was arrested, the crew were driven over the side into the boats, and the *Thompson* was taken into Callao. Here she was sold as contraband of war. The government, now back in power, claimed that the insurgent general had stolen its property and that any ship loading under his license was also involved in the theft. After much diplomatic correspondence with no agreement the ministers of both countries received their passports. At last the matter was referred to the King of Belgium as an arbitrator. When he declined to act, the matter was dropped.

Gradually the Cincha Islands' deposits were worked out, and in the seventies cargoes were sought in the so-called Southern Guano Ports, with loading points at Pabellon de Pica, Punta Lobos, and Huanillos. These were situated seventy-five to a hundred miles south of the nitrate port of Iquiqui on the straight north-and-south coast of Chile. The days spent in taking in cargo at these open roadsteads were an anxious time for the captains. At anchor they were in far more danger than when under sail, for nowhere in the world was shipping more exposed to danger. There might come without warning the furious "norther" or the even more dreadful earthquake with its attendant tidal waves.

On the night of the ninth of May, 1877, there occurred here a disaster without parallel in the annals of maritime Maine. On that day thirteen Maine-built vessels and one other owned in the state were loading. Four—the *Geneva* of Bath, *Benjamin Sewall* of Brunswick, *C. F. Sargent* of Yarmouth, and the *Resolute*, owned in Searsport, were at Huanillos, the most southerly loading point. At Pabellon de Pica to the north lay the *St. Joseph* and *Carrollton* of Bath and the *John Bryce* of Thomaston, while the *North Star* of Bath, *Shamrock* of Belfast, *Uncle Toby* of Freeport, and the bark *I. Sargent* of Machias were at other anchorages.

At about half-past eight in the evening came the earthquake. The ships shook like leaves. It was difficult to stand on deck. The shocks lasted one or two minutes and were accompanied by a deafening roar as loosened boulders came rolling down the steep mountainsides into the sea. The terrifying scene was heightened by the fires that broke out ashore and the shrieks of the townspeople—"La Mar! La Mar!" as they scrambled to higher ground for safety.

At the anchorage there came the clank of windlasses as the ships payed out their chains readying for the inevitable tidal wave. Then it came in roaring like a boiling cauldron, tossed the great vessels like chips, taking anchors and chains with them, and spun them round and round. There was crashing and groaning as masts and jibbooms were carried away or timbers crushed as the ships collided and twisted their anchor chains into a hopeless tangle.

Only one Maine ship was a complete loss. This was the Houghton's *Geneva*. With a full cargo of 2300 tons, she had been ready to sail the following morning. She sank in fifteen fathoms of water, but Captain Charles H. MacLoon and the crew were saved. The *Uncle Toby* also had nearly a complete cargo aboard. She was so badly damaged that she was sold after being towed to Callao. The Hitchcock's *St. Joseph* suffered to the extent of $20,000. The *John Bryce, Carrollton, Benjamin Sewall, Resolute,* and *I. Sargent* had rigging and hulls so injured that they provided a grist of work for the shipwrights of Callao. The *C. F. Sargent,* having but just arrived, was light, with only 150 tons aboard. Also she was anchored at some distance from the others. She lost her rudder stock, anchors, and chains and like the others had to run in for repairs, but she was able to serve as a refuge for some of the more unfortunate victims.

★   ★   ★

Although the long Pacific voyages were often made tedious by calms or contrary winds, there was never any lack of occupation for captain and crew. In a letter to a friend Captain David H. Rivers tells how the time was spent in the Bath ship *A. G. Ropes* on her outward voyage:

> In addition to sailing we have made upper and lower mizzen top-sails and repaired several sails in the sailmaker's department. We have scrubbed all the paint work, cleaned and oiled the decks and the tops of the houses, set up the fore rigging, repaired all chafes aloft and are pumice-stoning the ship on the outside and tarring the rigging.

In inspecting the work of his men Captain Rivers often climbed to the skysail yard. He continues:

> Because there is about twenty-five thousand dollars worth of sails, spars and rigging above the ship's deck and I think these things worth looking after, we have the yards scraped bright and as we have twenty-one of them ranging from

thirty-five to ninety feet in length and from seven up to twenty-one inches in diameter you can see what the job has been. I have had the pins and sheaves of every block in the ship brought to the poop deck for my inspection and as there are about twenty blocks connected with the cross-jack and the cross-jack yard alone you can see it was no small undertaking. I have every piece of rigging brought aft and pass every foot of it through my own hands. We have begun painting the ship today, white inside, and I have had the lower masts pumicestoned so that they are as smooth as a table top.

Despite all this activity the captains especially had many lonely hours. To while them away many often developed hobbies. Joanna C. Colcord, the author of *Songs of American Sailormen*, tells us:

> Captain Andrew S. Pendleton was a master hand at making net lace; he finished a bedspread each voyage. Captain David A. Scribner's specialty was macramé lace. Captain Joseph P. Sweetser became more than an amateur painter of marines. Captain Walter M. Mallett was a camera fan away back in the gelatine-negative days. . . . The hobby of Captain John Drew of the *Sea Witch* was writing—he was a regular contributor to the Maine papers under the pseudonym of "The Kennebecker." Captain H. A. Starrett in command of the first ship *Frank N. Thayer* during a period of seven years labored over a large rigged model of the vessel which he kept set up in the cabin.

Another captain of a religious turn of mind made a handsome scale model of Solomon's temple from the measurements given in the Bible. Others who did not care to work with their hands had special interests they followed in their reading—medicine, law, agriculture, and even bee keeping. One with a taste for history determined to master some classic each voyage. For one he chose Gibbon's *Decline and Fall of the Roman Empire* and for the next Josephus' *Complete Works*.

The Down-Easters

One of these hobbies deserves more than passing notice. It was that of Captain Edward Payson Nichols of Searsport. On each voyage he composed, set up, and printed on his own hand press a breezy little sheet called the "Ocean Chronicle." This he mailed to his friends to avoid, so he said, the trouble of writing letters. Its masthead states that he published it "for friends, not for critics. . . . Terms One letter." In it there were news of the voyage, political and maritime articles, witty comments, and under the headings "Hashed Meat" and "Mixed Pickles," jokes, original or selected. It also had an abundance of humorous advertisements. A volume of facsimiles of these papers has been published by the Penobscot Marine Museum.

From the earliest days wives had sometimes accompanied their husbands on their voyages. But in the days of the down-easters, when the captain and his family often owned a controlling interest in the vessel, family life on shipboard was the rule, not the exception. Not even the expectation of a baby kept the wife at home. A midwife was taken on at some port of call, or if necessary the father officiated. Many a birthplace is marked on the family record by latitude and longitude alone. In his history of the Nichols family of Searsport, Charles J. Nichols lists the names of thirty-five members of that family who were born at sea or in a port of call. In an incomplete list of the births of the children of Searsport parents at sea, there are seventy-five names with but one fatality.

The given names sometimes indicated the place of birth. There were Mindoro, Iona, and in one case Oceanica. Captain F. C. Duncan of Bath reared a family of five in the cabin of the *Florence*. Captain Joseph Sweetser had with him on his voyages his son Joseph D. from the time he was eighteen months old until he reached his majority. Joanna C. Colcord has described the domestic life on the ships in several delightful articles, and from these we draw heavily. She herself was born aboard her father's ship in the South Seas off the coast of New Caledonia, as was her brother Lincoln Colcord off Cape Horn.

The after cabin in which the family lived was sunk part way below the quarter deck and was reached by a companionway leading down from forward of the wheel. It was lighted by square windows near its top which were protected by heavy shutters, and by a large raised skylight in the center of the main saloon. In the starboard corner aft was the captain's stateroom. Across the companionway from this were the bath and toilet. Two doors led to the forward cabin. This was long and narrow, for along its sides were the steward's and officers' staterooms. Here was the dining table, equipped with "fiddles" to prevent the dishes from sliding off in rough weather. The custom was that first the captain, his family, and the first mate were served, and after them the other officers.

Many of these cabins were beautifully finished. Cabinetmakers vied with one another in their decoration. Some were all white embellished with gold leaf, carvings, paneling, and pilasters. In others there had been chosen the hard woods—bird's-eye maple, satinwood, or mahogany trimmed with ebony. There were carpets. There was often a piano. Easy chairs and a center table covered with knickknacks and pictures made it all very like home when the vessel was in port. At sea the deck coverings would be taken up, the furniture screwed down, and all loose ornaments stowed. Even then the cabins were very pleasant living rooms in calm weather. But when the seas were heavy, the water always got in and they became damp, dark, and gloomy.

All the household work as well as the preparation of the meals was done by the steward and cook. Chinese were preferred by American captains, for they were clean and extraordinarily capable. The food was excellent. Some captains took hens along, a pig, sometimes a cow, or if there were young children, occasionally a goat. The meat staple was the good old salt beef of the forecastle, which was equally relished in the cabin. There was condensed milk for the coffee and tinned Danish butter, supplemented by a variety of tinned fruits, vegetables, meats, and fish. The bill of fare would sometimes be varied when a bonito or dolphin was caught or a porpoise grained. The steaks and liver of the latter were quite a delicacy. Near the end of a long voyage shortages sometimes occurred, but they were rare. Nevertheless the fresh meats, fruits, and vegetables of the port were always eagerly looked forward to—"cocoanuts and whole bunches of bananas at the islands of the Pacific, grapes and peaches in Chile, pink fleshed pomeloes and mangosteens in Singapore, lychees and green skinned sweet oranges in China!"

Even the children did not find the days monotonous. They must play quietly, for almost always someone was trying to sleep in his watch below. But during pleasant weather there was no lack of interesting things to watch on deck. In heavy weather and at night there were all manner of games to be played on the cabin floor—cards, dominoes, or authors, and others, quite as ingenious, invented by the children themselves. There was knot-tying and splicing to be learned by the boys and sewing for the girls. Then there were always books, both the family's own and those in the ship's library supplied by the Seamen's Friend Society. Lessons went on daily. The parents always consulted the teachers at home, and the same subjects were studied from the same books as in the home-town school. Geography was learned through the eyes. Mathematics came alive as they watched and sometimes had a share in finding the ship's position, casting the day's run and laying off on the chart the run of the previous day. Miss Colcord mailed her final high-school examination from Hong Kong and received her diploma in Searsport six months later.

In the ports there was no lack of social life, both among those in the fleet and with those engaged in shipping activities ashore. By day the ladies made shopping, calling, sightseeing, and rickshaw trips. In the evening the masters and their families with guests from on shore gathered on one or another of the ships to sit under the awning on the quarter deck, smoking and talking in the soft darkness while white-jacketed stewards passed refreshments.

We should not give the impression that these voyages on the "West Coast" and "Out East" were all in ways of pleasantness and the paths of peace. Tragedy struck in the cabins of the down-easters just as it did in homes on shore. The *Phineas Pendleton* came into port from one voyage with her lower masts painted black. This was in token of mourning for the captain's three children, who had died of diphtheria off the Peruvian coast. Husbands were washed overboard, as was William York of the *Don Quixote*. Then a wife—like his—must navigate the vessel. Maine women of the sea showed themselves the captain's mate in the fullest sense of the word and of the same tough fiber as their men.

The record is replete with the unusual experiences of Maine captains. Captain Herbert Humphrey took the *El Capitan* from Sydney to Calcutta by the Great Barrier Reef route, which was used only by steamers. His was the only square-rigged vessel that ever went through. Captain F. A. Duncan, not finding a tug at the mouth of the Hoogli River, sailed the *Charles Davenport* up to Calcutta. This was a feat not accomplished since the days of the smaller East Indiamen. William Morey, second mate of the *Grey Feather*, was left behind in Colombo, sick, when his ship sailed. He decided to go into business there. He married a Singhalese princess and was appointed the first United States Consul to Ceylon.

★　★　★

The tales of adroit resource by which the Maine shipmaster got his ship out of trouble once she was in it should not eclipse the fact that he was even more adept in keeping clear of it. Indeed, from July 1881 to July 1884, which were the boom years of the California grain trade, William Bates, the United States Commissioner of Navigation, estimates that out of the 423 American wooden vessels employed, there were but 2 losses. Percentage-wise this was minute—.5 per cent. The property loss, including vessel, cargo, and freight for the same period averaged only $442,116 a year.

Competition was so keen that owners and builders could not afford to use anything but the best in construction. Moreover, not only were the down-easters built on more practical lines than their predecessors, the clippers, but they were sailed in a more rational manner. No longer was it necessary to carry three sets of spare spars and use them all. Nor was the captain's watchword "What she can't carry, she can drag." Although there were always drivers and sail carriers in the fleet, the sudden, unforeseen squall was ordinarily the reason for broken spars or for sails being blown out of the bolt ropes.

This greater care did not cause the down-easters to suffer much when we compare the speed of their voyages with those of the famous clippers. Frederick C. Matthews, who knew and studied both types, writes:

> The seven passages (from San Francisco to New York) made by Captain Wilbur in the *M. P. Grace* averaging 115 days and the five made by Captain Nichols in the *S. P. Hitchcock* in 111 days compare very favorably with the eight made by the *Mary L. Sutton* in 118½ days and the *Ocean Telegraph* in 121 days. The fourteen passages made by the *Henry B.*

Hyde in 124 days may be placed against the 125-day average made by the *Sea Serpent* and *Herald of the Morning* each making fourteen runs.[4]

The following runs are samples of the performance of the down-easters:

DATE	RUN	VESSEL	CAPTAIN	TIME
188–	SF to NY	*Henry B. Hyde*	John G. Pendleton	88 days
1892	SF to NY	*A. G. Ropes*	David H. Rivers	95 days
1892	SF to NY	*Benjamin F. Packard*	Zaccheus Allen	94 days
1887	NY to SF	*S. P. Hitchcock*	John R. Nichols	101 days
1889	NY to SF	*S. P. Hitchcock*	John R. Nichols	101 days
–	NY to SF	*M. P. Grace*	Robert P. Wilbur	102 days
–	NY to SF	*Roanoke*	Chadwick Thompson	102 days
1886	SF to Liverpool	*S. P. Hitchcock*	John R. Nichols	91 days
1886	SF to Liverpool	*Henry B. Hyde*	Phineas Pendleton	96 days
1897	SF to Liverpool	*Shenandoah*	James F. Murphy	102 days

On the whole, Maine shipowners made excellent profits with their down-easters. In lean years when the crop failed and ships might be laid up in port, sometimes for as long as two years, for want of a paying cargo, they were kept moving by their owners in the coastwise coal or lumber trade, or took cargo for Australia or "Out East." Sewall's *Carrollton* probably bears the palm as a paying ship. Launched in November 1872, she was immediately chartered for the San Francisco voyage at the lump sum of $31,900. There she loaded wheat for Liverpool at £4 and earned some $40,000. Shortly after her arrival, she was sold for $96,000. This was $15,000 more than her original cost. Thus in a short time she netted her owners a small fortune.

Examples might be multiplied. The *W. F. Babcock*, also owned by the Sewalls, is reported to have paid for herself twice over during her first eight years. The *William H. Connor* of Searsport in three voyages paid for the cost of her construction, and being kept going even when business was dull on the reg-

4 *American Merchant Ships*, Marine Research Society, 1930-31.

ular routes, returned to her owners 600 per cent on their investment. But these are extreme cases, and Basil Lubbock's estimate that they paid 15 or 20 per cent a year is perhaps nearer the truth. Running expenses were high, perhaps $2,000 to $2,500 a year for a vessel of 2,000 tons. To quote Lubbock again:

> No pinch penny 'pint and pound' policies ruled. Repairs were made promptly and sails, spars and ropes replaced with the best the market afforded as soon as they showed the least signs of wear. Food was excellent: preserves 'air tights' as the forecastle called them supplementing the excellent California hardtack and the salt beef of the harness cask. There were few rotten gaskets, cut rat lines or 'hungry ships' among the Maine Downeasters.

As the wheat fields spread over the Northwest, new shipping ports were developed and Maine ships were early arrivals at their docks. In 1876, Chapman and Flint's *St. Charles* was the first to load wheat at Martinez, near San Francisco, the event being celebrated by the enthusiastic inhabitants with an elaborate banquet. Five years later Captain Isaac F. Gilkey, rather than take his ship, the *Dakota*, up the Columbia River, had his cargo sent to him in Tacoma by rail from Portland. Thereby he saved over $50,000 for his owners. Other vessels followed his scheme, and Tacoma became a grain-shipping port.

Long before Paul Bunyan had turned from the white pine forests of Maine and commenced his long trek westward across the continent toward the mighty Oregon firs, Maine shipmasters had recognized great possibilities in the development of the woodlands of the Northwest. Indeed, the first commercial cargo of lumber to be carried out of Puget Sound in an American vessel was in the brig *Orbit* of Calais, Captain William H. Dunham. That was in 1850. Ten years later the first cargo of yellow fir spars was shipped to Atlantic ports in the *Lawson* of Bath.

The Maritime History of Maine

The beginning of things in a large way came in 1877, when Captain Guy C. Goss of Bath visited the Pacific coast. He was so impressed with the timber on the banks of Puget Sound that in order to test its value for shipbuilding purposes he sent a cargo home in the bark *William H. Besse*. The result proved the soundness of his judgment, and many cargoes were sent around the Horn to the yards in Boston, New York, Philadelphia, and Bath. One of these cargoes, carried out by the ship *Guy C. Goss*, contained 250 pieces suitable for masts or spars, many measuring 112 feet in length and 36 inches in diameter. Having neither knot nor blemish, each was worth $900. The building of the great ships and barks of the later period was made possible by the use of this heavy timber. The ship *Roanoke*, for instance, whose spars were massive sticks of Oregon fir, had lower masts 38 inches in diameter. The fore, main, and mizzen masts were 92 feet long, while the spanker was 98 feet.

As early as 1896 there came ominous signs that American wood was losing the California grain trade to English iron. Owners and builders in Maine began to turn with more serious attention to the fore-and-aft rig and to the rapidly increasing coast trade, which was secure from foreign competition. The shadows lengthened. By 1889 the grain fleet of 213 ships contained only 30 American vessels. For the five years from 1885 to 1890, no square-rigger left the ways anywhere on the Maine Coast.

The nineties brought a revival in world trade. The new kerosene trade with the Far East was calling for greater and greater ship tonnage and the promise of paying cargoes. Hope revived in Maine. The Sewalls, with their characteristic energy and enterprise, put off their famous fleet of four-masters—the *Shenandoah*, *Susquehanna*, and *Roanoke*. But the days of the *Granger*, *Reaper*, and *Harvester* had passed. And the end was at hand. For the square-rigged vessel the final word was said

The Down-Easters

in America in 1893, when Charles Minot launched the *Aryan* in his Phippsburg yard.

Square sails did not disappear from the sea with the passing of the California trade. For many years, in gradually decreasing numbers, they would gladden the eyes of their lovers watching from the deck of a steamer or from under the boom of a six-masted schooner. For a while there was case or barreled oil to carry from Atlantic ports to Hong Kong, Hiogo, or "Out East." There was coal, and there were government charters to be had for its transport to San Francisco, Honolulu, or Manila. And when these round-the-Horn voyages failed, the Pacific still offered a living in the west coast coal and lumber trade, until the great schooners took this away. Most important of all and a great boon to American shipping was the Hawaiian sugar business. This was a monopoly for American sailing ships until it was closed to them by the formation of the American-Hawaiian Steamship Company.

For a long time many vessels, when they became too old for longer and more strenuous voyages, found employment in the salmon fisheries. To the last the fleet of the Alaska Packers Association of San Francisco consisted almost entirely of old down-easters. The first ship bought by this firm in 1893 was the Brunswick-built *George Skolfield*. Her companions, among others from the home state, were Oakes' *Llewellyn J. Morse*, Houghton's *Bohemia*, Sewall's *Sterling* and *Indiana*, John Mac-Donald's *Santa Clara*, and Goss and Sawyer's *Tacoma*. Other Maine ships, such as the *A. J. Fuller* and *Benjamin F. Packard*, made themselves useful in the later days carrying box shooks, tin plate, empty cans, retorts, coal, and Chinese cannery workers north through the Unimak Pass to the fishing stations, returning when the canning season was over with full cargoes of "choice Alaska turkey."

To the lover of the tall ships the fate of the down-easters is

[235]

sad. Some went down where only latitude and longitude could record their burial, others went up in a holocaust of flame, and others still laid their bones on some coral reef or faraway shore. Many, however, were sold to the bargemen, Luckenbach or Sully. Then, shorn of their tapering masts and spars and with a ring in their noses, they were towed from port to port by a noisy tug. A few found a period of what passes for glamour in their old age as moving-picture ships. From these a generation that knew them not caught second-handed a little of their beauty and romance. The *Indiana* represented an old ship named the "Colonial Dame" in DeMille's picture *Splendid Road*. She also appeared with the *Bohemia* in *Yankee Clipper*. The *Llewellyn J. Morse* was seen as the *Constitution* in *Old Ironsides*, and the *Santa Anna* starred in the Metro-Goldwyn production, *Captain Salvation*.

Cremation was the end of many. Their ashes rest in many a "boneyard" on the west coast. That is all that is left after the shipbreakers dismantled them and then burned their hulls for the metal they contained. A few years ago the Pacific Marine Review published a copy of Charles R. Patterson's picture, "Their Last Harbor." In it four Maine vessels, the ships *B. P. Cheney*, *Pactolus*, and *Hecla* and the bark *St. Katherine* lie huddled together with their yardarms interlaced awaiting their passing in the boneyard at Antioch.

CHAPTER TWELVE

The GREAT SCHOONERS

> The great schooner was the last technical achievement of the
> builders of the wooden ships. Notable advances were made
> in model and rig, but particularly the latter. These made the
> American great schooner the most weatherly and economical
> sailing vessel in the world.—John G. Hutchins, *American
> Maritime Industries and Public Policy.*[1]

BY THE GREAT SCHOONER is meant the familiar fore-and-aft-
rigged vessel with four or more masts. Their day dovetailed with
and extended beyond that of the down-easter, and the story of
their use and decline is the last chapter in the history of the
wooden sailing ship and the old shipbuilding industry on the
coast of Maine. As with the clipper and the down-easter, the
Maine-built multi-masted schooners have a distinguished place
in the American merchant marine. Theirs is the well-justified
claim to have been "the most weatherly and economical sailing
vessel in the world."

Their evolution furnished an excellent example of the ease
with which Maine builders adapted themselves to new economic
conditions. Owing to foreign competition, the profits in long
ocean voyages began to diminish. Hence attention was turned
to the coastwise routes, which were secure from outside interference. Large-bulk cargoes—coal, ice, granite, lumber, and lime
—were demanding low-cost transportation. The economical
fore-and-aft rig was developed and improved to meet this de-

[1] Harvard University Press, 1941.

mand and pay a profit. Loading and discharge in these trades often occurred in shallow water. Hence for this a hull with solidly laid floors, heavy bottom, hard bilges, and little dead rise was moulded. Centerboard and keel models were designed to meet all conditions. The alertness of Maine builders in meeting and solving these problems and in taking advantage of every technical improvement kept their wooden sailing craft supreme in the coastwise trade from 1870 to 1905.

The origin of the term "schooner" and of the type is obscure. Moreover, the usage has changed. Prior to 1850 the word "schooner" betokened a two-masted vessel (though three-masters were by no means unknown) carrying in part square sails on the foremast—hence the phrase "tops'l schooner." In those days what has been known as a schooner since 1850, that is, fore-and-aft-rigged throughout, was generally termed a fore-and-after. This rig began its long career of popularity as a coastal carrier very early in American history.

These—the fore-and-afters, latterly known as schooners—were the errand boys of the coast. They averaged around a hundred tons and were to be found in every river, bay, and inlet along the shore from Quoddy to Cape Fear. To southern cities they delivered the products of Maine farms, shores, forests, and local industries—that is to say, butter and cheese, potatoes and dried fish, bricks and sawed lumber, screwed (that is, baled) hay and cord wood. In turn they brought back southern pine, pitch, tar, and turpentine to the yards in which they had been built. The brigs and the topsail schooners were preferred for the longer voyages to the Caribbean or to South America, but for the short haul up to five hundred miles the small schooner was supreme. Some idea of the amount of business they did may be gathered from the fact that in the year 1835 there arrived in Boston from Maine 574 schooners, in New York 328, and in Philadelphia 99.

The Great Schooners

Also in contrast with the great schooners of the latter part of the century which would bring their cargoes of coal north to feed the home fires of Maine were the little two-masters of the early days which carried high-piled loads of cordwood south to supply the fireplaces of Boston and Salem. In those days almost every coast town had its wood landing—the location now forgotten—a busy place where firewood was piled and laden. At one time Belfast, for example, had fifty or more wood schooners, and in April 1844 there was piled on its wharves awaiting shipment over 10,000 cords. A profitable cargo it was, too. Two dollars a cord was the cost in Maine of what would bring four dollars in Massachusetts. With an average lading of 50 cords the skipper might clear $100 a trip besides what he received for freight on merchandise brought home for the town merchants. He could make at least ten trips in a season.

The Maine town in which the three-masted schooner was "invented" is as various as the Greek towns where Homer was born. Chapelle says the "rig can be traced back to 1800 and earlier." The privateers in the War of 1812 had some modification of this rig. The *Dart* of Portland, which is referred to in her log as a "three-masted schooner," is an example. In the thirties and forties there were several in the state. Nahum Hall of Ellsworth built the *Aurora* of 147 tons in 1831 and two years later launched the 130-ton *Fame*. The same year Asa Clough launched the *Magnolia* of 109 tons at Bluehill, and in 1832 George Savage and others of Boston had the 140-ton *Horse* constructed at Joseph Day's yard in Damariscotta. Some of these craft crossed yards on one or more masts, and it is now generally agreed that the *Magnolia* was the first true-to-type, three-masted, fore-and-aft schooner in the state. The first example of the economical freighters of the later period did not put in an appearance until 1865, when Joseph Clark at Waldoboro built the *American Eagle* of 386 tons.

Handy, economical, and of comparatively low cost, the three-masted schooner soon all but monopolized the coastwise trade. Today she has survived her larger successors as an income-earning carrier. The name generally given the rig in the old days was "tern" schooner. The word means "a series of three." Never popular in Maine, the tern still survives in the "Bluenose fleet." In course of time a deep centerboard model was evolved which was extensively used in three- and four-masted craft. This entailed increased construction cost and loss of cargo space, and when tugboats and cheap towage became available it was gradually discontinued. In size the three-masters never attained as much as 1,000 tons. The largest ever constructed was the *Bradford C. French*, built by David Clark at Kennebunk in 1884. She measured 968 tons.

The success of the three-masters, coupled with the discovery that larger hulls could be sailed without any proportional increase in cost, led after 1880 to the building of four-, five-, and six-masters. The first of the "four-posters" was the *W. L. White*. She was launched in 1880 by Goss, Sawyer, and Packard at Bath for Jacob B. Phillips of Taunton, and registered 995 tons. At the time she was the largest vessel of her type in the world. She was followed in the Maine yards, especially those at Bath, by many of constantly increasing size. In 1882 the B. W. and H. F. Morse firm launched the *Augustus Hunt* of 1,200 tons, a notable vessel that paid large dividends. Four years later the New England Shipbuilding Company surpassed her with the *Sarah W. Lawrence* of 1,569 tons, and this was followed the next year by the Morse schooner *T. A. Lambert* of 1,630 tons. The rig culminated in size in 1897 when Nathaniel T. Palmer put afloat the *Frank A. Palmer* of 2,014 tons.

Maine builders and enthusiastic owners felt, however, that

the schooner had not yet reached its greatest possibilities. In 1888 Leverett Storer at Waldoboro launched the *Governor Ames,* the first five-masted schooner to be built on the Atlantic coast. The *Ames* did not prove a lucky boat, and it was not until ten years later that another five-master was built. This was the *Nathaniel T. Palmer* of 2,440 tons, which had the name of her builder and came off the stocks at Bath. She was followed the next year by the *John B. Prescott* from the yard of Holly M. Bean at Camden. Of the five-masted fleet on the eastern coast all but three were launched in Maine. In 1900 Mr. Bean built the first six-master in the world, the *George W. Wells* of 2,970 tons. Percy and Small also put off a six-master in 1900, the *Eleanor A. Percy* with a tonnage of 3,401. Thus rapidly did the schooners increase in size.

The economy of the great schooners lay in the extreme simplicity of their rig, which allowed the use of steam winches and other labor-saving machinery. On a full-rigged ship there were 204 running lines. The setting of a main topsail required the simultaneous handling of 11. By contrast the running gear on the principal sail of the fore-and-aft rig was reduced to three major lines which might even be handled by steam power. Not only did this demand less skilled sailormen—a considerable item in the later days—but much less manpower per ton. In his invaluable economic study of American maritime industries Hutchins shows this by means of a deadly parallel. The *Eleanor Percy,* whose crew numbered fifteen, was but five tons smaller than the great *Shenandoah,* for which a crew of thirty-three was necessary. The *Edward Cole* of 1,791 tons had a crew of eight, while the *A. J. Fuller* of 1,848 required twenty-one—nearly three times as many. His general conclusion is that the schooners were well manned with a man for each 200 or 250 tons, whereas the square-riggers needed one man to each 100 tons.

More money, more material, and greater efficiency were represented in one of the great schooners than in any of the old-time ships. Take as an example the *Edward B. Winslow*, a typical six-master built by Percy and Small in 1908. Into her construction went 1,150,000 feet of yellow pine, 350,000 feet of oak, 75,000 feet of white pine and spruce and 200 tons of iron. Each of her masts was a single stick of Oregon pine 120 feet long and 32 inches in diameter extended by topmasts 56 feet long, that on the foremast being 21 inches through. Her keelsons were one solid mass of heavy timber 8 feet deep running from stem to stern.

Wire rigging set up by turnbuckles was used in place of hemp. Steam winches handled cargo, sails, and anchors. Electricity furnished light. Steam heat, telephone connections in all parts of the vessel, the latest equipment in windlass, steering gear, pumps, submarine safety appliances, and sounding machines took much of the drudgery and peril from the sailor's life. Instead of being housed in a foul-smelling, dark forecastle, the crew now lived in a steam-heated deck house painted white and finished in hard pine. They ate meals, from oilcloth-covered tables, as good as those furnished ashore by first-class boarding houses. In fact, their comfort was superior to that enjoyed in the master's cabin in the days before the clipper ships.

One of these masterpieces of the shipbuilding craft cost over $175,000. But she could carry 4,500 tons of coal paying a freight of $2.00 a ton, thus earning a handsome profit for her owners. Twenty-four round trips a year was the average between Newport News and the Maine ports. Her speed, often as high as 12 or even 16 knots, rivaled that of the regular coastwise steamers. Many of the fore-and-afters could sail within five points of the wind, and, as one enthusiast has remarked: "Nothing but a hurricane can keep her in port; nothing but a flat calm can prevent her making headway."

The Great Schooners

Only a few of the old names appear among the builders of the great schooners. Not only was there a rising generation, but new families head up the firms of builders. Yet many of these firms are the descendants of the older yards where formerly only square-riggers were built. The New England Company of Bath was one of the largest and best-equipped yards on the east coast. Employing three hundred men, it was in direct succession to Goss and Sawyer, Goss, Sawyer and Packard, and the New England Shipbuilding Company. In the forty years of their activity these four companies put off 315 vessels with a grand total of 244,345 tons. Of these, 167 were schooners. In the twelve months of 1882 alone they launched 24 vessels, of which 16 were schooners. Their largest was the *Prescott Palmer* of 2,811 tons, which was built in 1902.

The Kelley-Spear Company, formed when the New England Shipbuilding Company was reorganized, was an offshoot of these firms. Their schooners were among the finest in workmanship, and though they built none larger than four-masters their output was in great demand. Their largest was the *Frontenac*, 1,701 tons, a member of the John S. Emery fleet. For many years they helped to keep the shipbuilding industry alive in Bath, usually employing as many as three hundred men. When they discontinued business in 1923 they had constructed over 400,000 tons of various types of vessels.

Percy and Small was the third of the three larger concerns in Bath. It employed two hundred men. From 1894 to 1920 they launched 44 vessels aggregating 81,689 tons—all but two of them schooners. They were pre-eminently builders of the great schooners and specialized in the construction of five- and six-masters. Of their great six-masters, the *Eleanor A. Percy, Addie M. Lawrence, Ruth E. Merrill, Alice M. Lawrence, Edward J. Lawrence, Edward B. Winslow,* and *Wyoming*, all but two, the *Eleanor A. Percy* and the *Wyoming*, were mem-

bers of the well-known Winslow fleet and are classic in the
annals of the American schooner. Some notion of the size of
the *Wyoming* may be gained from the statement of Colonel
Owen, Bath's historian, that her tonnage was greater by one ton
than that of the entire twenty-one vessels of the Jonathan Davis
fleet at the first of the nineteenth century.

Among other well-known builders of this era were Gardiner
L. Deering and William T. Donnell. Building together or separately they constructed 108 vessels—schooners for the most part.
Nathaniel T. Palmer in a short but distinguished career between
1894 and 1898 launched six large schooners. Down the Kennebec at Phippsburg Charles V. Minott with twenty-five men and
Frank S. Bowker with thirty kept up the reputation of that
town with staunch three- and four-masters until well into the
present century. Farther east at Birch Point in Wiscasset several of the J. Manchester Haynes fleet of three-masters were
built. Haynes built them for his own account to carry to
market the product of his brickyards, sawmills, and icehouses,
which formed one of the largest establishments of its kind in
New England.

At Waldoboro George F. Welt launched six of the great
five-masters of the William F. Palmer fleet—the *Fannie*, *Baker*,
Paul, *Dorothy*, *Singleton*, and *Harwood Palmer*. In Thomaston and Rockland there were the demands of the local lime
trade to meet as well as those of outside owners. Some three
hundred men were employed in the busy yards of Washburn
Brothers, Watts, Dunn and Elliot, Cobb, Butler & Co., and
others in the construction of three- and four-masters. After
Washburn Brothers bought out the Watts yard they added
22 great fore-and-afters to the fleet between 1887 and 1904.
Their largest was the *Washington B. Thomas* of 2,639 tons,
which could carry 4,000 tons of coal. She was wrecked on

her first voyage in a winter gale on Stratten Island, four miles off Old Orchard Beach.

Probably the largest individual builder of schooners was Holly M. Bean of Camden. His list totals 51 schooners, including 1 two-masted schooner, 17 three-masters, 20 four-masters, 12 five-masters and 1 six-master. He put afloat the second five-master, the *John B. Prescott,* and the first six-master, the *George W. Wells.* Mr. Bean employed 150 men, and it is said that the cost of his shipbuilding operations was over $2,500,000.

On the Penobscot, Fields C. Pendleton was building for the Pendleton fleet of Islesboro, which was the largest in Penobscot Bay. At Bucksport McKay and Dix on Verona Island launched at least two of over 1,400 tons, while at Brewer the Stetson yard was busy with sizable craft. The coast east of the Penobscot is especially the home of the small schooner. Of the 1,990 vessels registered in the District of Machias, 1,550 were fore-and-aft-rigged. On the rivers on this part of the coast smaller yards employing from twenty to thirty men and building a schooner a year were thinly scattered at Millbridge, Harrington, Cherryfield, Machias, Dennysville, and Calais. But by 1900 there were only twenty active yards along the Maine coast.

As they had in the days of the long voyages, builders often accumulated a fleet and took the profits of the cargo as well as of the yard. Thus in the coastwise trade many managed their own fleet of vessels. In 1891 there were twenty-eight Maine fleets of five or more schooners. To a great extent they were composed of two- or three-masters and generally engaged in carrying the products of their home ports to market. In 1900 there were but eight fleets of this size left. But their tonnage was very much greater, and the number of craft in each fleet had increased. The largest were the Dunn and Elliott fleet of Thomaston with 20, J. S. Winslow & Co. of Portland with 23, and Pendleton Brothers of Islesboro with 30 schooners.

Ten years later the great schooners predominated in the picture. In the number of vessels Pendleton Brothers still led with 30. But their rather small craft were not to be compared with Percy and Small's splendid group of 11, Gardiner Deering's 13, and J. S. Winslow's 27. In 1911 the Winslow fleet was increased by the addition of the vessels of the Palmer fleet. This accretion boosted the tonnage of its 34 vessels to 54,993. For several years the blue "W" on a white ground flew over the largest fleet on the Atlantic coast, if not in the whole North American hemisphere.

Other large New England firms drew on the Maine yards for their carriers. Crowell and Thurlow of Boston had schooners from a dozen different builders along the eastern coast. John S. Crowley was equally partial to the Maine product, and in his fleet in the Coastwise Transportation Company was Holly M. Bean's famous *George W. Wells*. The William F. Palmer fleet, John S. Emery and Company of Boston, and a few of the New York firms were good customers of the later yards.

The activities of firms such as these and of the larger Maine firms cannot be gauged by counting the number of their ships or reckoning up their tonnage. Many other vessels were controlled by them. Acting as managing owners, they promoted the vessels, obtained the charters, hired the crews, collected the freights, and divided the profits among the real owners—the merchants, schoolteachers, bookkeepers, and a hundred others who had purchased a share, in some cases as small as one two hundred and fifty-sixth. As payment for all this, they had a generous recompense in 5 per cent of the freight money. The returns in the heyday of the schooner were handsome. Even as late as 1907 Mr. Palmer boasted that his fleet of sixteen was earning 22 per cent on its cost.

The motive behind the remarkable increase in size and improvement of equipment of the great schooners was not competition among builders or the desire of the owners for a larger profit. A very real threat was present in the increasing numbers and keen competition of the ocean-going tug with its long string of barges.

The Morses of Bath are credited with having been the originators of the barge plan. At least they were one of the first firms to see its possibilities and to adopt it. Interested at first in Kennebec River towage and then in the ice business, this family kept a fleet of schooners busy carrying ice to the southern ports and returning laden with coal or ship timber. In and out of their ports of call and often up and down rivers they found that towage charges were eating into their profits. It was soon appreciated that great economies could be effected by towing all the way in strings of three or four vessels. At first old ships which had outlasted their usefulness as sailers were used as barges. They were stripped of all rigging and spars save the lower masts, which were schooner-rigged, and to provide more cargo space the hull was modified by removing the spar deck. As this plan proved successful and the supply of available old vessels became exhausted, the Morses began to build barges. With only a stump fore-and-aft rig, they required only about a third of the crew of a sailing vessel.

In the late eighties the Morses built three great ocean-going tugs. In 1889 they launched the 2,254-ton barge *Independent*. This was the first of a type that would become the last output of the wooden shipbuilding yards of Bath. The late nineties found the other yards busy with them. Kelly and Spear turned out eight a year from 1895 to 1899. William Rogers closed his life work by building four of 1,500 tons each, and the New England Shipbuilding Company, while not turning their attention exclusively to this type, put off nine in 1899.

The barge offered economies over even the great schooners. The lack of top hamper—that is, lofty rigging—made their upkeep much less. Tows could be kept constantly in motion, the tug leaving the loaded barges to be discharged while it took the empties back for another cargo. Thus with no port delays, very nearly a fixed schedule could be maintained. The crews were much smaller. That of the barge generally consisted of the master, two mates, two sailors, and a combination sailor and cook. With these advantages they were hard competitors.

Eventually freight on coal dropped from $2.00 to $1.00 and even to 60 cents a ton, while the charge for lumber from the Carolinas to Philadelphia dwindled from $5.50 to $2.40 a thousand. The schooners gradually surrendered to this economic pressure. Then the barges reigned supreme in the coal trade until they in turn were undercut and driven out by the steam collier, which could carry a cargo of 7,000 tons and make the trip from Hampton Roads to the Maine coast in a quarter the time.

For a while the schooners found some employment in the offshore trades, but their lean days had come. By 1910, instead of receiving dividends, many owners were paying as assessments the difference between the cost of upkeep and their vessel's earnings. With the first World War the Maine wooden vessel regained its position. For four years or so many formerly unprofitable vessels became veritable gold mines for their owners. Many yards again became active. At Harrington Edwin M. Frye put off six six-masters of about 1,100 tons each. The great schooners found handsome profits in the overseas trade to England, France, the Mediterranean, or Africa. Coastwise charters also jumped to a figure never before known. Coal rates, which in 1914 had been only 65 cents, rose in two years to $3.00, and in August 1917 to nearly $5.00. But the sun soon set and lucky was the owner who, noting the signs in the sky, sold out his holdings and taking his profits called it a day.

CHAPTER THIRTEEN

LUMBER *and* LIME,
ICE *and* GRANITE

Now the Kennebec ice houses are rotting and falling back
into the earth. The old piers are sinking into the water, no
ship comes up in tow of a tug through the first leaves of
May. For the Kennebec crystals, best harvest of Maine's
finest river have joined the white pine and the spruce, the
sturgeon and shad and salmon.—Robert P. Tristram Coffin,
The Kennebec.[1]

THE COASTWISE TRADE covered a multitude of activities. From
the outset it has been, and is today, the nursery of seamen and
the main prop of the American merchant marine. On the coast
of Maine, as this or that commodity came into large demand
there developed a regular pattern of activity. Ships were built
for the particular type of trade, used only in it, and more often
than not the proprietors built up their own fleets for the operation of that trade. These are the reasons why the cargoes of
lumber and lime, ice and granite call for consideration and
description.

The intimate tie between lumber and shipping has been
manifest from the earliest times. As a cargo for the ships of the
Pine Tree State it has had no peer from the day when the *Pyed
Cow* landed the first sawmill in America at the falls up the
Piscataqua in South Berwick, to the recent years when the mills
and gang saws along the Penobscot made possible yearly ship-

[1] Rinehart & Company, Inc., 1937.

ments of 250,000,000 feet of sawed lumber. While Maine was a District of Massachusetts the business had been relatively small, a matter for individuals or families.

The ascendency of Wiscasset in this trade was reached in 1815, when the tonnage of its shipping measured close to 20,000. Soon thereafter it ceased to be a boom town. Its resources, which were confined chiefly to the shipment of lumber, were limited by lack of capital and could not be adequately developed. The Kennebec, with the vast riches of two great river systems, was growing rapidly in importance. But the town on the Sheepscot had no rich hinterland on which to draw. In 1800 it had been second only to Portland among the customs districts of the state. Soon it was surpassed by Bath, Waldoborough, and Penobscot. After 1815 a rapid decline took place, and in six years the port slipped to sixth place among the twelve districts in Maine. In 1820, with the advent of the steam mill and co-operative effort along all the rivers from the Saco to the St. Croix, the logger, the riverman, the sorting boom, and the drive became an integral part of the picture.

Thus it is no accident that the period of greatest activity in the lumber business, from 1820 to 1880, should coincide exactly with that of shipping and that both should reach their climax in the burst of energy and initiative exhibited in the forties and fifties. Calais, Machias, Ellsworth, Bangor, Bath, and Portland were the most important shipping points. Each of these was the natural port of a system of lakes and rivers that tapped the virgin forests and furnished cheap transportation to the waiting ships. How busy these vessels were kept may be judged from some facts taken from the records of the period.

The farthest down east was Calais. The character of the St. Croix River determined the type of vessel employed. A vessel riding in twenty-three feet of water at high tide lay on the flats when the tide was low. Hence the demand was for small schooners. Calais was the boom town of eastern Maine in the second quarter of the nineteenth century. It more than doubled its population in the decade before 1820 and quadrupled it in the next ten years. The production from 36 saw mills was shipped out of this port. As early as 1842 there were 272 vessels employed here in the lumber trade. In the fifties these active yards supplied the demand for the small two-masted lumber schooners of the lumber shippers on either side of the St. Croix—the Murchies, Kings, Eatons, Barnards, Durens, and many others. The shipments in 1860 amounted to about 80,000,000 feet of long lumber shipped in the coastwise trade, and 5,000,000 to foreign ports, besides 115,000,000 laths. In 1874 there were 1,177 clearances.

The next to the westward was Machias. In 1762, "the year of the great drought," the men from Scarborough who sailed up the Machias River seeking hay for their cattle were so impressed by the stands of timber, by the magnificent falls, and by the depth of water at their foot that twenty-five of them came back the next year to make this place their home. It became a great lumber port. During two weeks in the year 1857 there was shipped out of here nearly 2,000,000 feet. In that year the little neighboring towns of Whitneyville, Columbia, and Cherryfield sent out 21,500,000 feet of long lumber, besides 28,000,000 laths and a million and a half shingles.

Ellsworth early became and long remained the lumber capital of eastern Maine. It lay on both sides of the Union River, which was navigable for good-sized schooners to the very foot of the first falls. Here the water came tumbling down over a succession of cascades, with a drop of a hundred feet in two and a quarter miles, providing excellent sites for lumber mills. From the four hundred square miles of forest reached by its waters, there came in 1853, the peak year, 35,000,000 feet of sawed lumber as well as 250,000 box shooks. To carry this to market many vessels were required. At that date 159 were owned in the town. At times as many as 60 could be seen lying four abreast taking in cargo at the eighteen wharves which fringed the river banks.

As a lumber port, Bangor on the Penobscot was without a peer. In the fifty-odd years from 1832 to 1888, a total of 8,737,628,202 feet was shipped from here. The peak year was 1872, when 246,453,649 feet were shipped. The yearly average was about 155,000,000 a year. The number of vessels employed may be judged from the fact that in 1860 there were 3,376 arrivals in this port. Coasters out of almost every port in the state carried on a busy trade to the towns of the Atlantic sea-board whose supplies of lumber had been exhausted. As an example, Col. John Black of Ellsworth, the agent for the Bingham interests in Maine, sent his vessels out with 103 cargoes during the sailing season of 1842.

The lumber cargoes were varied. Deals—that is, pieces of timber some 9 by 3 inches in section to be sawed at the destination into the dimensions required by the local market—planks, and boards were known as "long lumber." Clapboards, laths, fence posts and shingle bolts were "short lumber." Besides these there was great variety—ship timber of hard woods, knees of juniper or hackmatack, masts of pine and spars of pine or spruce, hemlock bark for tanning, box shooks for lemons, oranges, and sugar, piling and paving blocks, nests of casks, heading, shooks, hoops and hoop poles, and, after railroad construction began, cedar sleepers and posts. Deals, planks, and scantling went to England and northern Europe. Lemon and orange box shooks were in demand in the Mediterranean ports and in the Canary, Azores, and Cape Verde Islands. The lighter and well-seasoned timber found a market in South America, while the West Indies took lumber of all kinds as well as box shooks and cooperage stuff.

Almost as varied as these cargoes were the vessels that carried them. In *The Ark of Elm Island*, Elijah Kellogg tells a tale of the crude construction of the *Ark*. Laden with lumber, she sailed for the West Indies and was then broken up and sold with her cargo. Many of the lumber operators built their own. Especially was this true in the early days along the Androscoggin and Kennebec and later in the towns on the eastern rivers. In Bangor, at the head of navigation on the Penobscot and the shipping point for the enormous timber production of the East and West branches of the Penobscot, the Lakes, the Piscataquis and Mattawaumkeag rivers, a motley fleet, comprising sometimes as many as 250 at once, filled the river so that boys jumping from deck to deck could cross over from Bangor to Brewer.

There was a cargo for all, from the graceful *Belle of Bath* and the staunch *Phineas Pendleton* to the *Polly* of privateer fame, built in 1803, and "Old Liz" of uncertain age, now demoted to carrying slabs and refuse wood for the lime kilns at Rockland. There were also odd types such as the "Lake-built" schooners. Fastened with iron spikes, narrow and shoal with boxlike deck houses, they were known on the river as "canalboats under sail." Extreme freaks in marine architecture were the cheaply built, schooner-rigged scows. They were not intended to be seagoing, but they could carry astounding quantities of lumber to not too distant ports. The three-masted or tern schooner, which was trim, seaworthy, and easy to handle, in the later days became the standard equipment for this trade.

The long lumber was loaded through ports cut in the bows. It was brought down from the mills in great rafts which were either warped or sculled by skillful oarsmen. When it came to loading, the phrase "loaded to the gunwales" lost its meaning. A vessel with considerable sheer was sometimes so laden that even on an even keel the water stood several inches deep on

Lumber and Lime, Ice and Granite

her deck amidship. Tales are told of these vessels coming into port under their own sail with their hulls so submerged that the helmsman stood to his knees in water. The loading went on day and night. In later years many an old resident sensed a strange stillness. There was missing the slap of the planks and boards as the stevedores let them fall, and the tooting of the tugs as they made up the tow for down the river.

The Penobscot River was by no means easy to navigate in sailing vessels, with its sharp turns, mud flats, ledges, and tide runs. Yet myriads of craft made their way up under sail alone. Others, especially the larger craft, preferred a tow. Making up these great strings of vessels and guiding them safely down the crowded river was a difficult operation. Such tows often contained 20 to 30 loaded craft. There is one on record containing 36. Lashed three abreast with thick wooden fenders between them, they were an impressive sight as they passed down the river to separate in open water and then go their several ways to market.

In order to bring the lumber to the vessels, especially the short lumber, three railroads were built. The first of these, which was the first railroad in the state, was chartered in 1832. Until 1869 it transported lumber to Bangor from the mills at Milford, Old Town, and Stillwater. The second was chartered in 1836, and for over fifty years its twin locomotives, the "Lion" and the "Tiger," drew millions of feet of lumber from Whitneyville to Machias. The third, between Calais and Milltown, was completed in 1839, and for ten years its cars were horse-drawn. In 1851 it was extended to Baring and a few years later to Princeton, when two locomotives were placed on it.

★　★　★

Almost as old a cargo as lumber was lime. As early as 1733 William McIntyre erected the first kiln near the site of the present state prison in Thomaston. Here he burned lime in considerable quantities for shipment to Boston. At this time Brigadier Waldo also had two sloops carrying lime to Boston. After the Revolutionary War, as settlers came into the country, the business increased by leaps and bounds. Among them was General Henry Knox, whose various ventures, successful and unsuccessful, stimulated the development of Thomaston and its environs on the St. George's River. In his yard Captain Howland Rogers built the schooners *Quicklime* and *Montpelier* and a brig, the *Quantabacook*, in which the General's lime was carried to market and his lumber to the West Indies. In 1795 the Duke of Rochefoucauld when visiting Montpelier noted that in that year there were eleven vessels on the stocks on the banks of the St. George's. Farther upstream at Warren, founded in 1776, there were turned out during the next century some 269 small schooners and brigs designed to make quick coasting voyages and find a profit in the cargoes of lumber and lime. The development of this industry at Rockland and Camden came later.

By 1835 the kilns were burning 750,000 casks a year. In the fifties over five hundred sloops, schooners, and brigs supplied the voracious kilns with wood and carried the finished product to market. This was no inconsiderable fleet when it is realized that only the short strip of coast from Thomaston to Camden had been developed for this business.

In the days before the use of coal and oil it required thirty cords of wood to fire a single kiln. The harbors swarmed with the little vessels called "kiln wooders" from all along the eastern coast. Besides the cordwood cut for this purpose a market was to be had for the cast-off slabs and edgings of the sawmills. Thus the collecting of "skoots" in Bangor River became a business in its own right. As a rule these boats hailed from Maine, but among them were the famous St. John woodboats,

[256]

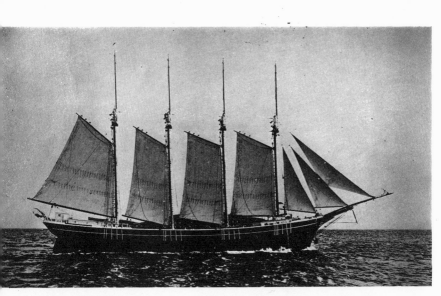

City of Georgetown—a four-master. *Courtesy Howard I. Chapelle.*

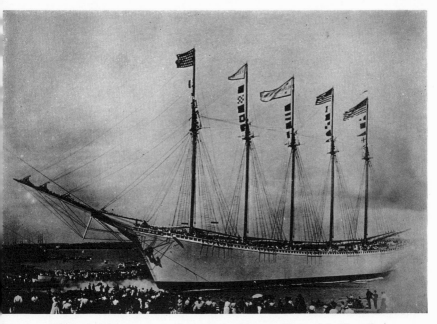

Elizabeth Palmer, 1903—a five-master. *Courtesy Howard I. Chapelle.*

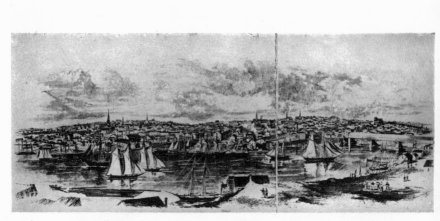

View of Bangor across the Penobscot from Brewer, about 1840.

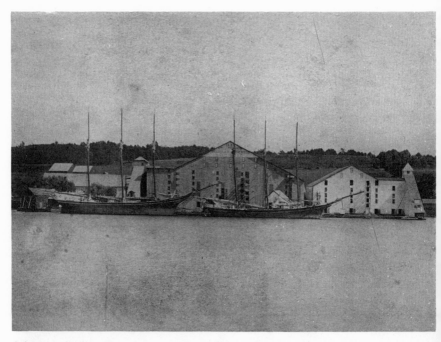

Schooners loading Kennebec ice at Cedar Grove, Dresden. *Courtesy Nat B. T. Barker.*

which were built of spruce and put together in the roughest possible manner with a cheapness which only the unsinkable character of the cargoes they were to carry allowed. The local wood boats were not much better. Many a one lacked a bowsprit lest it become tangled in the trees as she ran down some little river with her load. The foremast was stepped forward as far as possible, and topmasts were altogether lacking. They were broad of beam, and the wide stern had no overhang, so that the rudder hung "out of doors." So high was the wood piled on deck that the helmsman could not see over it. He would steer according to the directions bawled back to him by a man stationed forward on the top of the load.

The "Rockland limer," which carried the lime to market in rough spruce casks, was quite a different craft. She must be staunch and tight, for added to the other perils of the deep was the constant menace of fire. The slightest leak allowing the water to come in contact with the lime would cause a conflagration which could not be controlled by ordinary means. Schooners of moderate size were used. A stout platform would be built in the hold to avoid as far as possible any chance of contact with bilge water. Sometimes a deck load was carried, although this was regarded as a dangerous practice. For this purpose a second deck with open rails running well forward was built above the main deck.

The master needed a keen sense of smell. The odor of lime being slaked by water was an ominous danger signal. Smothering in short order was the only resort. Every crack and crevice through which air might get into the hold and the doors, ports, and smokestack were quickly sealed with plaster made from the lime. Then the craft was headed for the nearest harbor and anchored some distance from shore and away from other vessels. For at any time she might burst into flames. The schooner was stripped of all movables and the captain and crew sat down to await developments. Sometimes three months would go by before their patience was rewarded and the vessel saved.

If, however, the fire could not be smothered, the vessel was towed to some secluded place and scuttled. The rising tide entering through the holes cut in her bottom would put out the fire among the seething lime casks. But the swelling cargo would almost surely break the deck beams and hump the decks or burst out her sides beyond repair. Tales are told of the patching of the weakened hull by the plucky Captain, who by shoveling out the worthless cargo and working hard at the pumps brought his vessel home under her own sail. These days have now passed, and this dangerous cargo is towed to market in steel barges.

★   ★   ★

Sometime around 1820, William Bradstreet came up the Kennebec in his little 125-ton brig *Orion*. It was late in the fall, and she was frozen in at Dearborn's wharf in what was then Pittston. When the river broke up in the spring and the heavy cakes of ice floated about the brig, they were pulled aboard and stowed in the hold, and the *Orion* sailed for Baltimore with a cargo that cost nothing and sold for $700. This was the first shipment of "Kennebec River Ice," a name soon to be familiar the world over. It was a business which put millions of dollars into the pockets of Maine farmers, merchants, and shipowners. For years it was Maine's surest crop. In 1890, when the State House was remodeled, a picture of the ice cutter was placed on the stained-glass windows of the old senate chamber.

It was an enterprising shipbuilder and owner, Rufus K. Page of Gardiner, who erected the first ice house on the river, at Trott's Point in Richmond. There he stored some 1,500 tons, which he sold the next summer in the southern cities and the West Indies for the account of Frederick Tudor of Boston.

His plan was to give employment to his ship carpenters and their tools in the dull winter season. Plows to gouge lines across the ice fields were constructed by his shipsmiths, and the old whipsaw was taken from its pit to saw the cakes into four-foot lengths for storage. The speculation, however, did not show a sufficient profit, and for several years no ice was cut.

It was Frederick Tudor whose perseverance and ingenuity created a taste and a market for frozen dainties in almost every hot country. In 1831 he filled Page's building and also a temporary house he had put up on a Gardiner wharf, storing in all about 3,000 tons. Thereafter the business was carried on with success. When mild winters in the southern states left the rivers and ponds unfrozen, it was highly profitable. But when ice might be had near at home, there was a slump. In the winter of 1849 over 10,000 tons were cut on the river by Tudor and other independent operators.

The year 1860 and the entry into the business of James L. Cheeseman marks its beginning as a large industry. That year the crop was a failure south of Boston, but Kennebec ice was fifteen inches thick and clear as crystal. Cheeseman, who had hitherto operated on the Hudson, was so attracted by this that without delay he leased a lot on Bowman's Point, Farmingdale. Although it was February, he succeeded in stacking 30,000 tons before spring. In 1862 he bought the point and erected a permanent ice house. Here he introduced many improvements— steam for hoisting, endless chain conveyors, new plows, and other tools. Since much of his ice was taken by the government during the Civil War, his returns were large.

Soon both banks of the Kennebec, especially the reach extending twenty-five miles up river from Richmond, were lined with the houses of competing companies. Large operations were also begun on the Penobscot and the Cathance, and at a multitude of other points along the coast and inland. At one time there were 244 plants. The largest operators were the Knicker-bocker Ice Company of Philadelphia, who bought Cheeseman out in 1878, the Cochran-Ohler Ice Company of Baltimore, and the Independent and Great Falls Company of Washington. Besides these, many independent companies organized locally did a large business.

Only twice during the twenty years after 1870 did the cut fall below 1,000,000 tons. In 1880 it touched the 1,500,000 mark and paid an enormous profit. Ten years later 3,000,000 tons were stored, but a cool summer and lack of wisdom on the part of the speculators brought the operators a loss which more than ate up the profits of the ten previous years. Charles W. Morse of Bath in 1899 merged all the ice companies supplying Boston, New York, Philadelphia, Baltimore, and Washington into the American Ice Company. By enlarging the plants on the Hudson and cutting nearly all the supply in that river, great savings in transportation were made. In 1901 no ice was cut at all on the Kennebec, and in a few years the export ice business all but disappeared from Maine. In remodeling the State House in 1910 the ice cutter vanished from its windows.

These had been great days in the State of Maine. During the 3,000,000-ton harvest in 1890 at least 25,000 men and 1,000 horses were employed making ice. As they made hay in the summer, so they made ice in the winter.

A horse-drawn plowlike cutter marked out the strips and then scored them crosswise so that the field of ice to be cut came to look like a gigantic checkerboard. The sawyer then sawed down the line and cut off a strip—fifty feet and more in length. Tended by men with pick poles, these were moved through the open water toward the conveyor, which operated on an endless belt. There astride a platform stood a mountain of a man armed with a spade-ended crowbar. With a thrust and a blow as the strip passed beneath him he split off each block, which was then guided onto the endless chain and carried up to the chute leading into the ice house; there, tier upon tier, they were stowed and embedded in sawdust. Over all this scene was the contrast against the shining ice of the black forms of men and horses, and in the sharp air there resounded the shouted give and take of the trade.

Coffin has sung the saga of the ice harvest in *Kennebec Crystals,* but much is still left in the stories of the teamsters and workmen. To these fathers and sons the good money earned on the ice pushed back the margin between poverty and comfort or furnished a start toward a college education. Many a queer character drifted in to take part in what, along with the hard work, had in it much of a frolic. Their tall tales rival those told on the deacon seats in the lumber camps about Paul Bunyan.

The river was also busy during the summer season, though not with the same hectic activity. About the first of May the ice schooners began to come up the river in droves. Charles E. Allen, the historian of Dresden, counted as many as thirty vessels and three or four tugboats in sight from his river front at one time. He reports that he has seen more than sixty lying at anchor between Cedar Grove and Richmond Village, a stretch of some three miles. Thousands of men would find employment filling their holds with the chilly cargoes. In the early days they were limited to 300 tons, but later 1,000 tons were loaded. Three- and four-masted schooners were the craft first used, and this greatly stimulated the building of this rig. But the barges were at the last found more convenient.

The Knickerbocker Towage Company, headed by Captain Benjamin W. Morse, monopolized the towage business on the Kennebec. A fleet of from six to ten tugboats was kept busy towing the schooners in strings of from two to six up to the houses and then down again below Popham. In slack seasons this trade was a boon, especially to owners of old vessels too rotten to stand the strain of a deep-sea voyage. Some owners, however, would not allow their vessels to carry ice even on short coastwise trips. They believed that the fresh water from the melting ice and the constant straining of the cargo would permanently injure their ships.

On the Penobscot, in order to reach the channel where deeply laden craft could navigate, cribs built of heavy timber and ballasted with rock were placed many yards out from the shore and used as loading stages. These platforms, some forty feet square, were connected with the houses on shore by long chutes. The ice was shot down these into the holds of the waiting vessels. The sawdust from the Penobscot River mills, shipped along the coast and especially to Boston and used there for dunnaging the ice in the great square-riggers of Frederick Tudor for the long voyage to Calcutta and other far eastern ports, sometimes paid a better profit than a cargo of lumber.

★　★　★

Just as artificial ice and electric refrigeration has caused the disappearance of the ice schooner along the Maine coast, so artificial stone and concrete have almost put granite in the class of a vanished cargo. Granite quarrying was a leading industry for years. In 1890 Maine was first among the states in its production with a business totaling over $2,500,000. Its importance may be judged from the fact that one company alone, headed by Governor Bodwell at Vinalhaven, employed from twelve to fifteen hundred men and had a monthly payroll often amounting to $60,000.

Some of the finest qualities of granite are found on the headlands and islands along the Maine coast. With a product heavy to handle and of small value in comparison with its weight and bulk, Maine quarrymen had a distinct advantage over their competitors in the fact that cheap transportation could be conveniently had by water.

At many spots along the coast and rivers nature has provided granite with so lavish a hand that it lies almost on the surface ready to be taken. It was not even necessary to quarry deeply for it. When Dix, Hurricane, Fox and Crotch Islands, and Stonington in Penobscot Bay, Mount Waldo up the river, St. George and Spruce Head in Knox County to the westward, Hallowell on the Kennebec, and Jonesboro down east are mentioned, the Maine Coast man thinks of granite.

Little attention was paid to its possibilities until the third decade of the last century. The first cargo to be shipped from Vinalhaven on Fox Island is said to have been quarried by a New Hampshire man named Tuck and shipped by him in 1829 in the schooner *Plymouth Rock*. It was used to build the walls of a Massachusetts prison. In the building boom which followed the Civil War the business developed prodigiously. The list of public buildings, libraries, state capitols, city halls, churches, and residences built with Maine granite is a lengthy one. Not only building stone but paving and curbing stone and rubble were in such demand that many schooners and larger vessels were kept busy. As in the other trades, the quarry owners often owned and operated their own fleets.

It was rough and heavy work and the last resort of many an old vessel that had seen her best days. For example, the famous old *Bloomer* launched on the west shore of Mt. Desert Island was still carrying stone out of Penobscot Bay eighty-two years later. As George Wasson has remarked in *Sailing Days on the Penobscot:*

> It was a common remark that when a vessel got too old for even lumber coasting out of Bangor, or carrying wood for the Rockland lime kilns, she was considered none too ripe for

the stone business and was often loaded to scuppers with paving or huge blocks of granite.[2]

How huge some of the granite blocks were may be illustrated by the size of one quarried at Vinalhaven. The shaft was 60 feet long. It measured 5 by 5½ feet and in the rough weighed 185 tons. In order to set the column on board the vessel it was necessary to cut a hole in her bow and lay it in line with the keel on a bed of cross timbers. This is said to have been the largest monolith carved in modern times and to compare with the obelisks of the ancients. From the same town came the huge columns in the apse of the cathedral of St. John the Divine in New York City. Each of these was more than 54 feet high and weighed 120 tons.

A picturesque and important part of the stone fleet were the Chebeague Island rock sloops developed on that island in Casco Bay. They were employed in carrying stone and rock for use in wharfs, breakwaters, harbor retaining walls, and forts. At first they were small, and their chief occupation was carrying ballast for vessels in the yards up and down the coast. "Slooping" increased, and in the seventies half a hundred of them hailed from Chebeague alone. Their size had steadily grown, and when the *M. M. Hamilton* was built she carried the largest sloop sail afloat. Her mainsail measured 1,003 yards of canvas.

When the paper mills at Bucksport were built on the shore of the river from which the great Penobscot lumber fleet had formerly sailed, all the timber used in their construction came by rail from the west. Rockland lime now goes to market in steel barges towed by ocean tugs. Kennebec ice melts away harmlessly where it forms or piles up to work destruction in the

[2] Marine Research Society, 1932.

spring freshets. Only derrick booms stark against the sky, rusty boilers, and enormous cart wheels bear witness to the former importance of the granite quarries. The ships which were a part of all this too have gone, for there is now no more work for them to do.

CHAPTER FOURTEEN

The MAINE COAST FISHERMAN

As to the wealth which the colonies have drawn from the sea by their fisheries, you had all that matter fully opened at your bar. You surely thought those acquisitions of value for they seemed even to excite your envy; and yet the spirit by which that enterprising employment has been exercised ought rather, in my opinion, to have raised your esteem and admiration. And pray, Sir, what in the world is equal to it? . . . No sea but what is vexed by their fisheries. No climate that is not witness to their toils. Neither the perseverance of Holland nor the activity of France nor the dexterous and firm sagacity of English enterprise ever carried this most perilous mode of hardy enterprise to the extent to which it has been pushed by this recent people. . . .—Edmund Burke, *Speech on Conciliation with America*, March 22, 1775.

A fleet of three hundred vessels was seen off the harbor from the Observatory today catching mackerel. To the naked eye they presented the appearance of an immense city.—*Portland Reference Book*, October 21, 1850.

A TASTE FOR SALT CODFISH is well nigh an American national characteristic. In eighteenth-century Boston, no matter how luxurious or ceremonious the Saturday dinner party might be, it was not considered complete without a generous dish of dunfish at one end of the table. Nor was this alone a New England trait. President Washington was extremely fond of the fish. His

Saturday dinner, week in and week out, consisted of boiled potatoes, beets, and onions with "soaked-out" codfish all covered with sizzling fried pork scraps and egg sauce—the regulation down-east salt fish dinner. It is not surprising that one of the primary considerations of the First Congress in 1789 was the protection of the cod fisheries.

After the reduction of French Canada and the departure of hostile fleets from the fishing grounds, in the ten years after 1765 the District of Maine alone averaged 60 vessels a year in the fisheries. It gave employment to 300 men and brought in an annual revenue of $48,000 from a catch of 12,000 quintals of dried cod exported to the Mediterranean countries and the West Indies. At the peace conference after the Revolution the question of the fisheries was the first stumbling block encountered and the last obstacle overcome. Doughty John Adams persisted, and to the joy of the whole coast the treaty of 1783 secured to the fishermen their immemorial right to take fish anywhere in the sea where they "used any time heretofore to fish." Encouraged by this and by the bounty of five cents a quintal on dried or on a barrel of pickled cod granted by the First Congress, Maine fishermen by 1790, despite their lack of money and equipment, had won back half of their former prosperity. Thirty vessels were taking 120 men to the banks and bringing back some 4,500 quintals. Owing to the loss of their best markets in the British West Indies, these sold for only about $10,000.

In 1792 the first bounty was replaced by an allowance made to vessels engaged in the cod fisheries that were at sea at least four months of the year. This amounted to $1.50 a ton for vessels up to 30 tons and $2.50 for those of larger size, with a top limit of $170.00 a year. Three-eighths of this bounty went into the owner's pocket, and the remainder was distributed among the crew. Small boats under 20 tons might receive $1.00

a ton, provided they brought in twelve quintals for each ton of their measurement. These bounties, with some changes in scale, remained in force until after the Civil War.

In the period between the two wars with England little improvement was made in the models of the vessels. The off-shore Bank fisheries were carried on in barrel-bottomed schooners that were old-fashioned and clumsy. Only a small part of the Maine fleet was so employed. Most of the District fishermen sought the Bay of Chaleur, the Labrador shore, or the smaller banks nearer home—Old Man's Pasture, Matinicus, Sou'Sou' West, Spot of Rocks, Saturday Night Ledge, Kettle Bottom, Cashe's Ledge, or the Fippenies. For these grounds the Chebacco boat and the "Dogbody" were seaworthy enough. The Chebacco boat was so called from the parish in the present town of Essex, Massachusetts, where it originated. It was double-ended, pink—that is, sharp-sterned—and rigged with two pole masts stepped well forward. It had neither bowsprit nor jib. The Dogbody had the same rig, which was called "cat schooner," but it had a square stern.

Between 1797 and 1807 the tonnage of the Maine fleet more than doubled. The Portland district led with 2,927 tons, and the Penobscot and Frenchman's Bay districts, which grew rapidly after 1803, enrolled 1,726 and 1,011 tons respectively. The total tonnage of the state was 9,623, and this was the highest point it was to reach until 1820. Mr. Jefferson's embargo of 1807, although there was nothing in it to prohibit fishing, made the markets inaccessible, and the fleet was cut to a quarter of its former size in two years. At the close of Mr. Madison's War but 760 tons of the Maine fleet remained in existence. The stench of rotting fish in the embargoed vessels in the harbors suggested to the fishermen rotten politics in the ship of state.

After the war recovery was slow. By the treaty of 1818 American fishermen lost the right to take, dry, or cure fish within a three-mile limit of the shores of the British dominions except in unsettled places on the shores of southern Newfoundland and Labrador. Nor could they enter the bays or harbors to get bait—a most important item for the fishermen—but only for shelter, to repair damage, or to procure wood and water. Soon afterward the area was further restricted by England's adoption of the "headland theory," by which the three-mile limit was measured from a line drawn from headland to headland across bays and harbors.

To offset these restrictions in a measure, Congress increased the bounties so that $3.50 a ton went to vessels up to 30 tons and $4.00 to those from 30 to 96 tons. The response to this and the opening of many closed foreign markets was the beginning of the golden age of the Maine fisheries, a prosperity which would continue until the Civil War. By 1820 the fleet had increased to over 11,000 tons, with the Penobscot district leading and followed in order by Portland, Wiscasset, and Bath.

About this time there occurred Maine's only venture in the whale fisheries. In 1830 success of the whaling fleets of Nantucket, Provincetown, New Bedford, and Fair Haven suggested to the dissatisfied merchants of Wiscasset that here might be a way to retrieve their fortunes and build again the maritime prestige of the village. Accordingly the Wiscasset Whale Fishing Company was formed, and a hull on the Hitchcock ways at Damariscotta was bought and brought to Wiscasset. After being fitted out as a whaler and christened the *Wiscasset*, she sailed for the grounds under the command of Captain Richard Macy, an experienced whale fisherman. Forty months later she returned with 2,800 barrels of sperm oil. This was enough to clear the company of the cost of the ship and pay all the bills. Refitted, she sailed again, returning after a voyage of two years and a half with 900 barrels of sperm, $6,517 in cash, and 150 pounds of coffee. Although sperm oil was selling for over $1.00

a gallon, for some reason the company became discouraged and sold the *Wiscasset*.

Maine's venture in the seal fisheries was more tragic. In 1829 Samuel Hadlock, Jr., in command of the *Minerva*, in which he had gone "down to the ice after seals," was lost with the entire crew. He was one of five brothers, the sons of Samuel Hadlock, whom fortune had favored in the days of the long embargo. All of his brothers were sea captains, and all but one were lost at sea.

In the first six years after it became a state, Maine had about one-fifth of the tonnage of the fisheries of the United States. This gave employment to more than 2,600 men, and there was exported about $480,000 worth of fish a year. In addition to this, on the Maine coast were located over one-half the total number of fishing establishments on the Atlantic seaboard.

Each of the many little harbors had its fleet of fishing boats. Some were owned by merchants, others by neighbors who clubbed together to build them. Farmers and artisans could make one good trip "over the bay," that is, to Fundy or Chaleur, and return in time to finish their spring planting or take up their summer work. The full-time fishermen could go a second trip, generally to Labrador, Seal Island, or the Western or the Grand Bank. How this activity was carried on in the smaller centers has been described by Elijah Kellogg, who was personally familiar with the methods used in the town of Harpswell. In *The Fisher Boys of Pleasant Cove* he describes a voyage in one of the smaller vessels to Mingan, an island in the Gulf of St. Lawrence thirty miles northeast of Anticosti. The facts with which his stories were always heavily freighted provide a good picture of these early days in the "salt fisheries."

The fishermen were generally in very moderate circumstances—"poor yet making many rich." The cost of fitting out a vessel was from $800 to $1,500. To meet this situation many merchants in the coastal villages would furnish the vessel and outfit, undertake to supply the families of the crew while they were away, and then at the end of the voyage receive their return either in fish or in money. The skipper and his crew all fished on shares. No one received any money except the cook, who had monthly wages. If his duties permitted, he was expected to fish, and his catch belonged to the crew. If he was an exceptional cook he was sometimes allowed his share without any deduction from his wages.

The ancient custom was to fit the vessel "at the fifths," as it was called. It worked this way. The vessel, or, in other words, the owners, furnished one-fifth of the salt, provisions, lines, nets, bait, and so forth, and took one-fifth of the catch. The crew furnished the balance of the outfit and received four-fifths of what the fish brought when sold. Each man shared in proportion to the amount of fish he had caught. The phrase "high line" meant to catch the most fish. This meant more money and brought great reputation in the home village. The skipper, who provided his own charts and log book and took the responsibility for navigation, received as a bonus every sixty-fourth quintal. In like manner, the "salter," whose position corresponded to that of the mate on a merchant vessel, was customarily presented with a barvel (leather apron) and a pair of boots. The government bounty was divided on the same scale. In later years it became customary along the coast for the owners to take the whole bounty and fit out the vessel entirely, furnishing half the salt.

The pinky—a development of the Chebacco boat—came into use along the Maine coast sometime before 1820. Until 1840 it held the field against all others. They were of all sizes from 20 to 80 tons. The hull was very full forward, very sharp aft, deep, and of good breadth. Thus in heavy weather they could scud or work to windward, and in heavy seas they rode easily at anchor. Theirs was a simple schooner rig. The bowsprit was laid very high so that when lying at anchor with a long scope of cable the tremendous seas would not throw the cable over it. The timbers were gathered in at the stern, carried well abaft the sternpost, and brought to a point like those of a whaleboat. The false overhang thus provided a rest for the boom, and, being open on the underside, it formed a convenient seat for the crew. To the modest this was the pulpit; to the ribald, it was the seat of ease. When deeply laden, the sharp, smooth stern passed easily through the water, there was no pounding, and the pinky "steered like a pilot boat and did not leave a wake bigger than a shad."

For excellent sea boats, good sailers, and weatherly vessels, the model has, in the opinion of many, never been improved upon. Yet they have all but vanished from the seas. A few years ago Roger Sawyer reopened his grandfather's yard at Millbridge and built one for Howard I. Chapelle, the *Glad Tidings*. She was the first true pinky to be launched on the coast of Maine in over fifty years.

Below the narrow stern a bulkhead was built. This formed a bin for the salt which was taken in through a hatch under the tiller and taken out through a slide door into the hold when wanted by the salter. The cabin was well forward, with berths on each side and at the end with lockers beneath. The foremast rose up in the middle. Around this was built a circular table which, when not in use, could be slid up the mast out of the way. On the starboard side close to the ladder leading to the deck was a brick fireplace with a chimney of plank plastered on the inside to prevent fire. Inside the chimney was an iron bar on which was hung the Dutch oven. This was a deep iron pot with a flat bottom and an iron cover with a rim around it. When hot coals were piled on the cover as it hung over the fire, it would bake both at the bottom and at the top. A long-

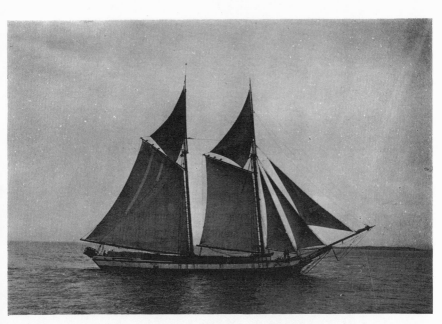

The *Lizzie D. Small* with a deck load of lumber. *Courtesy Peabody Museum of Salem.*

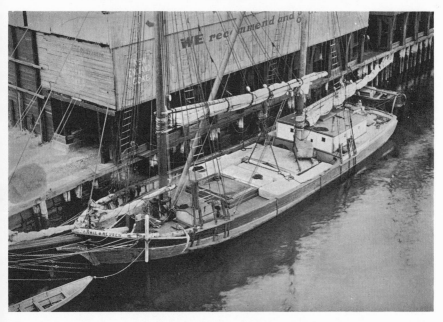

The *Annie & Reuben* deep laden with blocks of granite. *Courtesy Howard I. Chapelle.*

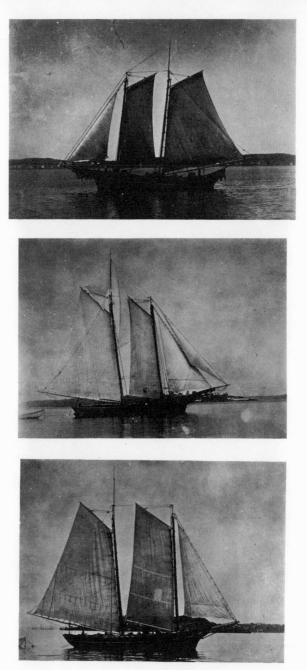

The Vanished Pinky

(Top) On her way to the fishing grounds with her nets over bowsprit and stern. (Center) Mackerel schooner *Oasis* out of North Haven about 1863. (Bottom) Herring schooner *Valiant* out of Friendship. *Courtesy Smithsonian Institution.*

handled frying pan, a kettle for stewing beans—they were not baked—and boards or tins on which to bake Indian cake comprised the cooking utensils.

Food was plentiful, if not in great variety. Fish and potatoes were the staples. There was plenty of salt pork, sometimes a little beef but oftener none, Indian corn meal, no butter except when it was brought as an extra, no sugar—the tea or coffee, if it was to be had, being sweetened with molasses. The bill of fare consisted of fish hash, beef hash, smoked halibut or herring, fried cod's tongues or a chowder of cod's heads, and, as a special treat, "scourer." This was corn meal mush with pork fat and scraps boiled into it and eaten with molasses.

On each side of the deck along the rail, pens were built. These "kids," as they were called, held each man's fish as they were caught. They were placed far enough apart so that a man could stand between them to handle his lines. Close by the main hatch was a very large kid crosswise of the vessel. This was to hold the whole day's catch. Into this, when the day's fishing was over, each man threw his fish, one by one, counting aloud while the captain recorded his catch in a book. When they were on the shoal chosen by the captain the pinky was anchored, her booms made fast with sheets hauled taut, and the helm lashed amidships that she might lie easy in the sea. A barrel of salted clams was then opened for bait and the lines, gaffs, and "killers" brought up. The captain having chosen the place where he was to fish, the rest of the crew "chalked" for berths by drawing lots. The midship berths were considered the best and the two forward ones the poorest.

When the day's fishing was over and the whole catch had been transferred to the large kid, dressing and salting began. This process differed in different times and places. As Kellogg describes it, it was like this. The "throater" cut the throat across and tore out the tongue, ripped open the belly and cut in on each side of the head. The "header" removed the liver, which was saved for the oil, drew out the entrails, and, breaking off the head, shoved the body along to the skipper. He was always the "splitter." With a wide-bladed knife he undercut and stripped out the backbone and then dropped the dressed fish into the hold. A fourth man, called the "idler," handed the whole fish to the throater, took away the tongues and livers, and when the cook was busy took his place tending the salter. When the dress gang got fairly at work a steady stream of fish was going down the hatch to the salter, who tiered or "kenched" them skin down, alternating napes and tails and with nice judgment sprinkled just the right amount of salt over them.

At the end of the voyage the fish were taken out at the flake yard and given into the care of the men who were to attend to the curing. In due time after they had been sold the captain and crew met to "settle the voyage." First the whole amount of the fish was reduced to dollars and cents. From this was taken the value of each sixty-fourth quintal—the captain's perquisite. Next the value of four-fifths of the salt, provisions, and everything the skipper and crew were to pay, including the cook's wages, was deducted. All bills having now been paid, the remainder was divided in proportion to the number of fish each man had caught as shown by the captain's record book. For their share of the bounty they must wait until the next January, when it would be paid out at the Custom House.

Although the Marblehead fleet had for a few years included two or three hand-line dory fishermen, the interest of Maine fishermen in this method was not aroused until 1858, when the *American Eagle* of Southport with some eight thirteen-foot dories came home with a full fare in about half the usual time. Soon hand-lining from the vessel's deck was practically given up and the new method became all but universal among the

The Maine Coast Fisherman

salt cod fishermen. Most Maine vessels sailed for the Western Bank on the spring trip in April, coming home in June. Then, if they did not go mackereling, they made a second trip, this time to Banquereau, getting back in September. The usual time for a trip to the Western Bank was about ten weeks, but some more skillful skippers "wet their salt" in less time. Captain George William Pierce made a record in 1875, having got a full fare in only six weeks and four days.

In the fifties, although the Maine fleet had in it many pinkies, a newer model with sharper bows and more dead rise was gradually finding a place. These were known to the fishermen as "Sharpshooters." Each vessel carried from eight to fifteen dories. They were nested on the main deck when making the passage but on top of the cabin when on the fishing grounds. Having arrived at his chosen berth on the bank, the skipper first assured himself that he could get "good school fish" by catching a cod and examining it critically. He then dropped his anchor and set his riding sail. Then, in the language of the fishermen, he was ready to "go to housekeeping"—that is, to catch fish.

At sunrise the dories were hoisted out. The fishermen rowed off in different directions, anchored, and threw over their lines. The gear consisted of two reels and codlines rigged with 3½-pound leads, with snoods and ganglings and two hooks bent on each line. The fisherman stood up in the boat. This was a feat in itself. With a line in each hand, he moved them up and down a few feet clear of the bottom. When he got a bite he quickly fastened one line and hauled in the other, often finding two cod on his hooks. They were pulled into the dory with the gaff. Throwing back his rebaited line, he quickly turned to his second line. By this time he generally had a fish on it.

The men worked hard and fast until the dory was full—sometimes with as much as 1,700 or 1,800 pounds of cod. The boats were called in around three o'clock, and after supper the

[275]

day's catch was dressed, the deck washed down, and the vessel pumped out. Then after having worked seventeen hours or more the crew turned in, calling it a day. Most of the Maine skippers were known as "Sunday keepers," as they fished only on weekdays.

The same year that Maine fishermen started hand-line dory fishing, the first down-east trawler, the *Albatross* of Boothbay, brought in 900 quintals of very large cod from the Gulf of St. Lawrence. The trawlers at first carried large Hampton boats, but they soon changed to dories, which could be nested. The trawls were merely strong ground lines with short lines or ganglings three feet long bent on at intervals of six feet and each carrying a hook. At one end of the ground line was attached an anchor and at the other a buoy. Each dory carried two men and from four to six tubs of trawl already baited and neatly coiled. This was thrown out as the boats rowed to leeward. When sufficient time had passed, the trawl was either under-run—that is, it was pulled across the dory and the fish were removed—or taken in. In Maine this method was employed on the inner banks along the shore, only a few trawlers going to the offshore banks. But the majority of those in salt fishing from 1870 to 1890 were hand-line dory fishermen.

By 1860 Maine had climbed to second place in the nation in the value of its fisheries. They now amounted to over a million dollars a year, having nearly doubled in the fifties. There were also twice as many fishing establishments as in any other state. They were not all small, as the average capital of about $2,000 invested in each indicates. Indeed, some were very large. The little town of Southport with just over 700 population had 59 bankers and mackerel vessels. Portland had 75, and Bucksport, Castine, and Lamoine several each in the salt cod business. In Lamoine in the seventies the annual catch came to 8,000 quintals of Gravel Bank cod and 100,000 of Magdalen herring.

The Maine Coast Fisherman

At Vinalhaven and North Haven, first known as the Fox Islands—the name survives in Fox Island Thoroughfare—on the western side of Penobscot Bay, there were owned in the half century between 1820 and 1870 at least 75 vessels which brought in their catches to the thirteen curing yards. Four freighters were kept busy carrying the salted product to Boston, and in the palmy days it exceeded 75,000 quintals a year. In like manner in the islands in the eastern part of the Bay, Swan's Island and Deer Isle, there was owned in 1860 a total of 10,000 tons of shipping. The bulk of it was engaged in the fisheries—"Bay men, Labrador men, and Bankers." So prosperous was this fleet that during the fifties, it is said, one-twelfth of all the fishing bounty paid in the United States went into the pockets of the Deer Isle fishermen.

It was about 1820 when Maine fishermen got the knack of catching mackerel. Up to that time the mackerel had been taken in nets or by trailing large hooks through the water. Between 1815 and 1820 some unknown genius invented the mackerel jig. This is a small hook with its shank enclosed in a shining sinker of lead or pewter. Then another nameless benefactor of the race discovered that by scattering bait on the surface as the vessel drifted to leeward, the hungry fish could be "tolled" up and would take the hook.

Mackerel are of very uncertain habits. Old Maine fishermen illustrate this by telling of two consecutive years. In the first one Blue Hill Bay was alive with mackerel, while Union River, which is separated from it only by Newbury Neck, had not a single fish; the next year the reverse was the case. They appear from some unknown place south of Cape Hatteras about the first of April and move northward. One body passes along the shore of Maine as far as the Bay of Fundy during July and August and returns south in the late fall. The best fishing grounds in the old days were off Mt. Desert Rock, Matinicus

Rock, Monhegan Island, Seguin, Casco Bay, and Cape Elizabeth. Another body of the mackerel swings offshore outside of George's Bank and reaches the Cape Shore of Nova Scotia in the latter part of May. These were known as "bay fish" and were also very important to Maine fishermen.

The introduction of the jig and the increasing market for mackerel, together with plentiful schools of fish, brought great prosperity to the hand-line fishermen from 1820 to 1831 and gave employment to a large fleet of various kinds of vessels. Indeed, 1831 is the banner year of all time for this method of fishing. The Maine fleet landed 386,548 barrels. This amount was not equaled until fifty years later, after the seine had come into use, when the catch, both fresh and salted, was over 400,000 barrels. After 1831 it fell off somewhat but was still large with many vessels engaged. For some years in the thirties and forties all varieties of fish were scarce off the Maine coast, and many mackerel fishermen went to the Bay of Chaleur and the Gulf of the St. Lawrence to find them. Some made the voyage in pinkies as small as 25 tons, the skippers showing remarkable skill in being able to navigate their small craft safely.

Jigging for mackerel was done in this wise. When the vessel was "on fish" it was allowed to drift. The men lined the rail, each in his allotted three feet of space and each with an empty barrel behind him into which to slat his fish. The skipper then threw the toll bait, menhaden with a few clams added, which he had ground all together in a bait mill, alongside fore and aft. This tolled the mackerel up and kept them near the surface. With remarkable skill and quickness the fishers "jigged" the shining fish over the rail and with a deft slat flipped them over into his strike barrel behind him. After the school stopped biting the catch was dressed, salted, and barreled, each man affixing thereto his own private mark. The business was very profitable, the price rising rapidly from $5.00 a barrel in 1830 to $19.00 in 1856 and $30.00 in 1864.

These high prices were an incentive to seek improvement in equipment and warranted greater investment in gear. A company of ten retired fishermen in Southport clubbed together and bought a purse seine in Boston. It was a crude affair, only about a quarter as large as those now used. Made of coarse twine, it was heavy, bulky, and hard to handle, and its cost was considerable—$2,400. They stored it at Cape Newagen, and having procured a seine boat and a small fishing boat, the *Niagara,* they gave it a trial near the Ark outside the harbor in September 1865. Their catch of large mackerel was remarkable. It took all the available men in town to handle the fish, and the net stock— that is, return—was about $8,000. Thus these pioneers netted about $800 each from the experiment. This was the beginning of mackerel seining along this part of the coast, which in the seventies and eighties brought such large returns.

Purse seines in the eighties were often 1,300 or 1,400 feet long and 30 feet deep. They were equipped with corks along the top to keep the head up and lead sinkers on the bottom to hold down the foot. Around the bottom through iron rings ran the purse line. This was hauled up after the fish had been enclosed. Like the action of a puckering string, it draws together and shuts up the bottom of the net, thus forming a purse to hold the silver fish. In prosperous years one haul might take and hold from 300 to 700 barrels of fish, filling the vessel full "from rail to rail and from windlass to wheel box."

At such times it was impossible to dress and salt the mackerel before they spoiled. In consequence, a bag net to hang alongside was devised. There they might be kept until the crew could handle them. One of the first of these was invented by skipper Hanson B. Joyce of Swan's Island. Later an improved one was patented by H. E. Willard of Portland. When the fish were dressed and salted at sea, the barrels were first packed tight full of clean, white fish, then headed up, and finally filled up through the bunghole with strong salt pickle. When the vessel came in to its home station, these "sea barrels" were opened and the mackerel sorted and culled into "tinkers," "threes," "twos," "ones," and "extras" and packed for the market, 200 pounds to the barrel.

Portland, Southport, Boothbay, and the Penobscot Bay Islands, particularly those of the Burnt Coat group, were the chief centers of the mackerel purse-seining business. The Swan's Island skipper Hanson B. Joyce was high-liner of the New England fleet for seven years from 1875 to 1881. In 1881 he landed from his schooner, the *Alice*, the largest catch of mackerel ever brought in by a single skipper. The 4,900 barrels gave his vessel a stock of $28,000, which was also the largest amount made in the fleet up to that time. Each of his crew earned $1,000 to $1,200 for the eight months' work. Another Maine skipper, Eben L. Lewis of Boothbay Harbor, was high-liner for a year or two in the eighties.

Among the early cod fishermen the despised "white-eye" or haddock was thrown back into the water in disgust. After the introduction of the delectable "finnan haddie" in the seventies and the marketing of freshly caught fish, the popular taste rapidly changed. Haddock became more popular as a table fish and brought a higher price than cod. The "shore haddock," generally regarded as the best fish, were taken in winter on the inside banks and ledges by trawling. These "haddockers" usually made short trips of not much over twenty-four hours. Larger vessels came in from George's Bank sometimes with fares of 100,000 pounds caught in three or four days. Winter haddock catching is the extreme of hardship. The men in their small boats must endure freezing winds, snowstorms, angry,

The Maine Coast Fisherman

choppy seas, and constant labor while on the grounds. One who has seen a banker come into her wharf in a thick snowstorm, her sails sheeted with ice from the flying spray, her running rigging frozen stiff, and every spar encased in ice, will never object to the high price of fresh haddock.

The rapidly increasing demand for fresh fish called for faster vessels to bring the catch more quickly to market so as to secure the top prices. A mania for speed characteristic of merchantmen of the fifties took possession of the fishermen, and the clipper schooner came into being. The models were increasingly more shoal with less and less dead rise, long, concave bows and very large sail plans. These changes produced speed but made them easy to capsize when they heeled in a stiff breeze. Although the loss of life and property was appalling, the model was popular well into the eighties.

One of the more famous of the Maine smart sailers was the *Georgie Willard*, built at Bath and commanded by George Willard, for whose daughter she was named. Skipper Willard was acknowledged all along the coast to be the greatest sailing master of his day. During the ten years before his death that he held the *Georgie's* wheel, very few could beat her as she led the mackerel seiners into New York and Fulton Market. The model of the *Georgie* was so sharp that when she fitted out for her first voyage a part of her crew backed out and would not go. They were afraid of her, called her a "diving bell," and predicted her loss in the first heavy gale. She proved to be one of the finest sea boats, riding out the gales like a gull, and was especially fast when close-hauled.

In 1880, A. M. Smith, who was one of the largest individual owners of fishing craft in Portland, had built in Kennebunk, on a model furnished by Joseph Dyer, the *Elizabeth W. Smith* of 82 tons. She has been claimed to be the first of a new type of fishing vessel. The next of this model was the 80-ton *Fannie O.*

Spurling, built in 1882 for Captain Benjamin Spurling. She proved to be a very fast sailer and in the mackerel fisheries stocked $24,000 in four months. The same year, also in Kennebunk, on the same model enlarged to 110 tons, he had constructed the famous *Elsie M. Smith*. The *Elsie* was built for young Captain Lincoln Jewett, and as her skipper he made a national reputation.

As the greatest sail carrier and most skillful helmsman of the down-east fleet, he has become a tradition. In two trips to the Bay of Chaleur, within the compass of ten weeks, which included coming and going, he stocked $13,000. Skipper "Linc" handled the *Elsie* as if she were a small boat or yacht, pushing her under whole sail in heavy winds and rough seas and slapping her without mishap into a dock full of vessels—a feat few would care to attempt. It would be hard to persuade some of the older Maine fishermen that it was not the competition of such vessels as the *Elsie* and her sisters that caused Massachusetts fishermen to call in the young yacht designer Edward Burgess to model for them the notable *Fredonia*.

The Civil War marks the close of an era in the Maine fisheries. The bounty which for nearly three-quarters of a century had eked out the scanty returns received by the fishermen was removed by Congress. The result was that the salt cod fisheries decreased over one-half in five years and steadily dwindled so that in 1900 only six Maine vessels were thus engaged. This brought disaster not only to the men and vessels engaged but also to merchants along shore. Many, who had built great salthouses and maintained large general stores to supply the bankers and seiners, found their profitable business gone.

Up to this time Castine, the wealthiest town in Maine in proportion to its population, had been the great salt depot of eastern Maine. Sometimes as many as five hundred fishermen assembled in the capacious harbor in the spring waiting to take in salt and other supplies for the four-month voyage to the Grand Banks or the Bay of Chaleur. During the summer would come the salt fleet from Cadiz or Liverpool, Castine ships with great cargoes of coarse salt, to be stored in the staunch salthouses and sold by the ton to the fishermen coming from all quarters. Of this trade the town had almost a monopoly. In the fall the fishing fleet would return with the harvest of the sea and dispose of their cargoes. Again in January, they returned to collect the bounty with which the United States encouraged them in their labors.

After 1857 Castine's importance as a fishing and shipping center rapidly decreased. Great losses were sustained by the principal merchants during the Civil War, and the once numerous fleets of fishing schooners became smaller and smaller as such ports as Portland and Gloucester gained an advantage, being nearer the market. There were only left the fine old homes and the massively framed salthouses on the wharves to testify to the importance of the trade in the salt cod era.

As has been the case not once or twice in the history of the industries of the state, so with the Maine fisheries, the variety of the resources and the enterprise of the citizens held her place as second in the nation. By this time the railroads were penetrating down the entire coast. This brought about a great increase in the fresh fish business. Ice pens quickly replaced the salt bins on the bankers. Also the war had increased the demand for many products.

Perhaps the richest of these "war babies" was the increased market and high price of fish oil. The menhaden, mistakenly called the "pogy," is a fish much like the herring. It finds its best food along the Maine coast and becomes very fat here, yielding nearly twice the oil it does south of Cape Cod. It had long been used for bait, and as early as 1855 its oil had been tried out in numerous small establishments along Blue Hill Bay. This oil, which brought only 25 cents a gallon in 1863, soared to $1.25 during the war. An abundance of the fish appeared off the coast at this time, and oil factories were built on a more elaborate scale. The first large establishment was that of W. A. Wells & Company at Bristol in 1864.

This fishery developed rapidly from small seine boats fishing just offshore to schooners with fleets of small boats attached and finally to fleets of steamers which swept the seas far and wide. By 1876 over 2,000,000 gallons of oil were produced along the Lincoln County shore alone. The fish were cooked by steam and the oil extracted by hydraulic pressure. The residue was profitably used in place of Peruvian guano by fertilizer factories which were built alongside the oil works. In 1876 this product amounted to 21,414 tons. Many a comfortable home along the shores of Boothbay, Bristol, and Bremen is the result of these fisheries. The prosperity was of short duration. After 1878 the menhaden deserted the Maine coast and have never returned with enough regularity to make the business profitable again.

Herring, from time immemorial the people's greatest food fish, abound all along the coast but especially in Passamaquoddy Bay. Anciently they were taken by driving the schools into narrow bays or inlets or by attracting them by fires on the boats —that is, "torching"—and then dipping them from the water with nets. Weirs of brush or twine followed, and later seines. At Eastport as early as 1808 the Scotch method of smoking was adopted, and all along the shore smokehouses sprang up. This business as late as 1900 amounted to nearly 6,000,000 pounds a year. In the same year 2,500,000 pounds were pickled for bait or food and 72,000,000 were kept fresh by freezing to be used as bait or canned as sardines. The sardine-packing business which was commenced at Eastport in 1875 expanded to such an extent in twenty-five years that it was occupying 68 factories, employing 6,000 people, and producing a product worth $3,500,000. In this business Maine has a natural monopoly. There are no small herring suitable for this purpose south of the state line.

Shipbuilding up and down the coast has since the earliest times been stimulated by the demands made upon it by the fisheries. The town of Bristol will serve as an example. From 1801 to 1895 there were put off her 275 vessels—the greater part of them fishing schooners. The Forbeses and McFarlands built a goodly number of fishing schooners, but the largest and perhaps the best-known fishing schooner builder on the Maine Coast was the A. and M. Gamage Shipbuilding Company of South Bristol. In the half century of their activity they launched 77 schooners of the finest type.

Moreover, it is the fisheries which keep the art alive at the present time. The proof is to be had in the notices in any waterside journal of the hulls of all types of fishing craft which are in course of construction for both local, out-of-state, and even foreign accounts such as the sardine fisheries of Bordeaux. Just as at any time in the three centuries since the launching of the first wooden ship, the yards on the Maine coast, from the Piscataqua down east to the St. Croix, are still active and busy.

CHAPTER FIFTEEN

The MAINE SEACOAST TOWN

It was a dog's life but it made men out of those who followed it. I see a change for the worse even in our town here; full of loafers now, small and poor as 'tis, who would have followed the sea, every lazy soul of 'em. There is no occupation so fit for that class of men who never get beyond the for'cas'le. I view it, in addition, that a community narrows down and grows dredful ignorant when it is shut up to its own affairs, and gets no knowledge of the outside world except from a cheap, unprincipled newspaper. In the old days, a good part of the best men here knew a hundred ports and something of the way people lived in them. They saw the world for themselves and like's not their wives and children saw it with them. They may not have had the best of knowledge to carry with 'em sightseeing; but they were some acquainted with foreign lands and their laws and could see outside the battle for town clerk here in Dunnet; they got some sence of proportion. Yes, they lived more dignified and their houses were better within and without. Shipping's a terrible loss to this part of New England from a social point o' view ma'am.—Captain Littlepage in *The Country of the Pointed Firs,* by Sarah Orne Jewett.[1]

IN THE YEAR 1860 there were 11,375 mariners in the State of Maine. They comprised almost one-fifth of the population. Of these, 759 were masters of ships. In turn nearly half of these were in command of "Cape Horners."

The little town of Searsport with 1,700 inhabitants will

[1] Houghton Mifflin Company, 1896.

serve as an example. It was known in every deepwater port in the world. Over a hundred and fifty masters of full-rigged ships knew it as home. In the seventies and eighties it is estimated that 10 per cent of all the shipmasters in the American merchant marine had Searsport as their hail. In 1889, 33 captains out of 77 were in command of Cape Horners.

Many of their vessels were built for their own account in the Matthews, Merrithew, Carver, and McGilvery yards at the head of the harbor. In later years, when the shoal waters precluded the launching of the larger ships, the Searsport captains had their ships built up the Penobscot at Brewer and Bangor. Out of twenty full-rigged ships built there, Lincoln Colcord lists at least eight for Searsport accounts. Or they turned to Bath, and Ebenezer Haggett at Newcastle on the Damariscotta was a favorite.

Before the railroads thrust their lines down the Maine coast in the fifties, the only outlook for many of the towns east of Portland was toward the sea. The harbor mouth was a door leading out into life. To them in reality it opened up the world. Many a man built his home facing the sea with its back to the village street. And from the front door a shell-bordered walk led down to the family wharf or shipyard. The inhabitants of a seacoast town in Maine in their customs and habits, hopes and fears, ambitions and disappointments, language and institutions, and even their loves and hates, "followed the sea."

The shipmaster had an assured place in the community. He took precedence over all save the members of the "learned professions." They were his peers. Even more than the clergymen, he decided the character of the community and gave tone to its style of living. Generally he retired from the sea at an early age--fifty or thereabouts, having acquired a competence that assured gracious living. His was a broad outlook on life, and his seasoned judgment and business efficiency were often a boon to his neighbors. With half of his mature life still before him he often found a second career—in business, as ship's husband for his own or agent for his neighbor's vessels; in politics, as selectman, mayor, or member of the state legislature; and in public service as president of the village bank or trustee of its academy. His opportunities for useful activity were many and varied, and he had no fear of the woes of idle retirement.

Although Maine's retired shipping men had no Charles Bulfinch or Samuel McIntyre to design their houses, their homes in Wiscasset, along Summer Street in Kennebunk, State Street in Portland, High Street in Bath or Belfast, and in fact in all the coastal villages, have a charm as enduring as that which characterizes Boston's Beacon Hill or Chestnut Street in Salem. Massachusetts architects such as Alexander Paris and Nicholas Codd of Boston and Aaron Sherman of Duxbury may in some instances have contributed their skill, but in large measure these houses are the work of local ship joiners, wood carvers, and cabinetmakers. They acquired a nice appreciation of line and form in that finest school of design, the modeling of vessels. Not only the great square mansions of the merchants and shipmasters but also more modest homes possess this same sense of proportion and simplicity which give to them an unmistakable dignity and charm.

The walk to the front door was bordered with queen conch shells. Inside were many other shells picked up on tropical beaches and used as ornaments—murex, nerita, cowry, spiny oyster, and an abundance of coral. China tea sets, Japanese screens, satinwood and lacquer boxes, teakwood chests, and many another curio were to be seen. Out in the pantry there were delicacies no longer familiar—curry powders, guava jelly, preserved tamarinds, and blue jars of Canton ginger in syrup. On the parlor mantelpiece were artistically arranged bouquets of the feathers of tropical birds or the silky white clusters of pampas grass.

Even the common articles of daily living bespoke foreign lands. The head of the house cut his morning newspaper with a sandalwood paper knife. He cast up his accounts at a desk of camphorwood. When his wife went calling, she wore her beautifully embroidered shawl of Japanese silk and carried her cards in their case of filigreed ivory—a miracle of Chinese carving. The children spent many a rainy day over ingenious puzzles devised by Eastern minds or turning over brilliantly colored Chinese pictures. The ever-present whatnot was a museum in miniature. It was laden with curiosities from every corner of the world—ostrich eggs, Japanese trick fans, coral beads, queer necklaces, scrimshaw work (which is the curious carving done by sailors at sea), pieces of jade, lumps of pumice, and even bottles of volcanic ash swept up from the deck of the vessel a hundred miles away from the volcano.

The favorite gathering place in a Maine Coast community of the boys of today is the neighborhood garage. There, in the gas-laden atmosphere, if you listen, you will hear intelligent debate as to the relative merits of every automobile under heaven, and the talk reveals considerable technical knowledge of differentials, transmission or ignition, crank shaft, carbureter, and choke. All these are part and parcel of the vocabulary of the present generation.

Had you sat with the grandfathers of these boys under the willows near the building yards, breathing in the fresh salt air driven upriver by the flooding tide and sweetened with the odor of the spruce and hard pine chips lying all about, the conversation would have been equally intelligent. But barks and brigantines, ships and topsail schooners would have been the subject of debate, and words all but meaningless to this genera-

[289]

tion, such as futtock, apron, timber strake, stemson, keelson, mizzen, spanker, and jibboom would have fallen on your ears. For all these were a part of a boy's vocabulary in the old ship-building days.

As the boy grew older he found that even his school curriculum followed the sea. His Greenleaf's National Arithmetic had sections devoted to subjects now no longer of common interest. There were pages given to definitions, tables, and problems in "Custom House Business," "Reduction of Currencies," "Tare and Tret," "General Average," "Duodecimals," "Tonnage," and "Gauging." All these were to fit the young captain to transact business in any part of the world. The last year in the local Academy always offered a course in navigation with Bowditch as the textbook. Many of the schools in towns with a West India or South American trade added Spanish to the regular course of studies. Geography was a living subject. The inadequate descriptions of foreign countries and ports given in the textbooks were made vivid by the graphic descriptions of uncles, cousins, and neighbors to whom the city of Cadiz or the harbor of Shanghai was as familiar as the home town and the bay out front.

Before the growing size of the vessels and lack of native timber or insufficient financial resources led to consolidation of the building industry in the larger centers with deepwater harbors, nearly every town on the Maine coast or along the tidewater rivers had local building yards. The economic life of the whole community centered about them, for they provided the livelihood of a large proportion of the inhabitants. Besides the common labor needed in the work, every town had its experts in the varied skills. In Kennebunk in 1874 Captain Nathaniel Lord Thompson was at the height of his career and his powers. In the thirty-five years that he built on the Kennebunk River, he constructed, either on his own account or as principal owner or on contract for others, 101 vessels—41 ships, 11 barks, 5 brigs, 39 schooners, and 3 steamers. All this gave employment to 8 master carpenters, 5 carpenters, 6 smiths, 5 joiners, 5 painters, 3 fasteners, 2 calkers, a spar maker, a brass founder, and a tin "knocker." The main support of all of these was shipbuilding.

Thus the construction of a vessel was a community affair. As the saying went, "all the parish" had an interest in it. The captain for whom she was being built would take a goodly number of shares, and also he would lay off a voyage to oversee her building and especially her rigging. The contracting builder and the merchant for whose fleet she was being built would each be responsible for a part. Then the remainder would be taken up in small blocks by the joiner, the calker, the smith, the lumberman who had furnished the frame, and the ship chandler who fitted her out, not to mention farmers, lawyers, doctors, and village storekeepers. A large proportion of the citizens of the town had an interest in its vessels. The usual division of shares was into sixteenths, thirty-seconds, or sixty-fourths, but the registers show that they were often split up into many more. One Machiasport schooner was divided into three hundred sixty-fourths among thirty owners. Shares in the local shipping were the securities of those days along the coast.

This made for a widespread interest in the vessel's fortunes. In the later days she was seldom seen off the little town where she was launched. Rather she saw and was seen in the great deepwater ports of the world. None the less her career was followed with anxious interest. Turning the faded pages of the files of that gone but not forgotten institution of seventy-five years ago, the "weekly family journal of literature, news, etc."—for example, the *Portland Transcript*—one realizes with what care its contemporary readers scanned the column under the heading "Marine Journal." The sight of a well-known name under

"Arrivals" caused how many prayers of thanksgiving! Or again mention of another ship under the head "Spoken" lifted a heavy load of anxiety that was oppressing another. Last in the column, withholding ill news until all good news was told, comes the heavy black line "DISASTERS"—the cause of how many heartaches and tears!

World news was of local interest. It was minutely and intelligently discussed on the post office steps, around the pot-bellied stove in the village store, and at the dinner table in the home. This was especially so during the hectic days when the fortunes of war might make or break the family fortune. Revolution in South America might seem of small import to a Maine town but to Kennebunk it meant the loss of one of her finest ships. Whether the English cabinet was liberal or conservative would seem a matter of no concern on the Maine coast, but it was the cause of casual negligence that allowed the *Alabama* and her sister cruisers to get to sea and deal a tragic blow to American shipping in the loss of some two hundred magnificent ships. Thus were the people of the smallest seacoast town brought into contact with the wide world. As Captain Littlepage said, it "gave them perspective," and lifted them above the petty commonplaces that too often stultify small-town life.

This seafaring folk had other wide interests. There were the many pleasant personal relationships with people of different nationalities and background. Especially was this so in the West India trade. Skippers made friends of the island merchants and planters with whom they did business, and this resulted in agreeable social exchanges and mutual understanding. Boys were brought home to live in the captain's family and attend the local academy. The catalogue of one school in a single year shows five pupils from Cuba, one of whom was a Garcia, as well as two others from Liberia. Merchants from New Orleans, Mobile, and other cotton ports came to the villages with their families to spend the summer while their "kettle-bottom" was being built in the local yard. The relationships which were thus established made especially tragic the final break between the North and the South.

A tang of salt touched and seasoned the religious life of the community. Not all Maine ships were christened with a bottle of rum. It was not unusual to have a religious ceremony or at least a prayer before the blocks were split out. This was the unvarying custom in the Russell yard at Pembroke. When in Brunswick the Pennells' last and largest vessel, the *Benjamin Sewall*, was launched, General Joshua Chamberlain, the president of Bowdoin College, spoke and Professor John S. Sewall led in prayer as a thousand heads were reverently bowed. In Kennebunk it was once the custom for the crew of a vessel to come to church in a body on the Sunday after they came home.

Often a popular preacher, one who "knew the chart of a sailor's heart," was asked to speak to the mariners at a special service. In 1821 Dr. Edward Payson was invited to address the seamen of Portland. There was no Bethel church at the time, and the "Old Jerusalem" was packed with sailors. There were many vessels in the harbor, and all the boardinghouse keepers lined up everyone in their houses. They made a long and remarkable procession as they marched up from the "black wharves and the slips." Dr. Payson was a pulpit orator second to none in New England and his sermon was replete with references to ships and the sea. So tense was the attention that as he described the last judgment, saying, "Then our world driven by the last tempest will strike and be dashed in pieces on the shores of eternity," an excited sailor leaped to his feet and cried out, "She has struck!" and caused a near panic in the crowded meetinghouse.

[293]

The same year the mariners of Yarmouth asked the Rev. Stephen Chapin to preach to them. This good pastor's skillful blending of nautical and theological terms in his closing exhortation may be of interest. He asks:

> What is your present character and condition? Have you been launched from the stocks of nature into the ocean of grace? Have you on board all things necessary for your passage to eternity? Where is your pilot? Are you furnished with chart and compass? Is the Bible your support and guide? Is it by this book you ascertain your position, your course and your bearings? Are you supplied with ships stores to last the voyage? When you make harbor and enjoy temporary rest and peace from the storms of life do you preserve an anchor watch lest you be assaulted and robbed by enemies or drift from your ground and be carried upon rocks and quicksands? Do you often try the lead and heave the log to know your bottom and rate your run? If so, happy men, happy mariners, spread all sail and the winds of mercy will soon waft you into the port of eternal rest.

How close these "sky pilots" were to the lives of their people may be judged by Elijah Kellogg's introduction of himself as he took up his work as the pastor of the Mariner's Church and chaplain of the Boston Sailor's Home. Referring to his pastorate in Harpswell, he said:

> The greater portion of my life has been spent among seamen, either at sea or on shore. The first personal effort, to any extent, I made for the salvation of souls was while teaching in a community of sailors. The first sermon I preached was to sailors. The first couple I married were a sailor and his bride. The first child I baptized was a sailor's child. The first burial service I performed was over the body of a seaman. The society with which I have been connected during the last eleven years is with scarcely an exception composed of sailors and their families. There is not a house in the parish in which the roar of the surf may not be heard, and in many of them the Atlantic flings its spray upon the door stone.

The Maine Seacoast Town

Two popular hymns have a Maine coast background. Although the words of "Jesus Savior, Pilot Me" were written by Edward Hopper while he was pastor of the Mariner's Church in New York Harbor, the music was composed by John Edgar Gould, a native of Bangor. The other is a famous old nautical hymn which fifty years ago was a universal favorite—"Throw Out the Life Line, Someone Is Sinking Today." Both words and music were written by the Reverend Edward S. Ufford, a Baptist preacher, lecturer, and evangelist. For many years he conducted the Bethel Mission, near Snow's shipyard at Rockland. It is said to have been written after the pastor had seen the drill of the crew of the Coast Guard Station on Whitehead Island.

The talk in a Maine seacoast village seventy-five-odd years ago was enriched by many a salty word or phrase that had come ashore with its seamen. This seafaring usage formed almost a dialect. Dean Chase in his entertaining monograph on *Sea Terms Come Ashore* tells a story also quoted by Joanna C. Colcord in her equally delightful volume on the same subject:

> An exasperated mother was chasing her twelve-year-old son in a gale of wind. The mother with her wide spread of skirts was bearing down on him and fast overtaking him when his eight-year-old brother sang out,
> "Take her on the wind, Jimmy!"

And Miss Colcord comments, "Only a longshore boy could have said that." An old sailor writing of seafaring language in *Scribner's Magazine* some years ago entitled his article, "An Elegy for a Dying Tongue." In the days of the wooden ship it was a living language along the Maine coast.

Today we use many of the terms, but their original setting has been lost. We speak of "running afoul" of someone or something. To our grandfathers the expression conveyed not a mere chance encounter but rather a not too pleasant entanglement of rigging and spars. We say we are "taken aback." This phrase derived from the decided shock of sails which a moment before had been full and drawing suddenly blown flat against the masts. When they claimed they "hadn't room to swing a cat" this meant no cruelty. It had reference to the boatswain's cat-o'-nine-tails. We speak of a vacillating person as "backing and filling." While we may not be as ignorant as the inland-bred English teacher who explained it to his class as the process of backing into and filling a dumpcart in a gravel pit, we cannot appreciate the complicated operation in navigation which it describes. When in an extremity one refers to his predicament as "the bitter end," one uses the "bitter" as an adjective. But consider the hazardous situation of a ship with all her cable out up to the windlass-bitts, with no reserve to ward off disaster. We do not realize that we are using sea language when we speak of an honest man as "aboveboard," of a penniless one as "hard up," of a thrifty soul as having "an anchor to windward" or a well-informed one as "knowing the ropes." In the morning we "turn out" and "turn to," and at night we "turn in."

To the sailor and coast villager certain place names, as Dean Chase points out, had peculiar connotations. To the skipper of the coasters "The Cape" meant Cape Cod, but to blue-water men it always meant the Cape of Good Hope. Although the Atlantic lay to the east of New England, it was, by ancient usage inherited from European mariners, always known as the "Western Ocean." Similarly the Azores, even as in Columbus' time, were known as the "Western Islands." Any Mediterranean port beyond Gibraltar was "up the Straits." The "Middle Passage" referred to the westerly course in the days of the slave trade through the trades from Africa to the West Indies. It was the middle leg of the triangular voyage from New England to

The Maine Seacoast Town

Africa, the West Indies, and home. "The Horn," of course, referred to Cape Horn, but the "West Coast" always meant the west coast of South America, while the corresponding part of North America was known as the "Pacific Coast." "Out East" was any voyage to the Orient, and by "the River" sailors signified the Rio de la Plata.

Very little attention was paid to the native pronunciation of foreign place names. They were approximated to something as near to English as possible. Hilo in Hawaii became High-Low; Buenos Aires was Bunny's Ears; Montevideo, Monty-vée-dio; Talcahuano in Chile, Turkey-wanna; Porto Rico, Portyreek; and Rio de Janeiro was shortened to Rio. In no way did a landlubber betray his inland origin so surely as by his pronunciation of nautical terms. Even Webster had to come to his assistance and give a second pronunciation of the word as it would be heard on shipboard. To say nothing of the careful phonetics which nautical usage requires in boxing the compass properly, if the inlander would not provoke the derision of the seacoast folk he must disregard the spelling of forecastle and say "fok's'l," studding sail must be "stun's'l," and even so innocent-appearing a word as leeward must be pronounced "lū-erd." And so on *ad infinitum.*

The description of life on the Maine coast in *The Country of the Pointed Firs*, by Sarah Orne Jewett, has the contour and quality of a true classic. In our own time Mary Ellen Chase has written of the seagoing tradition not only as a part of the goodly heritage but as a vital force in the lives of the people. Even now in the quiet villages and towns of the Midwest and West to which Maine-bred people have scattered there are men and women who have, as it is said along the coast, "salt in their blood." Although the wharves have crumbled and the building yards are grass-grown, although the ships, barks, brigs, and even the great schooners are now to be seen only in pictures and their captains sleep on the hill overlooking the ocean they loved so well, they have the sea woven into the fabric of their lives.

BIBLIOGRAPHY

GENERAL

MANUSCRIPTS

The Custom House records of the old Maine customs districts are now in the National Archives. A list of registers, enrollments, and licenses issued at Maine ports and now in the National Archives is given in an article by Forest R. Holdcamper in the *American Neptune* of July 1941.

A very complete list of manuscripts relating to Maine shipping may be found in Part II of *A Reference List of Manuscripts Relating to the History of Maine*, compiled under the direction of Elizabeth Ring, published as University of Maine Studies, 2nd Series, No. 45, Orono, 1939.

Badger, Neal and Pray, papers—The Misses Locke, Kittery, Maine
Clapp, Asa and A. W. H., papers—Maine Historical Society, Portland, Maine
Colcord, Capt. T. R., Sixteen Track Charts—Penobscot Marine Museum, Searsport, Maine
Fernald and Pettigrew papers—Peabody Museum, Salem, Mass.
King, William, papers—Maine Historical Society
Knox, Gen. Henry, papers—Maine Historical Society
Lord, Albert, papers—Maine Historical Society
Marks, Lionel Peabody—Maritime History of Maine, Maine Historical Society
Pepperell papers—Maine Historical Society
Pote, Samuel, papers (1731–1789)—Maine Historical Society
Preble, Commodore Edward, papers (1761–1807)—Maine Historical Society

[299]

Sewall Family papers—Arthur Sewall, Bath
Thornton papers—Maine Historical Society
Witherle Family papers—Miss Amy Witherle, Castine

NEWSPAPERS AND PERIODICALS

Bangor News
Bangor Weekly Courier
Bath Anvil
Bath Daily Times
Belfast Republican Journal
Eastern Argus (Portland)
Eastport Sentinel
Hallowell Gazette
Lewiston Saturday Journal
Lincoln County News
Old Eliot
Old Times in North Yarmouth
Portland Advertiser
Portland Board of Trade Journal
Portland Daily Press
Portland Gazette
Portland Sunday Telegram
Portland Sunday Times
Portland Weekly Transcript
Rockland Courier-Gazette

STATISTICS

American State Papers—Commerce and Navigation
Business Directories
Commerce and Navigation Reports, Treasury Department
Greenleaf, Moses—*A Statistical View of the District of Maine*, Boston, 1816
—— *A Survey of the State of Maine*, Portland, 1829
Hunt's Merchants' Magazine and Commercial Review, New York, 1840–1869
Maine Registers, Portland, 1819 *et seq.*
Niles Weekly Register, Baltimore, 1811–1849
Pitkin, Timothy—*A Statistical View*, New Haven, 1835

Bibliography

Ship Registers and Enrollments of Machias, Maine, 1780–1930. National Archives Project, Rockland, 1942

Ship Registers and Enrollments of Saco, Maine, 1791–1915. National Archives Project, Rockland, 1942

BY SUBJECTS

COLONIAL MAINE—CHAPTERS III AND IV

Albion, Robert G.—*Forests and Sea Power*, Cambridge, 1926

Burrage, Henry S.—*Beginnings in Colonial Maine*, Portland, 1914

—— *Maine at Louisburg*, Augusta, 1910

Cushman, D. Q.—*History of Ancient Sheepscot and New Castle*, Bath, 1882

Lounsbury, Alice—*Sir William Phipps*, New York, 1941

Mayo, L. S.—*John Wentworth*, Cambridge, 1921

Parsons, U.—*Sir William Pepperell*, Boston, 1855

THE WAR YEARS—CHAPTER V

Adams, Henry—*History of the United States during the Administration of Thomas Jefferson*, New York, 1921

Coggeshall, G.—*History of American Privateers*, 1812–1814, New York, 1856

Dictionary of American Biography, New York, 1928–1937

Gould, William—*Portland in the Past*, Portland, 1886

Kellogg, Elijah—*Live Oak Boys*, Boston, 1882

Logs of the Privateers—*Dash, Teazer, Partridge, Lilly, Young Teazer, Fly, Dart, Rover, St. Michael*, and *Favorite*—in Maine Historical Society

Maclay, E. S.—*A History of American Privateers*, New York, 1899

Naval Documents Relating to the Quasi War between the United States and France, Washington, 1935 *et seq.*

Naval Documents Relating to the Barbary Wars, Washington, 1935 *et seq.*

Rowe, W. H.—*Shipbuilding Days in Casco Bay, 1727–1890*, Yarmouth, 1929

Smith and Deane's Journals (With Notes by William Willis), Portland, 1849

State Street Trust Company—*Some Famous Privateers of New England*, Boston, 1928

Sturgis, William—*The Northwest Fur Trade*, Old South Leaflets #219

THE WEST INDIA TRADE—CHAPTER VI

Collins, Daniel—*Narrative of the Shipwreck of the Brig Betsey*, Wiscasset, 1825

Elwell, Edward H.—*Portland and Vicinity*, Portland, 1881

Impost Book of Port of Kennebunkport

Kellogg, Elijah—Pleasant Cove and Elm Island Series, Boston, 1890

Wells, Theodore—*Narrative of Life and Adventures*, Biddeford, 1874

LOCAL SHIPBUILDING

Adams, Silas—*History of Bowdoinham*, List 1796–1877, Fairfield, 1902

Allen, Charles E.—*History of Dresden*, Dresden, 1931

Barker, Fen G.—*A Complete Schedule of Vessels Built, Registered or Enrolled in District of Bath, Maine* (1783–1888), Bath, 1888

Barry, William E.—*A Stroll by a Familiar River*, Kennebunk, 1908

Bourne, E. E.—*History of Wells and Kennebunk*, Portland, 1875

Bryant, S. E.—*List of Vessels Built in District of Kennebunkport, 1800–1874*, Kennebunk, 1874

Chase, Fannie S.—*Wiscasset in Pownalborough*, Wiscasset, 1941

Davis, Albert H.—*History of Ellsworth*, List 1831–1890, Lewiston, 1927

Eaton, Cyrus—*History of Thomaston*, List 1787–1864, Hallowell, 1865

—— *Annals of Warren*, List 1770–1850, Hallowell, 1870

Edmunds, J.—*Portsmouth City Directories, 1839, 1851, 1854, 1857, 1860*

Hichborn, Faustina—*Historical Sketch of Stockton Springs*, List 1845–1875, Waterville, 1908

Lermont, Levi P.—*Historical Dates of City and Town of Bath*, Bath, 1874

Limeburner, Grace L.—*Tradition and Records of Brooksville*, Bangor, 1924

Bibliography

Littlefield, Ada D.—*An Old River Town* (Winterport), New York, 1907

Locke, John L.—*History of Camden*, Hallowell, 1859

Miller, Samuel L.—*History of the Town of Waldoboro*, Lists 1829–1904, Wiscasset, 1910

Nason, Emma H.—*Old Hallowell on the Kennebec*, Augusta, 1909

Owen, H. W.—*History of Bath*, Bath, 1936

Plummer, Edward C.—*Reminiscences of a Yarmouth Schoolboy*, Portland, 1926

—— *Bath the City of Ships*, Bath, 1907

Reed, Parker McCobb—*History of Bath*, Portland, 1894

Remick, Daniel—*History of Kennebunk*, Kennebunk, 1911

Rice, George Wharton—*The Shipping Days of Old Boothbay*, Boothbay Harbor, 1938

Robinson, Reul—*History of Camden and Rockport*, Camden, 1907

Rowe, William Hutchinson—*Shipbuilding Days in Old North Yarmouth*, List 1796–1890, Portland, 1924

—— *Shipbuilding Days in Casco Bay*, Yarmouth, 1929

—— *Ancient North Yarmouth and Yarmouth, Maine*, List 1796–1890, Yarmouth, 1937

Saltonstall, William G.—*Ports of Piscataqua*, Cambridge, 1941

Sidelinger—*List of Vessels Built in Newcastle, Damariscotta, Nobleboro and Bristol (1782–1895)*

Thompson, Margaret J.—*Captain Nathaniel Thompson of Kennebunk and the Ships He Built 1811–1889*, Boston, 1937

Thurston, Florence G. and Cross, Harmon, S.—*Three Centuries of Freeport, Maine*, Freeport, 1940

Turner, Walter F.—*Historical Souvenir of Bath*, List 1762–1899, Bath, 1899

Wheeler, George A.—*History of Castine, Penobscot and Brooksville*, Bangor, 1875

Wheeler, George and Henry—*History of Brunswick, Topsham and Harpswell*, Boston, 1878

Wasson, George S.—*Sailing Days on the Penobscot*, with a Record of Vessels Built There, compiled by Lincoln Colcord, Salem, 1932

Williamson, Joseph—*History of City of Belfast*, List 1796–1901, Boston, 1913

The Maritime History of Maine

THE STATE OF MAINE CLIPPERS—CHAPTER IX

Clark, Arthur H.—*The Clipper Ship Era*, New York, 1910
Cutler, Carl C.—*Greyhounds of the Sea*, New York, 1930
Howe, Octavius T., and Matthews, Frederic C.—*American Clipper Ships, 1833–1858*, Salem, 1926, 1927, 2 vols.
Kittredge, Henry C.—*Shipmasters of Cape Cod*, Boston, 1935

THE CONFEDERATE COMMERCE RAIDERS—CHAPTER X

Adams, James Truslow—*The Adams Family*, Boston, 1930
Alabama Claims Dockets, No. 1–5770
Court of Commissioners of Alabama Claims. List of Claims. Washington, 1883
Hale, Clarence—*The Capture of the Caleb Cushing*, Portland, 1901
Hunt's Merchants' Magazine, Vol. 53, pages 449–457
Porter, David D.—*Naval History of the Civil War*, New York, 1886
Schaff, J. Thomas—*History of the Confederate States Navy*, Albany, 1894
Semmes, Raphael—*The Cruise of the Alabama and Sumter*, New York, 1864
—— *Memoirs of Service Afloat During the War between the States*, Baltimore, 1869
Soley, James Russel—*The Commerce Destroyers in the Blockade and the Cruisers*, New York, 1883
Meriwether, Collyer—*The Life of Raphael Semmes*, Philadelphia, 1913

THE DOWN-EASTERS—CHAPTER XI

Carter, Isabel Hopestill—*All Sails Set*, London, 1934
Coffin, Robert P. Tristram—*Captain Abby and Captain John*, New York, 1939
Colcord, Joanna C.—"Domestic Life on American Sailing Ships," *American Neptune*, July, 1942
Humphrey, Omar J.—*Wreck of the Rainier*, Portland, 1887
Lubbock, Basil—*The Downeasters*, Boston, 1929
Matthews, Frederic C.—*American Merchant Ships, 1850–1900*, 2 vols., Salem, 1930–1931
Nichols, Capt. E. P.—*The Ocean Chronicle*, New York, 1941

Bibliography

Ranlett, L. Felix—*Master Mariner of Maine*, Portland, 1942

Reynolds, Lucy Brown—*Drops of Spray from Southern Seas*, Waterville, 1896

Webster, Benjamin—*Autobiography of Captain Benjamin Webster and Diary of Mrs. Benjamin Webster*, Portland, 1900

FISHERIES—CHAPTERS II AND XIV

Baxter, James Phinney, Editor—*The Trelawney Papers*, Portland, 1884

Bishop, W. H.—"Fish and Men in the Maine Islands," *Harper's Magazine*, August, 1880

Bureau of Industrial and Labor Statistics for the State of Maine Reports

Commission of Sea and Shore Fisheries. Biennial Reports

Collins, Joseph W.—"Evolution of the American Fishing Schooner," *New England Magazine*, n. s. XVIII:336, 1898

Green, Francis B.—*History of Boothbay, Southport and Boothbay Harbor*, Portland, 1906

Kellogg, Elijah—*Fisher Boys of Pleasant Cove*, Boston, 1874

Maddocks, Luther—"Looking Backward." Unpublished manuscript in Maine State Library

Pierce, Wesley George—*Goin' Fishing*, Salem, 1934

Rich, George A.—"The New England Fisheries," *New England Magazine*, n. s. X

Thornton, Mrs. Seth S.—*Traditions and Records of Southwest Harbor*, Southwest Harbor, 1938

United States Census, Eighth, 1860

MISCELLANEOUS

Briggs, Thomas J.—"Cruise of the Caribee," *Harper's Magazine*, October 1907

Buxton, Henry—*Assignment Down East*, Brattleboro, 1938

Chapelle, Howard I.—*History of American Sailing Ships*, New York, 1935

—— *American Sailing Craft*, New York, 1939

Chase, George Davis—*Sea Terms Come Ashore*, Orono, 1942

Chase, Mary Ellen—*A Goodly Heritage*, New York, 1932

Coffin, Robert P. Tristram—*Kennebec*, New York, 1937

Colcord, Joanna C.—*Songs of American Sailormen*, New York
———— *Sea Language Comes Ashore*, New York, 1945
Eckstorm, Fanny Hardy, and Smith, Mary Winslow—*Minstrelsy of Maine*, Boston, 1927
Emery, William M.—*Peleg Talman*, privately printed, 1935
Hutchins, John G. B.—*American Maritime Industries and Public Policy*, 1789–1914, Cambridge, 1941
Hennessy, Mark W.—*The Sewall Ships of Steel*, Augusta, 1937
Jones, Herbert G.—*Maine Memories*, Portland, 1940
———— *Old Portland Town*, Portland, 1938
Johnson, Daniel—*American Shipmaster's Daily Assistant*, Portland, 1807
Johnson, Lewis C.—*Voyages from 1847 to 1883*, Portland, 1885
———— *Johnson's Original Progression*, Portland, 1886
Morison, Samuel E.—*The Maritime History of Massachusetts*, Boston, 1921
Nevens, William—*Forty Years at Sea*, Portland, 1860
Norton, Lemuel—*Autobiography*, Portland, 1862
Oakes, Charles C. and Abbie Buxton—*The Old Sea Chest*, privately printed, 1932
Picking, Sherwood—*Sea Fight off Monhegan*, Portland, 1941
Pinckney, Pauline A.—*American Figureheads*, New York, 1940
Plummer, Edward C.—*Shipping Scene*, Bath, 1926
———— *True Tales of the Sea*, Portland, 1930
Preble, G. H.—*History of the Navy Yard Portsmouth*, Washington, 1892
Roberts, Kenneth—*Trending into Maine*, Boston, 1938
Snow, Edward Rowe—*Great Storms and Famous Shipwrecks on the New England Coast*, Boston, 1943
Sterling, Robert Thayer—*Lighthouses on the Maine Coast*, Brattleboro, 1935
Todd, John M.—*Reminiscences*, Portland, 1906
Willard, Benjamin J.—*Captain Ben's Book*, Portland, 1895
Wood, R. G.—*A History of Lumbering in Maine, 1820–1861*, Orono, 1935

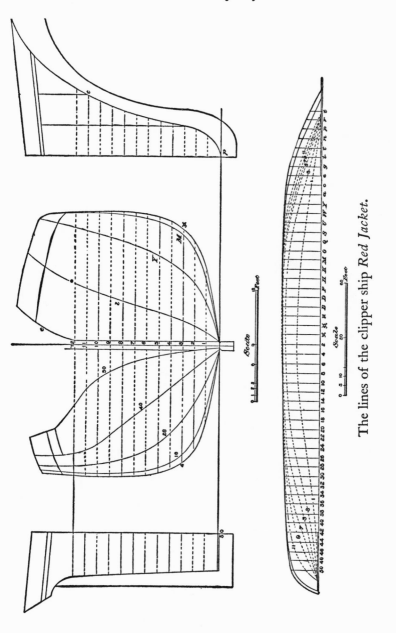

The lines of the clipper ship *Red Jacket.*

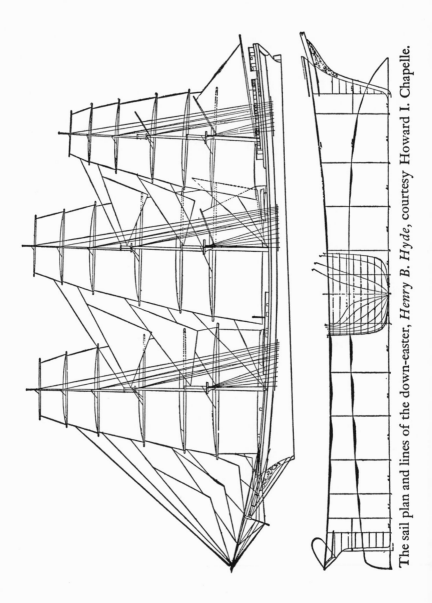

The sail plan and lines of the down-easter, *Henry B. Hyde*, courtesy Howard I. Chapelle.

APPENDIX

I. A LIST COMPRISING THE PLACES WHERE THE MAINE
CLIPPERS WERE BUILT, FROM THE PISCATAQUA TO
THE ST. CROIX, THEIR BUILDERS, AND THEIR MASTERS
1850-1856

KITTERY
Fernald and Pettigrew
Typhoon, 1851—Charles H. Salter
Red Rover, 1852—William O. Putnam
Young Australia, 1852—
Water Witch, 1853—Washington Plummer
Dashing Wave, 1853—John B. Fiske
Midnight, 1854—James B. Hatch
Express, 1854—T. M. Weeks
Noonday, 1855—W. B. Gerry

ELIOT
Captain Samuel Hanscom
Nightingale, 1851—John H. Fiske
Josephine, 1852—William Jameson

KENNEBUNK
Bourne & Kingsbury
Roebuck, 1851, Walden

CAPE ELIZABETH
————
Warner, 1851—Luther Ripley, Jr.
Alfred Butler
Bk. *Black Squall*, 1850—John Codman
Snow Squall, 1851—Isaac Bursley

[309]

Thomas Knight
  Phoenix, 1853—John Hoxie
J. W. Dyer
  Portland, 1853—William Leavitt

CUMBERLAND
  David Spear, Jr.
  Bk. *Grapeshot*, 1853—E. J. Parker

FREEPORT
  Enos Soule
  Quickstep, 1853—Cook

BRUNSWICK
  G. Schofield
  Rising Sun, 1856—Orr

BATH
  Trufant and Drummond
    Monsoon, 1851—L. Winsor
    Emerald Isle, 1853—Henry Scott
    Viking, 1853—Zenas Winsor
    Flying Dragon, 1853—Judah P. Baker
    Windward, 1854—Whiting
    Mary Robinson, 1854—Frederick Crocker
  Hall, Snow and Co.
    Carrier Pigeon, 1852—Azariah Doane
    Undaunted, 1853—William Freeman
  Houghtons
    Pocohantas, 1855—

RICHMOND
  T. J. Southard
    Gauntlet, 1853—Sam G. Borland
    Wizard King, 1854—J. Cobb
  Patten and Sturdevant
    Peerless, 1852—Caleb G. Babson
    Pride of America, 1853—Hawthorne

Appendix

Strelna, 1853—Thomas Leach
G. H. Ferrin
Wild Wave, 1853—Josiah N. Knowles

FARMINGDALE
Grant
Miss Mag, 1853—Josiah S. Arey

HALLOWELL
J. Rideout
Dashaway, 1854—

PITTSTON
William Stevens
White Falcon, 1853—Ryan

ALNA
D. Weymouth
King Phillip, 1856—Gardner

NEWCASTLE
William Hitchcock and Abner Stetson
trading as William Hitchcock and Company
Flying Eagle, 1852—W. Parker
Western Empire, 1852—Chas. F. Winsor
Golden Rule, 1854—
Criterion, 1855—

DAMARISCOTTA
Metcalf & Norris
Alert, 1850—Francis Bursley
Queen of the East, 1852—Freeman Bartlett
Levanter, 1852—William A. Follansbee
Flying Scud, 1853—Patten, Warren H. Bearce
Talisman, 1854—Francis Bursley
Austin and Hall
Wild Rover, 1853—Hamilton

Austin & Co.
  Black Warrior, 1853–Murphy
Col. Cyrus Cotter
  Ocean Herald, 1853–Spencer

BRISTOL

  Sparkling Sea, 1854–Nehemiah Rich

WALDOBORO
  Edward Achorn
    Wings of the Morning, 1852–H. A. Lovell
    Woodcock, 1853–Frederick M. Ranlett

  Spark of the Ocean, 1853–Willard J. Treat

THOMASTON
  Chapman & Flint
    Oracle, 1853–Charles E. Ranlett
  J. C. C. Morton
    Hyperion, afterwards *Golden Racer*, 1852–Benj. M. Melcher
  Thorndike
    Empire, 1851–E. A. Thorndike
  Hon. Joshua Patterson
    Crest of the Wave, 1854–William S. Colley

WARREN
  Burgess & Clark
    Stephen Crowell, 1855–Burgess

ROCKLAND
  George Thomas
    Bk. *Springbok*, 1851–S. L. Hurd
    Defiance, 1852–Robert McCerron
    Rattler, 1852–Richard Brown
    Red Jacket, 1853–Asa Eldredge
  Horace Merriam
    Live Yankee, 1853–Thorndike
    Euterpe, 1854–George W. Brown

Francis W. Rhoades
  Anglo Saxon, 1853—John Leeds
  Progressive, 1853—
  Young Mechanic, 1856—H. Freeman
Trowbridge
  Yankee Ranger, 1854—

BELFAST
  Carter & Co.
    Seaman's Bride, 1856—A. B. Wyman
  David, John & Hiram Pierce
    Sportsman, 1856—William Thompson

ORLAND
  Samuel B. Keyes
    Stornaway, 1853—

FRANKFORT
  George Dunham
    Flying Arrow, afterwards called
      Wings of the Wind, 1852—Charles T. Treadwell
    Ocean Spray, 1852—Charles A. McLellan
    Nonpareil, 1853—Edward Dunn
    Speedwell, 1853—
  James Arey & Sons
    Spitfire, 1853—John Arey
  Williams & Arey
    Arey, 1856—Samuel J. Sewall

TRESCOTT
  ————
    Sea Lark, 1852—Charles L. Willcomb

EASTPORT
  C. S. Husten
    Grey Feather, 1850—Daniel McLaughlin
  George Fountain
    Crystal Palace, 1854—Benj. F. Simmons

PEMBROKE
  S. C. Foster
    Western Continent, 1853—Stephen Higgins
  Isaac Elwell
    Queen of the Pacific, 1852—William Reed

———

  Bk. *Comet*, 1852—

ROBBINSTON
  James W. Cox
    Bk. *Francis Palmer*, 1852—
    Red Gauntlet, 1853—Thomas Andrews
    Dictator, 1855—T. Everett

———

  Juniper, 1853—Parsons
  Thomas Vose
    Virginia, 1854—Freeman G. Sparks

Appendix

II. MAINE-BUILT VESSELS TAKEN BY CONFEDERATE COMMERCE RAIDERS

	NAME	TONS	BUILT	CAPTURED BY	DATE	WHERE	DISPOSAL
Bg	A. Richards	274	Columbia Falls	Tallahassee	Aug. 11, 1864	Fire Island	Burned
Sp	A. B. Thompson	800	Brunswick	Lady Davis	May 19, 1861	Savannah	Sunk
Sc	A. J. Bird	178	Rockland	Olustee	Nov. 3, 1864	39:30 N-74 W	Sunk
Sc	Agricola	195	Ellsworth	Freely	Aug. 25, 1861	Cape Ann	Released
Bg	Albert Adams	573	Dennysville	Sumter	July 5, 1861	Cienfuegos	Released
Bk	Alina	999	Searsport	Shenandoah	Oct. 29, 1861	16:40 N-26:45 W	Sunk
Sp	American Union	900	Bath		May 26, 1861	New Orleans	Confiscated
Sp	Anglo Saxon	800	Rockland	Florida	Aug. 20, 1863	Florida	Burned
Bk	Anna F. Schmidt	237	Kennebunk	Alabama	Jan. 2, 1863	26:14 N-37:51 W	Bonded
Bg	Albion Lincoln	293	Harpswell	Chickamauga	Oct. 31, 1864	300 M. S. E. New York	Burned
Sc	Arabella	121	Frankfort	Tacony	June 12, 1863	New England	Burned
Sc	Arcade	90	Hampton	Sumter	Nov. 26, 1861	20:27 N-51:15 W	Retaken
	Archer		Essex	Tacony	June 24, 1863	Cape Sable	Confiscated
	Ariel		Bath	Pickens	May 21, 1861	Mississippi	Burned
	Atlantic	1330	Addison	Tallahassee	Aug. 11, 1864	Fire Island	Burned
Sc	B. K. Eaton	156	Searsport	Sally	Oct. 30, 1861	Abago	Destroyed
Bg	B. T. Martin	198	Bristol	York	July 23, 1861	Hatteras	Bonded
Sc	Baron de Castine	293	Castine	Alabama	Oct. 29, 1862	39:18 N-69:12 W	Released
Bg	Ben Dunning	270	Falmouth	Sumter	July 5, 1861	Cienfuegos	Bonded
Bg	Bethia Thayer	284	Thomaston	Alabama	Mar. 1, 1863	39:50 N-38:31 W	Confiscated
Sp	Betsey Ames	900	Wells	Sally	Oct. 17, 1861	Bermuda	Retaken
Bg	Billow	180	Gardiner	Tallahassee	Aug. 12, 1864	Off Gay Head	Burned
Bg	Carrie Estelle	173	Cutler	Tallahassee	Aug. 11, 1864	Sandy Hook	Burned
Sc	Carroll	248	Machias	Tallahassee	Aug. 11, 1864	Fire Island	Cartel
Bg	Chas. A. Farwell	138	Rockland		May 26, 1864	New Orleans	Confiscated
Sp	City of Bath	1298	Bath	Georgia	June 28, 1863	Trinidad	Detained
Sp	Constitution	736	Bath	Georgia	June 26, 1863	Off Brazil	Burned
Bg	Corris Ann	997	Machiasport	Florida	Jan. 22, 1863	Cardenas	Burned
Bg	Cuba	366	Millbridge	Sumter	July 4, 1861	Cuba	Retaken
Sp	Delphine	236	Bangor	Shenandoah	Dec. 29, 1864	59:20 S-69 E	Burned
Bk	Dictator	705	Robbinston	Georgia	Apr. 25, 1863	25 N-25 W	Burned
Bk	Dorcas Prince	1293	Yarmouth	Alabama	Apr. 26, 1863	7:35 S-31:40 W	Burned
Sc	E. F. Lewis	700	Cape Elizabeth	Olustee	Nov. 3, 1864	Barnegat	Burned
Bk	Elsinore	182	Bangor	Sally	Oct. 29, 1861	Abago	Burned
Sp	Emma Jane	284	Bath	Alabama	Jan. 14, 1863	Malaba	Burned
Sp	Emma L. Hall	1200	Millbridge	Chickamauga	Oct. 31, 1864	Off New York	Damaged
Bk	Emily Fisher	492	Pembroke	Retribution	Feb. 19, 1863	Guantanamo	Burned
Bk	Estelle	330		Florida	Jan. 1, 1862	No. of Cuba	Burned
Bg	Etta Caroline	31	So. Bristol	Tallahassee	Aug. 10, 1864	Seal Island	Sunk
Sc	Floral Wreath	54	Georgetown	Tallahassee	Aug. 14, 1864	Monhegan	Burned
Bk	Glenavon	795	Thomaston	Dixie	Aug. 13, 1864	Nantucket	Sunk
Bk	Blen	287	Freeport		July 23, 1861	Off Florida	Burned
Sp	Golden Rocket	607	Brewer	Sumter	July 3, 1861	Isle of Pines	Burned

	NAME	TONS	BUILT	CAPTURED BY	DATE	WHERE	DISPOSAL
Bg	Grenada	255	Cape Elizabeth	Sally	Oct. 12, 1861	31 N–72 W	Confiscated
Bk	Greenland	549	Brunswick	Florida	July 9, 1864	Off Hatteras	Burned
Sp	Investigator	595	Searsport	Sumter	Jan. 18, 1862	Gibraltar	Bonded
Bg	Itaska	299	Orrington	Winslow	Aug. 4, 1861	Hatteras	Sunk
Sp	John A. Parks	1250	Hallowell	Alabama	Mar. 2, 1863	29:25 N–37:47 W	Burned
Sp	John Carver	599	Bath	Jeff Davis	Aug. 11, 1861	Off Florida	Burned
Sp	James Littlefield	177	Brewer	Tallahassee	Aug. 14, 1864	42:20 N–66 W	Sunk
Bg	Joseph	244	Rockland	Savannah	June 3, 1861	Charleston	Burned
Bg	Joseph Park	123	Stockton	Sumter	Sept. 25, 1861	6 N–42 W	Burned
Sc	Josiah Achorn	207	Rockland	Tallahassee	Aug. 17, 1864	Nova Scotia	Burned
Sp	J. P. Ellicott	1160	Bucksport	Retribution	Jan. 10, 1862	Cuba	Retaken
Bk	Lafayette	279	Freeport	Alabama	Oct. 23, 1862	Seal Island	Burned
Bk	Lamplighter	284	Calais	Alabama	Oct. 11, 1862	Off New York	Burned
Bk	Lauretta	853	Damariscotta	Alabama	Oct. 28, 1862	Off New York	Burned
Bk	Louisa Hatch	374	Rockland	Florida	Apr. 4, 1863	3:13 S–26:12 W	Burned
Sc	M. J. Colcord	245	Prospect	Sumter	Mar. 13, 1863	28:30 N–33:26 W	Burned
Sc	Machias	26	Machias	Tallahassee	July 4, 1861	Cienfuegos	Released
Sc	Magnolia						Burned
Bk	Marcus	398			Aug. 14, 1864		Sunk
Bk	Mark L. Potter	577	Stockton	Yorktown	Mar. 6, 1862		Confiscated
Sc	Martha Wenzell	198	Brewer	Chickamauga	Oct. 30, 1864	Monhegan	Released
Sp	Mary E. Thompson	181	East Deering	Alabama	Aug. 7, 1863	Off Sandy Hook	Burned
Sp	Mary Alice	717	Searsport	Jeff Davis	July 9, 1861	Cape of Good Hope	Released
Sp	Mary Goodell	621	Machias	Winslow	July 9, 1861	Nantucket	Confiscated
Bg	Milan	1083	Searsport	Jeff Davis	May 18, 1861	39:10 N–68 W	Bonded
Bk	Montmorenci	290	Bath	Calhoun	Nov. 28, 1861	Mississippi	Confiscated
Sc	Ocean Eagle	284	Bath	Sumter	May 18, 1861	18:30 N–84:40 W	Burned
Sc	P. C. Alexander	41	Rockland	Calhoun	Aug. 16, 1864	Gulf of Mexico	Burned
Bg	Pearl	59	Harpswell	Tallahassee	Aug. 16, 1864	Monhegan	Sunk
Sc	Restless	127	Boothbay	Tallahassee	Aug. 15, 1864	Monhegan	Burned
Sc	Roan	198	Harrington	Tallahassee	Aug. 20, 1864	Cape Sable	Burned
Sc	Santa Clara	974	Eastport	Jeff Davis	Aug. 6, 1861	Off Halifax	Burned
Bk	Sea Lark	126	Trescott	Alabama	May 3, 1863	Off Florida	Burned
Sp	Spokane	339	Tremont	Tallahassee	Aug. 12, 1864	9:35 S–31:20 W	Confiscated
Bg	State of Maine	267	Machias	Calhoun	May 12, 1861	40:15 N–71:45 W	Bonded
Sp	Suliote	1250	Belfast	Tallahassee	Aug. 12, 1864	Mississippi	Burned
Bt	Talisman	196	Damariscotta	Alabama	June 5, 1863	Off New York	Burned
Bg	Umpire	1100	Sullivan	Tacony	June 14, 1863	14:45 N–32 W	Burned
Sp	Vigilant		Bath	Sumter	Dec. 3, 1861	20:12 N–42:20 W	Burned
Bk	Village	198	Cape Elizabeth	Archer	June 25, 1863	Damariscove	Confiscated
Bg	William McGilvery	1226	Prospect	Jeff Davis	July 25, 1861	Hatteras	Bonded
Sp	Washington	350	Pittston	Alabama	Feb. 27, 1863	30:19 N–40:01 W	Burned
Bk	Whistling Wind	299	Blue Hill	Clarence	June 6, 1863	Gulf Stream	Burned
Bg	William B. Nash	199	Millbridge	Florida	July 8, 1863	33:38 N–71:29 W	Burned
Sc	Windward		Stockton	Jeff Davis	Aug. 4, 1861	Turk's Island	Released

III. SHIPPING TONNAGE OWNED IN THE CUSTOMS DISTRICTS OF MAINE, 1798–1890 [1]

DISTRICT	12/31 1798	12/31 1800	12/31 1807	12/31 1810	12/31 1820	12/31 1830	9/30 1840	6/30 1850	6/30 1855	6/30 1860	6/30 1870	6/30 1880	6/30 1890
Passamaquoddy	777	2,599	6,929	5,801	5,508	10,486	12,171	19,985	44,505	25,270	26,038	23,510	20,205
Machias	7,796	1,025	2,720	2,259	3,797	4,099	11,847	21,318	34,215	34,921	15,237	19,354	17,654
Frenchman's Bay	3,576	3,958	5,110	4,828	8,005	6,090	20,365	32,168	47,977	35,794	15,778	14,849	13,371
Penobscot	7,768	8,029	15,368	18,019	14,048	19,177	37,130	36,950	53,965	49,414	24,075	19,082	13,998
Belfast					8,128	13,245	38,218	45,595	70,762	80,785	39,431	47,064	18,710
Bangor								25,268	40,297	36,302	27,124	26,686	23,402
Waldoboro			18,268	19,041	21,754	21,789	25,997	96,330	148,896	187,215	59,406	84,016	59,861
Wiscasset	11,653	11,303	16,349	17,911	10,636	7,949	13,469	18,241	26,929	28,167	7,846	9,851	5,590
Bath	8,144	8,563	21,758	20,344	21,612	26,668	64,035	103,625	175,258	165,318	87,621	135,975	126,273
Portland	19,134	26,379	41,241	32,599	33,619	42,717	174,935	86,502	137,317	131,825	77,819	118,699	70,942
Saco	11,396	9,320	5,854	7,719	3,364	3,340	3,358	2,723	7,167	4,956	3,647	654	687
Kennebunk			8,296	8,808	8,571	4,789	7,132	11,349	17,420	20,421	9,209	8,672	3,012
York	3,013	2,890	3,155	3,723	1,326	957	1,200	6,361	1,891	1,547	708	311	218
Total	66,257	73,985	148,048	141,052	140,368	161,306	409,857	501,415	802,389	801,935	803,999	598,729	373,929

[317]

[1] From American State Papers, Commerce and Navigation, Vols. I and II, and Commerce and Navigation Reports.

IV. THE ESTIMATED NUMBER OF VESSELS AND THEIR AGGREGATE TONNAGE BUILT IN THE YARDS ON THE MAINE COAST—1820–1890 [1]

YEAR	NUMBER	TONNAGE	YEAR	NUMBER	TONNAGE
1820	149	14,248	1851	254	77,399
1821	104	12,278	1852	354	110,047
1822	118	17,500	1853	351	118,916
1823	124	18,845	1854	348	168,631
1824	159	25,138	1855	396	215,904
1825	248	34,558	1856	316	149,908
1826	247	36,245	1857	240	110,933
1827	168	26,000	1858	167	55,959
1828			1859	125	40,905
1829	140	14,658	1860	172	57,868
1830			1861	161	57,343
1831			1862	75	26,264
1832	180	40,000	1863	99	48,867
1833	316	51,687	1864	180	73,754
1834	174	28,505	1865	193	79,291
1835			1866	226	73,921
1836	162	27,021	1867	280	89,014
1837	149	23,475	1868	214	59,946
1838	144	24,322	1869	177	61,537
1839	181	27,706	1870	202	74,322
1840	181	38,937	1871	228	48,545
1841	131	26,874	1872	149	32,420
1842	164	38,040	1873	276	89,817
1843	71	15,121	1874	353	122,548
1844	96	20,200	1875	223	113,988
1845	160	31,105	1876	153	69,118
1846	289	49,748	1877	131	72,696
1847	346	63,549	1878	117	41,060
1848	449	89,975	1879	93	42,628
1849	342	82,256	1880	78	36,009
1850	326	91,252	1881	94	41,374

Appendix

YEAR	NUMBER	TONNAGE	YEAR	NUMBER	TONNAGE
1882	168	75,085	1887	38	13,336
1883	174	74,708	1888	52	20,723
1884	97	46,402	1889	125	74,467
1885	57	23,054	1890	96	56,319
1886	47	22,251			

[1] From American State Papers Commerce and Navigation, Vol. I and II, and Commerce and Navigation Reports.

INDEX

Index

Index

Index

Index

Index

Index

Index

Index

Index

Index

Index